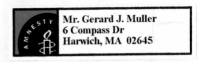

10/08

Outpatient Management of Advanced Cancer

J. B. Lippincott Company
Philadelphia

London
Mexico City
New York
St. Louis
São Paulo
Sydney

Outpatient Management of Advanced Cancer

Symptom Control, Support, and Hospice-in-the-Home

J. Andrew Billings, M.D.

Assistant Clinical Professor of Medicine,
Harvard Medical School;
Assistant Physician,
Massachusetts General Hospital;
Director, Hospice–Home Care Program,
MGH–Chelsea Memorial Health Care Center;
Medical Director,
Harbor Hospice of Massachusetts

With 4 Contributed Chapters

Acquisitions Editor: Micaela Palumbo
Sponsoring Editor: Sanford J. Robinson
Manuscript Editor: Helen Ewan
Indexer: Sandra King
Art Director: Tracy Baldwin
Design Coordinator: Anne O'Donnell
Designer: Arlene Putterman
Production Supervisor: Kathleen P. Dunn
Production Assistant: Susan Hess
Compositor: University Graphics, Inc.
Printer/Binder: R. R. Donnelley & Sons

6 5 4 3 2 1

Library of Congress Cataloging in Publication Data

Billings, J. Andrew.
    Outpatient management of advanced cancer.

    Includes bibliographies and index.   1. Cancer--
Treatment.   2. Cancer--Patients--Home care.
3. Cancer--Patients--Family relationships.   4. Terminal
care.   I. Title.   [DNLM: 1. Home Care Services.
2. Neoplasms--therapy.   3. Terminal Care.   QZ 266
B598o]
RC270.8.B55   1985   649'.8   85-6747
ISBN 0-397-50648-1

The author and publisher have exerted every effort to ensure that the
drug selection and dosage set forth in this text are in accord with current recommendations and practice at the time of publication. However, in view of ongoing research, changes in government regulations,
and the constant flow of information relating to drug therapy and drug
reactions, the reader is urged, when using each drug, to check the package insert or product information sheets for any change in indications
and dosage and for added warnings and precautions. This is particularly important when the recommended agent is a new, unfamiliar, or
infrequently employed drug.

    Additionally, individual variations in medication requirements
must be respected, especially when treating debilitated patients. Differences in drug tolerance may be of major significance in properly prescribing narcotic analgesics.

To Susan and Joshua

Contributors

Margaret Adams–Greenly, M.S.
  Administrative Supervisor, Department of Social Work,
  Memorial Sloan–Kettering Cancer Center

Susan D. Block, M.D.
  Instructor in Psychiatry, Harvard Medical School;
  Director of Psychiatry—Primary Care Training,
  Acting Director, Consultation Liaison Service,
  The Cambridge Hospital;
  Former Medical Director, Hospice of Cambridge

Edwin H. Cassem, M.D.
  Associate Professor of Psychiatry,
  Harvard Medical School;
  Chief, Psychiatric Consultation–Liaison Service,
  Massachusetts General Hospital

Grace H. Christ, M.A.
  Director, Department of Social Work,
  Memorial Sloan–Kettering Cancer Center

Rosemary T. Moynihan, M.S.
  Administrative Supervisor, Department of Social Work,
  Memorial Sloan–Kettering Cancer Center

Harriet Slivka, M.S.W.
Social Worker, Department of Social Work,
Memorial Sloan–Kettering Cancer Center

Reverend Thomas Welch, M.Ed.
Director, OMEGA—A Program of Hospice and Bereavement Support,
Somerville, Massachusetts

Preface

Outpatient Management of Advanced Cancer is written for clinicians as a guide to the palliative care of advanced cancer patients in the office and home. It describes the common physical and psychosocial problems of these patients and their families, especially as they face the terminal phases of the illness, and offers a practical approach to clinical management.

Part One, Symptom Control, provides a detailed manual for understanding and managing pain and the other common symptoms of advanced cancer. Guidelines are suggested for the difficult decisions about appropriate treatment limits in far-advanced illness. Part Two, Psychosocial Support, describes supportive care for the patient and family, including the children: managing the burden of physical care in the home, promoting security and coping, and recognizing the psychosocial problems that require special intervention. The task of truth-telling is also discussed, and existential and spiritual concerns are briefly presented. Part Three, Hospice-In-The Home, begins with a review of why home-based care may be desired by dying patients and their families, and then provides instructions on managing a death in the home. The Afterword is a personal essay on the physician's experience of working with the dying and their families.

Practitioners in different medical settings encounter different clinical problems. A few words about myself may put into perspective my vantage on the care of advanced cancer patients, and my choice of topics for the book. For the past 10 years, I have practiced general internal medicine as a member of a multidisciplinary group practice that is affiliated with a large teaching hospital and medical school. While most of my time as a practitioner is spent in the office setting, home care has been a major interest. For the past 7 years, I have been involved intensively in the care of the terminally ill, and have served as the medical director of a hospice/home-care program in a relatively poor, ethnically heterogeneous group of communities within metropolitan Boston. Because of my special interest in terminal illness and home care, I have had the opportunity to care for patients with advanced cancer, largely with solid tumors, in the home, office, and hospital, and to act as a consultant on individual cases or as a lecturer or discussant for groups of physicians, nurses, and others interested in this field.

The scope of this book has been defined by my own experience as a primary-care physician, consultant, and teacher. The topics that I have selected are those that I have had to master in order to care well for my own patients, or that I have been called on to share when advising others. Collaborators have covered four important areas, which seemed best discussed by specialists.

I have not reviewed the management of problems that are familiar to the general physician, especially those problems that are similarly handled for advanced cancer patients as for others. I have also generally avoided many subjects that are common concerns in oncology and hospital-based medicine: the evaluation and treatment of cancer in its earlier stages; the choice, administration, and toxicity of chemotherapeutic agents; the management of hospital-acquired infections; and the care of the compromised host. These topics are treated well in standard textbooks of oncology; some are surprisingly rare concerns for a community-based physician. Many other topics—the management of pain, nausea, pruritus, pressure sores, confusion, normal fear, and home support—are covered here in depth, since they are often neglected in training and in textbooks. These topics are important in the care of cancer patients in all stages of the disease, and often of non-cancer patients as well, and so the book should prove useful in many areas of medical practice.

I have addressed this book to physicians. The physician-reader is envisioned as a "jack-of-all-trades," who supervises every detail of the care of the patient and family. In reality, responsibility for excellent care must fall on a team of health-care professionals, as well as on the patient and his or her family and community. I hope that non–physician-readers, especially medical students, nurses, and mental health and social workers, will find the text valuable. My own understanding of medical care has been greatly enhanced by contributions of non–physician-caretakers and of persons outside the health professions, and I have often wished while writing that I might share my clinical viewpoint with the various sociologists, anthropologists, ethicists, mental health workers, nurses, social workers, hospice workers, administrators, patients, family members, and others who share an interest in this field. I have integrated material from a variety of medical, psychological, and social science studies into my own daily clinical practice, and have tried to present such material in a form that is useful and intelligible to the clinician. For physicians and nonphysicians alike, I have tried to indicate those areas in which good clinical data are lacking, while at the same time providing a manual of practical advice to the clinician who must act with incomplete information and must make immediate decisions about the best care for the patient.

The Selected References offer reliable summaries and bibliographies, interesting or original contributions to the literature, support for major assertions in the text, or reports of new forms of treatment. Exhaustive documentation has not been attempted. Where many citations could have been offered, a few favored references have been chosen.

J. Andrew Billings, M.D.

Acknowledgments

As a physician, I have had many teachers, and in writing this book, I have enjoyed much encouragement. First, I acknowledge the many patients and family members who have shared their lives with me. In a curious tradeoff, they have enriched my life and my understanding of the problems of the dying, spurring me on in my work, while simultaneously benefiting from my inquisitiveness and expertise. I particularly thank the 350 families for whom I have been the primary physician in the home over the past 10 years. Their stories and their words—hastily recorded during my daily rounds and later altered to protect their privacy—have been used throughout the book.

Second, I thank the colleagues who have helped me find and enjoy this field and who have deepened my appreciation of the care of patients and families. When I was a fourth-year medical student, John Stoeckle showed me the pleasures and excitement of primary-care medicine; he continues to provide irreplaceable inspiration, appreciation, support, and criticism. Harrison Sadler at the University of California, San Francisco, helped me pursue my interests in psychosocial aspects of medicine and find the vocation I enjoy. Roger Sweet introduced me to the care of the dying at home, starting me along the path that led to this book. Many colleagues at the Massachusetts General Hospital—especially Ned Cassem, Sherman Eisenthal, and Aaron Lazare in the Department of Psychiatry, and Sue Fisher and Joanne O'Brien in the Continuing Care office—enriched my understanding of patient care. Pam Marron, John Van Wye, and many other medical students have joined me in making housecalls, have visited my patients or participated in my teaching seminars, and have added greatly to my knowledge and pleasure in this work. For the past 7 years, the members and speakers at my weekly seminar on the Doctor–Patient Relationship have also enhanced my appreciation of the psychosocial aspects of daily medical care. I am also indebted to many of the staff of the MGH Cox Cancer Center for consultation and referrals.

At the MGH–Chelsea Memorial Health Center, Lorraine Capistran, patient care representative, has been a model of kindness to patients, while many other co-workers there—too many to name—have taught and encouraged me. The physicians, nurses, and other members of the Adult Medicine team have been valued comrades in the often exhausting practice of community medicine, and have made my work humanly possible by taking a portion of night, weekend, and vacation coverage of hospice patients and by allowing me to shut off my beeper with the assurance that my patients were being cared for well. The staff has also covered my practice while granting me leave to work on this book. Terry O'Malley and Fred Rubin have shared longest in these tasks.

Alexander Leaf and the Department of Medicine at Massachusetts General Hospital have provided moral encouragement and financial support for this work. Additional funds have been furnished by the MGH Primary Care Fund and the MGH–Chelsea Memorial Health Center Adult Team Funds. Harrison Schreppell and his "friendly" Morrow Micro-Decision computer gave welcome technical assistance.

My wife, Susan Block, has patiently participated in the preparation of this book and has been a regular source of encouragement and enthusiasm. I have enjoyed her support and companionship during many late hours of work. On all our vacations and summer weekends, she has cheerfully helped me stuff our car full of the books, papers, and computer components I needed for my writing. She is a favorite consultant, especially over dinner, as well as a valued reader of early versions of the book.

Helpful readers of preliminary drafts have included Paul Billings, Betsy Bishop, Tad Campion, Gil Daniels, Suzanne Deutsch, Sherm Eisenthal, Barbara Gilchrest, Pablo Gomery, John Goodson, Donna Greenberg, Alex Leaf, Maury Martin, Helen O'Malley, Ruth Palumbo, and James Richter. Micaela Palumbo, formerly my editor at J. B. Lippincott, understood the importance of the hospice concept and was an essential advocate for this book when it was first conceived.

I extend my gratitude to the many authors, cited in the Selected References, who have contributed to my understanding of patient care through their research, critical reviews and essays, textbooks, and fictional works. The act of writing a book has heightened my sense of indebtedness to these teachers.

Finally, my colleagues in the hospice movement have provided companionship and inspiration for pursuits that were otherwise often solitary. I am particularly grateful to the staff, volunteers, and members of the Board of the Harbor Hospice of Massachusetts, and to our marvelous hospice coordinator, Mary Gesek. Cicely Saunders, Robert Twycross, Balfour Mount, Richard Lamerton, and their associates also deserve particular thanks for pioneering good works and writings.

Contents

8.
Existential and Spiritual Concerns   260
Thomas Welch

9.
Helping the Children When a Parent Is Dying   269
Margaret Adams–Greenly, Rosemary T. Moynihan, Grace H. Christ, and Harriet Slivka

Part Three   Hospice-in-the-Home

10.
Why Dying People and Their Families Seek Home Care   285

11.
Death in the Home   293

Afterword.
On Being a Reluctant Physician—Strains and Rewards in Caring
for the Dying at Home   309

General Index   319

Drug Index   335

Introduction

.
.

CONCEPTUAL BACKGROUND

Four contemporary themes, reflecting both societal and professional pressures to improve medical care, are embraced in this text.

"Death and Dying" and the Hospice Movement

"Death and dying" has recently received increasing attention among both popular and professional audiences. The treatment of the terminally ill has been widely criticized, and improved methods of care have been suggested. While "death education" has been slow to enter the medical school curriculum or the postgraduate training of physicians, doctors and other health professionals now regularly recognize that the care of the dying poses special problems. More recently, the hospice movement has contributed many useful notions about the medical and psychosocial management of terminally ill patients and their families, and has offered intriguing institutional solutions to problems in the care of the dying in the modern hospital. Indeed, hospice care offers a model or ideal, which should not be applied solely to patients with a particular medical condition or prognosis; many lessons from the hospice will be valued long after a cure for cancer has been discovered.

Unfortunately, the blend of biomedical and psychosocial expertise that physicians recognize as an essential feature of good medical practice is treated rather unevenly in the literature of the "death and dying" movement, particularly in some writings portrayed as "holistic." In a field where attention to details is essential, the richness of clinical practice has often been reduced to cookbook formulas or has been distorted by a lopsided, often idiosyncratic, view of patients' needs. In addition, a number of clichés and problematic concepts have been promulgated: "caring versus curing," "terminal care," "a good death," "stages of dying," "the family as the unit of care," and "death with dignity." While steering away from such well-meant but often simplistic and misleading terms, this text extracts many valuable notions embraced by the hospice and "death and dying" movements, and attempts to present them in an intelligent and clinically useful form.

Home Care

Home care has been increasingly recognized as a valuable method for improving the well-being of the growing numbers of aged and chronically ill in the population and for perhaps reducing the costs of their care. Indeed, rival elements in the health policy arena—the "cost-containers" and the "service-expanders"—have, at times, been allies in promoting home care. In the United States, the hospice concept has flourished as a community-based program, reminding us that many patients with chronic and progressively debilitating or fatal conditions prefer to live outside institutions.

This book presents a perspective on the optimal management of advanced cancer, developed by the author while attending to patients and families in the home. The home is the site where most patients manage their illnesses—major and minor, acute and chronic—and almost every clinician, whether or not he or she makes housecalls, is responsible for care in this setting. When a full range of health services is available, many seriously ill patients can achieve the highest quality of care in the community.

The text describes an approach to patient management that recognizes the potential for excellent care in the community and that stresses the special skills, knowledge, attitudes, and services needed to promote such care. Unfortunately, few physicians in this country have been trained in home visiting, yet physician housecalls may, at times, be invaluable for good home-based care, especially for preventing unnecessary emergency ward visits, hospitalization, and nursing home placement. On the other hand, nurses can provide the bulk of professional management in the community, and many terminally ill outpatients who are cared for in the home may see their doctors in ambulatory care facilities. The term, "home-based care," is occasionally used in this book with the hope of tempering the notion, sometimes associated with the term, "home care," that patient management in institutional settings must be strictly avoided.

Primary Care

The primary-care movement has reasserted the value of the personal physician—the provider of readily available, comprehensive, integrated, and continuous biomedical and psychosocial services. Subspecialists, as well as generalists, strive to meet the primary-care needs of their patients. The primary-care movement is attempting to delineate the intellectual and organizational basis for a modern practice of general medicine. This text is written in the belief that the advancement of the art and science of clinical care requires fuller descriptions of common acts of practice, such as supporting patients in the home, providing reassurance, and promoting a sense of security during a serious illness. Foremost, the patient's experience of illness must be appreciated, and thus some sections of the book present a naturalistic study of the life of the patient with advanced cancer. Some clinical methods have been painstakingly elaborated upon. Daily medical acts have been unravelled and laid out so that the reader has the opportunity to share in and understand the process of care, to criticize and, it is hoped, improve on the assumptions and behaviors of one physician in practice. In many of the chapters, the reader should recognize Erik Erikson's prescription: "The new doctor thus must translate an old person-to-person commitment into modern methods of communication."[1]

Advances in Oncology and Medical Technology

Finally, in the past few decades, three relatively new disciplines—the subspecialties of radiation oncology, medical oncology, and surgical oncology (the last of which, as yet, is only informally recognized as a specialty within surgery)—have vastly transformed our understanding of the cancer patient. Concurrently, the technology of medicine has blossomed. Approaches to the clinical management of malignant disease are rapidly changing and improving. Cancer has become a much less hopeless condition. Increasing numbers of patients are living longer and better lives with their cancer, and many patients are enjoying complete cures. Greater interest in and attention to this illness have contributed to the heightened awareness of a longstanding failure to provide excellent symptom control and psychosocial support to cancer patients, especially to those persons—still the majority of cancer victims—who succumb to their disease.

Advanced technologies, as usual, present mixed blessings. New problems have emerged. With improved prospects for managing cancer, unrealistic expectations may develop about the value of treatment. When a hoped-for cure fails, when the doctor says "nothing more can be done," the patient and family face profound disappointment and, sometimes, bitterness. Patients are also encountering the hazards of zealous treatment, finding that the aggressive measures that can prolong or sustain life may occasionally diminish the quality of life or even cause great harm. Ironically, as aggressive comfort measures (such as those promoted in this book) become more effective, treatments that previously seemed merely to prolong suffering may now be appreciated as useful for sustaining a life that still can be valued and enjoyed.

Diagnostic and therapeutic measures are increasingly being scrutinized for their "appropriateness"—their usefulness in terms of goals such as comfort, prolongation of life, convenience, cost, and various other personal, professional, and societal values. Defining a patient as terminally ill, declaring an illness as irreversible, or placing a patient in a hospice or palliative-care program does not solve the difficult problem of determining the best form of care for that individual. Much of the popular rhetoric about the care of the dying—the antitechnology bias, the hostility toward modern medicine, the nostalgic invocations of "death with dignity"—obscures the difficult task for the patient, family, and medical staff of finding "appropriate care" through an appreciation of both medical facts and personal goals. Moreover, while the cost of services is rarely addressed in this book, the task of defining good care for each patient has become even more difficult in recent years, as enthusiasm over the accomplishments of modern medicine has been tempered by a growing awareness of the financial burden of health expenditures. The aged and terminally ill are commanding an enormous share of scarce resources, and the vast expenditures on their behalf sometimes yield disappointingly little benefit. Physicians now are increasingly subject to social and economic sanctions to limit expensive efforts on behalf of their patients, further redefining the notion of "appropriate care."

This text emphasizes attention to comfort, support, and the personal values of the patient with far-advanced cancer, viewing "invasive measures" and some life-pro-longing measures with a good deal of skepticism. Nonetheless, the text recognizes the constant tensions in clinical work between overtreating and neglecting, and between professional (or technical) and personal (or subjective) methods of evaluating care. These tensions will not be readily resolved. Indeed, a recurrent theme in the history of American medicine has been the dispute between "mainline medicine" and those "sects" that have found standard care either overly heroic (*e.g.*, excessive in drugging or bleeding patients) or lacking in a psychological perspective.[2]

SELECTED REFERENCES

1. Erikson EH: On protest and affirmation. Harvard Med Alum Bull 4:30–32, 1972
2. Starr P: The Social Transformation of American Medicine. New York, Basic Books, 1982

Outpatient Management of Advanced Cancer

Symptom Control

Part One

Pain Control 1

No death need be physically painful. . . . There are no circumstances contradicting the practice of Thomas Fuller's good physician: 'when he can keep life no longer in, he makes a fair and easy passage for it to go out'. Nowadays, when the voice of Fate calls, the majority of men may repeat the last words of Socrates: 'I owe a cock to Asclepius'—a debt of thankfulness, as was his, for a fair and easy passage.

William Osler[70]

THE PROBLEM OF CHRONIC PAIN

The word "cancer" raises the specter of chronic pain and suffering. Unrelieved physical distress is the foremost concern of the dying patient. The control of pain is a prerequisite for successful management of a terminal illness in the home.

Unlike the familiar phenomenon of acute pain, the devastating and demoralizing qualities of chronic pain may be inadequately appreciated by the untrained observer.[15,55] Chronic pain sufferers often appear relatively well, and they communicate their distress poorly. The pain seems to tie its victim's tongue; cries for help may be ineffectual groans. Once relieved, chronic pain, like a nightmare, is vaguely recalled.

A fine description of chronic pain was provided by Leo Tolstoy in "The Death of Ivan Ilych," a remarkable story that recounts the effects of unrelieved bodily suffering and a lonely dying on a 45-year-old judge.[87] Pain seems to fill up every bit of the judge's awareness, grossly distorting his personality and leaving him no mind or energy for living. Tolstoy describes the experience as like "being thrust into a narrow, deep black sack."

The life of the chronic pain sufferer becomes organized around avoiding or treating pain, rather than making the most of the remaining time. The patient may feel that the discomfort will never go away and is constantly reminded of impending deterioration and death. The sufferer cannot sleep, is constantly anxious, and becomes worn down, withdrawn, whining, helpless, and defeated before the meaningless aching that invades and takes over the body. Emily Dickinson described the distortion of time and consciousness provoked by chronic pain[22]:

3

Pain—expands the Time—
Ages coil within
The minute Circumference
Of a single Brain—

Pain contracts—the Time—
Occupied with Shot
Gamuts of Eternities
Are as they were not—
                    [circa 1864]*

Pain—has an Element of Blank—
It cannot recollect
When it begun—or if there were
A time when it was not—

It has no Future—but itself—
Its Infinite contain
Its Past—enlightened to perceive
New Periods—of Pain.
                    [circa 1862]†

In this setting, death becomes a wished-for and welcomed end, a relief from suffering.

Bonica has pointed out how pain control is neglected in oncology textbooks.[14] A similar charge could be brought against general medical textbooks and medical training. While there need be no apology for the emphasis in contemporary health-care training on precise diagnosis and specific treatment, the lack of attention to the goal of comfort (sometimes disparaged as merely covering up the problem) is unfortunate.

In Cartwright's study, 87% of cancer patients had pain in the last year of life.[17] Only about half of cancer patients, however, will have a significant problem with pain during the course of their illness, and pain will be difficult to control in roughly 10%.[92] Among patients hospitalized at a cancer center, 9% were referred to a pain service, and 38% were noted to have significant pain; 60% with terminal cancer had pain.[29,30] Parkes noted that 20% of the spouses of patients who died of cancer in a hospital reported "severe or nearly continuous pain."[72] Thus, despite all the resources available in such institutions, the perpetual aggravation of chronic pain is allowed to continue.

The quality of pain control at home has not been systematically studied. Parkes reported from Great Britain that 28% of terminally ill patients at home suffer "severe and mostly continuous pain" in the final phase of the terminal period, compared with about 20% in the hospital and 8% at St. Christopher's Hospice.[72] (Since the patient groups are dissimilar, no conclusions can be made that one site of care is better than another.) Cartwright reported that about half of patients who went home to die had cancer and that 84% suffered "very distressing symptoms"; discharge from the hospital also led to increased pain, insomnia, vomiting, anorexia, constipation, bedsores, dyspnea, and depression.[17]

The reputation and success of the hospice movement lie, in great part, on the ability of hospice staff to provide comfort to patients with chronic pain, especially those with the so-called "intractable pain" that other clinicians have failed to eradicate. The success rates in hospices are most impressive. St. Christopher's in London now boasts that less than 1% of its patients have pain that is "difficult to control."[4] Equally remarkable is the testimony that comes from walking on the wards at St. Christopher's Hospice. Many of the patients have been referred there because of intolerable pain, most of them will die within days or a few weeks, and many of them are on high doses of narcotics, yet they look bright, comfortable, alert, even cheerful—not restless, withdrawn, or sedated.

Wondrous as the achievements of St. Christopher's Hospice may seem, miracles or secret formulas are not required for such success. When straightforward principles are applied, patients with pain can live well until they die. The first set of principles, outlined in this chapter, bears on the clinical pharmacology of analgesics, particularly the intelligent use of narcotics to free patients from the "narrow, deep black sack" of chronic pain. A second set of principles, outlined especially in Chapters 2 (The Management of Common Symptoms) and 6 (Coping with Loss), deals with careful attention to and aggressive management of all the discomforts that may accompany advanced cancer—symptoms such as nausea, anxiety, depression, dry mouth, and itching. A final set of principles, touched on in this and subsequent chapters, regards the development of the proper environment for the patient: a secure, comfortable, familiar setting, which offers appropriate physical and emotional supports and an atmosphere of encouragement and hope, and which, furthermore, provides continuity with the distractions and pleasures of a normal life, so that the patient does not focus on suffering and slip into the "black sack." These principles define an ideal of care, and the physician who grasps them will find them widely applicable to the practice of medicine, not just to the care of the dying.

Cancer patients, regardless of their current medical condition, will be concerned about pain and the prospect of suffering. Early on in their illness, they should be reassured about the infrequency of pain and of the ready availability of excellent pain-control techniques. They do not need to tolerate discomfort. They should expect and demand relief.

A GENERAL APPROACH TO PAIN CONTROL

Whereas this chapter focuses on the use of narcotics, optimal pain control entails a great deal more than knowing how to prescribe medication. Good treatment begins with understanding the cause of the pain and with appreciating the patient's perceptions of being ill and receiving care.

The Diagnosis of Pain

Acute pain is a useful warning signal of tissue damage or irritation. The sensation commands attention, telling the sufferer to take his or her hand away from the hot stove or to get help for a broken bone or an inflamed appendix. For the patient with chronic cancer pain, however, the continual alerting has no ongoing value. Once the warning message has been heeded, the pain should be erased.[66]

New or changed pains, however, must be carefully noted, especially in situations where the patient's sensitivity to discomfort has been diminished by drugs. Accelerated pain should suggest new diagnoses, particularly when the patient does not describe the discomfort as merely a worsened version of an old pain.

Even in the last stages of cancer, a proper diagnosis of the cause of pain can be valuable. Discomfort from impaction should not be treated with narcotics, nor ulcer pain with aspirin. Specific diagnoses often imply specific treatments: steroids for the headache of increased intracranial pressure; anti-inflammatory drugs and radiation for bone pain; psychotropic agents for complaints that reflect anxiety or depression; drainage and antibiotics for infectious processes; muscle relaxants for spasm; and so on.

Unfortunately, most of the pain experienced by cancer patients comes from the disease itself. Some pains may result from paraneoplastic processes (*e.g.*, hypertrophic osteoarthropathy, myalgias, arthralgias, arthritis, and neuropathies), but most reflect local tumor processes. In a review of oncology inpatients at the Sloan–Kettering Institute for Cancer Research, only 3% of the diagnosed pains were unrelated to cancer, although 19% were due to the treatment for cancer.[29] Twycross found 303 distinct pains in 100 patients with far-advanced cancer; 80% had more than one pain, while 34% had four or more.[94] Ninety-one percent of patients experienced pain caused directly by the cancer; 12% had discomfort that could be attributed to treatment; and 19% had pain indirectly related to cancer but attributed to chronic disease or debility (*e.g.*, the pain of constipation), while 39% of patients had discomfort unrelated to cancer, usually myofascial in origin. Table 1-1 reviews pain syndromes caused by cancer treatment.

TABLE 1-1
Pain Syndromes Associated with Cancer Therapy

POSTSURGICAL PAIN
>   Incisional pain after thoracotomy, mastectomy, neck dissection, amputation
>   Phantom pain (*e.g.*, "phantom limb" or "phantom breast" pain)
>   Lymphedema, especially after mastectomy

POSTCHEMOTHERAPY PAIN
>   Polyneuropathy—symmetrical dysesthesias with vincristine, vinblastine, procarbazine
>   Steroid pseudorheumatism from withdrawal of steroids (myalgia, arthralgia; sometimes
>   fever, joint swelling, and worsened neurologic symptoms)
>   Aseptic necrosis (of the head of the femur or humerus) with steroid therapy
>   Mucositis (lips, mouth, pharynx, nasal passages)
>   Gout
>   Phlebitis, necrosis from extravasation at site of injection
>   Second primary tumor

POSTRADIATION THERAPY PAIN
>   Fibrosis around nerves
>   (*e.g.*, brachial or lumbosacral plexus, often appearing late [8 mo–3 yr] with
>   lymphedema)
>   Radiation myelopathy
>   Radiation burns
>   Mucositis (often with secondary infection) including radiation cystitis
>   Second primary tumor

(After Bonica JJ: Cancer pain. In Bonica JJ [ed]: Pain, pp 335–362. New York, Raven Press, 1980)

Psychosocial Components

Pain is not solely a reflection of tissue damage. The significance of the psychological component in the experience of pain can hardly be exaggerated. Attempting to understand and eradicate pain without respecting its affective component is like trying to win at poker without being dealt a full hand.

A striking example of the effect of emotions on pain perception is provided by Beecher.[11] He compared a series of soldiers who were wounded on the battlefield with a group of civilians brought to an emergency ward with injuries from car accidents and other civilian trauma. On the whole, the degree of tissue injury was greater among the soldiers, yet only about a third of them complained of pain or requested or required narcotics, while about four fifths of the civilians required pain medication. Beecher suggested that the soldiers were living in great fear of dying and that they experienced their calamitous wounds with some sense of relief, knowing that they would now be removed from battle and sent home. The civilians encountered an unexpected and totally unwanted disruption of their lives and hence seemed to suffer more from a lesser injury.*

Another instance of the importance of nonpharmacologic factors in the daily practice of medicine is provided by studies of the placebo effect.[27] Patient expectations and the nature of the doctor–patient relationship have a powerful bearing on the immediate outcome of treatment, including the response to analgesics. Unfortunately, our understanding of how to promote this effect and of its significance in the management of chronic cancer pain is meager. Indeed, the challenge to the clinician comes not in accepting the general importance of psychological factors but in recognizing their specific role in the individual patient's distress and in harnessing their enormous potential to promote well-being. This text assumes that the perceived competence and compassion of the physician and his or her ability to convey optimism and encouragement can be extremely important in comforting patients. Indeed, such qualities are valued regardless of whether they induce a helpful psychological effect on pain. Subsequent chapters on fear and insecurity, truth-telling, and coping with loss will underscore the importance of trustfulness and hopefulness, and will help the reader appreciate and enlist psychological factors that seem to be of major importance to the patient's well-being.

Five psychological issues in the perception and expression of pain deserve special mention here.

---

*The long-standing clinical observation that pain has both sensory and affective components is mirrored in recent neuroanatomical and neurophysiological studies. Research on the neural pathways of pain has led to a distinction between two systems within the ascending spinothalamic tract.[58] The first, the "neospinothalamic," transmits spacial localization and sensory quality from small, well-defined receptive fields; ascending pathways with few collaterals extend to topographically organized thalamic and cortical areas. The second, the "paleospinothalamic" tract, transmits from wide receptive fields and shows extensive collaterals with the brainstem and higher centers; it seems to carry the diffuse autonomic and emotional components of pain, *e.g.,* alerting and affective responses. Moreover, a descending analgesic system which originates in cortical and limbic centers seems to act on pain transmission at the level of the spinal cord, providing an endogenous pain inhibitory mechanism mediated partly by enkephalins. Research on endorphins has suggested a neurochemical basis for some psychologically-induced changes in pain threshold and perception, but has not yet led to a clinically useful method for turning on or adjusting this pain mechanism.

Depression and Anxiety

Two broad diagnoses, depression and anxiety, are worth keeping in mind with dying patients, since both conditions may contribute markedly to pain and may respond to a variety of therapies. Pain, of course, can produce anxiety and depression, and the use of drugs to produce physical comfort may lead to striking improvement in a patient's mood. On the other hand, narcotics will not treat loneliness, insecurity, or despair, nor alleviate depression that is not the result of physical pain. The difficulty of making the diagnosis of depression in cancer patients, especially when they are in pain, and the rudiments of treatment for both anxiety and depression are discussed in Chapter 6 (Coping with Loss).

The Meaning of Pain

The meaning of the pain may be more important to the patient than the associated physical distress. Ask what the patient makes of the symptom, the illness, and the treatment. Cancer patients are often fearful, and they anxiously monitor their bodies for evidence of disease. They may attribute mild, even normal sensations to the illness and may interpret unrelated sensations or the side-effects of treatment as evidence of progressive disease. A patient with a headache may fear a stroke, going blind, being crazy, not being able to work, or being prevented from attending an important social event. Once this personal meaning of the pain is understood, shared, and addressed, the patient may not even want to take an aspirin. Attention to treating pain, rather than to alleviating the underlying fear, may serve only to confirm that the anxiety is justified, that something is seriously wrong.

A number of studies have demonstrated the efficacy of providing accurate information in order to relieve pain.[23,84] Patients respond to unexplained discomforts differently than to understood ones. Thus, a patient who is put on narcotics for the first time may think he or she is being "put to sleep," "doped up," turned into a "junky," or made ready for the grave and may resist helpful treatment until these feelings are understood and the useful nature of the treatment is clarified.

To explain routinely the diagnosis and the treatment is not enough. The physician needs to listen carefully and to elicit the meaning of events for the patient:

> What do you think is wrong?
>
> What have others said?
>
> Do you know anyone with similar problems?
>
> What do you make of the diagnosis? The treatment?
>
> What are you thinking this means about the future?

Chapter 5 (Feeling Secure) offers an approach to understanding and managing common fears: anticipating problems, eliciting concerns, rehearsing what to do in a crisis, and reassuring. The resultant sense of security and confidence can be a great painkiller.

The Social Value of Suffering

Patients gain attention by complaining of pain. A complaint of pain sometimes may be the only way of obtaining care from others. Thus, the symptom may have a social function: ensuring assistance from the nurse and physician or from family and friends. In some cultures, people ask for help by saying, "I hurt." Also, care-seeking and dependency may be considered legitimate only when physical suffering has been demonstrated. As one patient noted, "You have to be dying before you can get any attention around here."

When offers of help are always contingent on the patient's report of physical discomfort, pain complaints may not be readily relinquished. Drugs will not cure this situation. The clinician should ask, "What would this person's life be like without the pain?" Complaining behaviors can be reduced by providing greater support, particularly by giving attention that is not contingent on the expression of distress. At times, the style of communication can be discussed by the family, and their responses modified. Alternately, when a complaint seems to serve a social purpose and has little physical distress attached to it, and especially when it functions as part of a longstanding, stable pattern of family behavior, the physician may choose not to try to treat it.

The usually benign "secondary gain" engendered by the sick role can be contrasted with an extreme form of manipulation seen in very unhappy, empty patients who seem never to get enough from the family or health-care workers and who may be endlessly demanding or angry. Some of these "problem patients" try to use narcotics to obliterate awareness, hoping to withdraw into a stupor that is more pleasant than reality. Awakened from sleep, they complain of unbearable pain. Such patients are usually very difficult to manage, regardless of how they use narcotics. They often produce feelings of rage, resentment, guilt, and frustration in the people who try to care for them. Such hateful feelings may be manifested as friction among health-care workers or family members or between these two groups. Psychiatric liaison or consultation should be considered.

The Patient's Environment

Terms such as the "patient's environment" or "milieu" refer to a host of physical, social, and psychological factors—people, places, objects, and activities—that may have potent effects on the perception of pain. The Palliative Care Service at the Montreal General Hospital noted that 90% of their patients in a special hospice unit achieved satisfactory pain control, but that similar pain patients on general medical or surgical wards, treated with the same approach and the same medications, were successfully managed only 75% to 80% of the time.[61]

Inpatient hospice units have emphasized the value of a warm, secure, cheerful atmosphere. The staff is familiar with the care of the dying and is confident that they can succeed in comforting any patient. They convey a sense of calm optimism. The staff is allowed the time to provide meticulous personal attention to patients. Such ready availability of help and such a sense of security, as discussed in Chapters 4 (The Task of Physical Care) and 5 (Feeling Secure), are important ingredients in optimal pain control.

Various features of the inpatient hospice help maintain the patient's self-esteem, feeling of personal control, and sense of an identity beyond that of being a sick or dying person. Ideally, hospice patients wear their own clothes rather than hospital gowns, and they surround themselves with personal possessions. Patients may administer their own medication. The family is welcomed and can participate in care, including cooking. Young children and pets may be brought to the ward. Food is warm, palatable, and prepared especially as the patient wishes, perhaps by the family. Alcoholic beverages are allowed. Music, games, television, hobbies, and other sources of recreation and pleasure are promoted.

For the hospice patient who wants to be with other people, perhaps to reminisce or share feelings or to join in everyday banter, the family and staff are on hand, available for befriending and listening. A sympathetic person, such as a trained volunteer, who attends to the patient's fears and concerns and who shares in common pleasures, makes life today more joyous and pain more bearable. As one voiceless patient wrote when asked by his physician if he needed anything, "Being here is enough." Training for hospice staff and volunteers focuses on the psychosocial aspects of living with a fatal illness, realizing that attention to all areas of distress—physical, emotional, social, spiritual, or existential—helps the patient feel better and makes the pain treatment more successful. A meticulous regard for the details of the environment and an ongoing commitment to addressing physical and psychosocial factors in the patient's experience of illness may make the difference between adequate and excellent pain relief.

The promotion of home care represents, in large part, an argument for the importance of these environmental factors. Some pains may vanish or diminish notably when a patient is transferred home (although an equally familiar phenomenon is the resolution of pain in the doctor's waiting room or the emergency ward). Many carefully designed and engineered aspects of inpatient hospice care are almost effortlessly available at home. Ingenuity still should be exercised to help the home-based patient adjust to a restricted life and to find meaningful activities that both give pleasure and focus attention away from symptoms. Distractions help all but the more severe pains and should be abundant—not the stereotyped "activities" of recreational therapy in the "old folks' home," but personally meaningful pursuits.

The Contribution of Other Physical Symptoms

Finally, just as anxiety, depression, insecurity, and fear make pain worse, so do other physical symptoms. The physician must pay careful attention to anything that causes distress—nausea, vomiting, shortness of breath, dry mouth, anorexia, bedsores, aching muscles, itching, malodorous wounds, insomnia, the discomfort of nasogastric tubes or injections, or feeling the need for a haircut or a shower—big problems and little ones. When these symptoms are relieved, life becomes less difficult, and mild pain can sometimes be ignored. Conversely, the patient who has been made physically comfortable is much better able to deal with the inevitable emotional crises of sickness and dying.

> There is far too much talk in death and dying circles in this country about psychological and emotional problems, and far too little about making the patient comfortable. Any group concerned with service to the dying must be talking about smoothing sheets, rubbing bottoms, relieving constipation, and sitting up at night. Counseling a dying person who is lying in a wet bed is ineffective. . . .
>
> If people are cared for with common sense and basic professional skills, with detailed attention to self-evident problems and physical needs, then patients and families themselves can cope with many of their emotional crises. Without pain, well-nursed, with bowels controlled, mouth clean, and a caring friend available, the psychological problems fall into a manageable perspective.[49]

A PHARMACOLOGIC APPROACH TO PAIN CONTROL

Common Problems in the Use of Analgesics

In 1973, a lead article in the *Annals of Internal Medicine* suggested that the most common form of "narcotic abuse" in hospitalized patients is *undertreatment of pain*.[57] Marks and Sachar examined 37 medical inpatients receiving meperidine (Demerol).

TABLE 1-2
Diagnoses, Distress Scores, and Drug Regimens for Medical Patients Treated with Intramuscular Meperidine (Demerol)—
Results of 12 most distressed patients

Diagnosis	Distress Score	Dosage of Meperidine Prescribed (mg)	Dosage of Meperidine Received (mg/day)
Coronary ischemia	18	100 q4h	300
Chronic cholecystitis	17	75 q4h	150
Diabetic neuropathy	17	50 q4h	100
Duodenal ulcer	16	75 q4h	175
Angina pectoris	15	75 q4h	75
Arterial occlusion of leg	14	75 q4h	85
Duodenal ulcer	14	50 q4h	100
RHD, congestive failure	14	50 q4h	50
Cancer of pancreas	14	50 q4h	25
Diabetes with cellulitis	14	50 q3h	25
Myocardial infarct	13	75 q4h	75
Pulmonary infarct	13	50 q4h	75

(Marks RM, Sachar EJ: Undertreatment of medical inpatients with narcotic analgesics. Ann Intern Med 78:173–181, 1973)

Pain was rated on a scale of 1 to 18. One third of patients had distress scores over 12, indicating "marked distress." The authors then looked at physicians' medication orders and at the medication sheets wherein nurses recorded the timing and the amount of drug given. Table 1-2 shows the results of the 12 patients with "marked distress." In reviewing these findings, it should be appreciated that 50 mg of parenteral meperidine is often an inadequate dose for the average patient. Effective doses are regularly in the range of 75 to 150 mg. Also, meperidine usually wears off in 2 to 3 hours. In this study, meperidine was prescribed in doses that were too low and too infrequent, and the actual amount given, even for patients in marked distress, was not only well below what should sensibly have been offered, but also well below what was actually prescribed.

This article, along with similar studies,[19,20,100] editorials,[1] and reports from hospice groups,[66,78–80] identifies four common and recurrent problems in the use of narcotics for the chronic pain of advanced cancer (and for other painful states): the prescribed dose, the prescribed interval, the delivery of medication, and inappropriate fears of tolerance or addiction.

The Prescribed Dose

Patients often get too little narcotic; sometimes they get too much. Low doses leave the patient in pain; high doses produce sedation. As shown in Figure 1-1, between these two "analgesic zones"—"inadequate effect" and "toxicity"—is a zone of "useful effect" in which pain is abolished.[96]

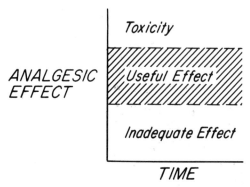

FIG. 1-1. Narcotic analgesic effect zones (After Vere DW: Pharmacology of morphine drugs used in terminal care. In Vere DW [ed]: Topics in Therapeutics 4, pp 75–83. Kent, England, Pitman Medical Publishing, 1978)

The appropriate dose provides adequate pain relief without sedation. On the one hand, patients do not need to suffer with pain; persistent discomfort implies too low a dose. On the other hand, patients do not need to be made drowsy or put to sleep in order to escape from pain; a clouded sensorium suggests an overdose of narcotics.

Contrary to widespread notions that narcotics do not obliterate pain but merely act on its affective component or cause patients not to care about their discomfort, properly medicated patients regularly report that their pain is entirely gone.*

Conscientious efforts are required to arrive at a dose within the proper analgesic zone, but patients under good medical supervision need never experience severe discomfort from chronic cancer pain. Relief from severe or moderate pain should be achieved rapidly. The patient may endure short periods of mild discomfort or drowsiness while the medication is further adjusted and, of course, may be subjected to brief pain in moments of crises (*e.g.*, when new pains develop or old pains change).

Figure 1-2 illustrates the difference between comparable orally and parenterally administered doses of narcotics. Oral medication is slower to take effect; it wears off more slowly, producing a sustained period of analgesia in the proper zone. Parenteral medication acts rapidly and has a likelihood of causing brief toxicity immediately after administration; it wears off more quickly, leaving the patient uncomfortable sooner than does the oral preparation.

*While overt sedation is not clinically evident in patients receiving appropriate opiate doses, mental status changes may occur. Smith gave standard doses of parenteral morphine to healthy young subjects, and noted impairment in their performance on a variety of tests of mental function.[82] The narcotics did not decrease the subjects' accuracy in performing tasks, but slowed their speed in completing them. Comparable data is not available for medical patients who use narcotics chronically for pain. In a study which relied on subjective reports, Lasagna observed that normal subjects receiving parenteral narcotics, especially at higher doses, noted more sedation, impaired mentation, and dysphoria than those receiving a placebo.[53] Increased drowsiness was not reported among chronically ill patients, however, leading the authors to emphasize that both subjective and objective effects of these drugs are dependent on the patient population and the situation in which they are administered. When narcotics are used chronically, the clinician usually will have little evidence of these drugs' potential subtle psychotropic actions: the possible satiation of aggressive, sexual, and other pleasure-seeking drives; the promotion of indifference and detachment; subclinical effects on learning, memory, and performance; and related psychosocial effects.

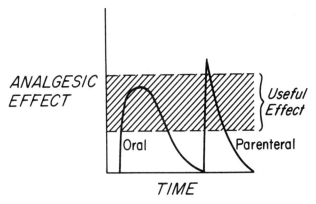

FIG. 1-2. Analgesic effect with oral and parenteral narcotics (After Vere DW: Pharmacology of morphine drugs used in terminal care. In Vere DW [ed]: Topics in Therapeutics 4, pp 75–83. Kent, England, Pitman Medical Publishing, 1978)

The Prescribed Interval

The interval between doses also requires careful adjustment. Analgesics are typically prescribed *prn* (as needed). Such a regimen may be sensible for managing acute pain (*e.g.*, for postsurgical patients whose physical distress and alertness may be fluctuating rapidly). For chronic cancer patients, however, the practice of waiting for a narcotic to wear off before giving the next dose ensures that the patient is subjected to recurrent periods of pain. With prn analgesic orders, the following sequence occurs repeatedly: the medication wears off, mild pain returns, pain becomes bothersome, the patient asks for medication, the medication is delivered, the medication is ingested, the medication is absorbed and begins to work, the pain gets better, and the pain is relieved. While waiting for the medicine to take effect, the patient may have 30 minutes (and usually more) of pain between every prn dose (Fig. 1-3). The patient becomes preoccupied with the regular recurrence of discomfort.

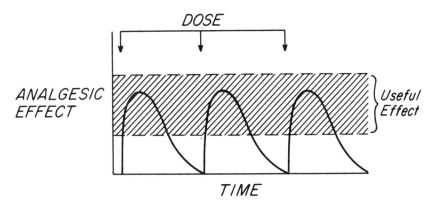

FIG. 1-3. Poorly timed (prn) dosage (After Vere DW: Pharmacology of morphine drugs used in terminal care. In Vere DW [ed]: Topics in Therapeutics 4, pp 75–83. Kent, England, Pitman Medical Publishing, 1978)

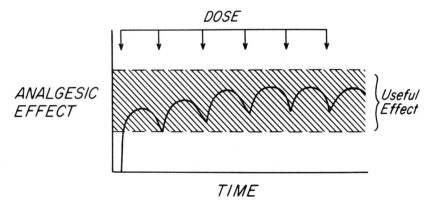

FIG. 1-4. Properly timed ("by the clock") dosage (After Vere DW: Pharmacology of morphine drugs used in terminal care. In Vere DW [ed]: Topics in Therapeutics 4, pp 75–83. Kent, England, Pitman Medical Publishing, 1978)

Do not wait for pain; anticipate it. Give the next dose before pain recurs. Do not prescribe prn; prescribe regularly by the clock (Fig. 1-4). This principle of treatment should be clarified with the patient and family, as well as with the staff, especially those who have been trained to hold off the administration of analgesics as long as possible.

A number of authors have stressed the importance of "erasing the pain memory," of freeing the patient from the fear of pain.[66] Pain itself seems to antagonize analgesia. Often, less medication is needed to keep pain obliterated than to erase existing pain repeatedly. When pain is treated prophylactically, the discomfort and anxiety associated with improper scheduling of medications is avoided, and the daily dose of narcotics may diminish.

The Delivery of Medication

Medicines are not always given as ordered. Understaffed wards and late-night nursing shifts are notorious for letting pain patients suffer. At home, some patients and families have difficulty following a prescribed regimen or may omit treatments because of misunderstandings. Some patients and families simply prefer prn regimens (and the attendant discomfort); their wishes should be respected. Commonly, improper delivery of medications is related to the fourth problem.

Inappropriate Fears of Tolerance or Addiction

TOLERANCE.[101]   Tolerance is the phenomenon whereby some drugs become less potent when used for a long period of time. (The term generally is used to reflect "cellular tolerance"—the response of the nervous system to the drug—rather than "metabolic tolerance"—changes in the metabolism of the drug, which necessitate increased doses to achieve stable levels at tissue or receptor sites.) Patients may be afraid to use a medicine now because they feel that they will have greater need for it later or that even higher doses will eventually not be effective.

Tolerance is, in fact, an easily managed problem when narcotic analgesics are used for chronic terminal cancer pain. In the first place, required doses often remain quite low. At St. Christopher's Hospice, for example, only 28% of patients needed more than 20 mg of oral morphine.[80] Mount reported average doses of morphine of 10 to 13 mg po.[65] Furthermore, Twycross has presented data suggesting that long-term cancer pain patients with stable conditions will escalate their narcotic requirements for 3 weeks to 6 months, then level off for subsequent months.[92] Figure 1-5 illustrates a typical patient's use of narcotics over many years.

Second, when tolerance develops, the narcotic dose merely needs to be increased slightly so that good pain control is reestablished. Stronger pain-killing effect is always available. Tolerance to the analgesic effects of narcotics parallels tolerance to toxic effects (*e.g.*, clouded sensorium and respiratory depression), and a zone of useful analgesic effect can still be identified (Fig. 1-6). Thus, a patient who initially requires morphine 20 mg po q4h and is sedated with 30 mg po q4h may eventually require 40 mg po q4h to be comfortable, but will not be sedated unless 50 or 60 mg po q4h is given. Some tolerant patients use over 100 mg of oral morphine (or equivalent parenteral doses) and yet are fully alert.

The only practical concern related to tolerance is the need for a greater number of pills or a larger volume of oral solution or injections. Most patients can be managed with oral morphine elixirs, which can deliver very high doses in small volumes. Low-volume injections are reviewed in a subsequent section of this chapter.

DEPENDENCE.[101]   Dependence (formerly called addiction) can be physical, psychological, or both. Many writers have stated that concerns about dependence in a patient near death are ridiculous and cruel, yet such worries are habitual and common among health-care workers. Moreover, such fears of dependence are misfounded for even the "terminal patient" who lives for months or years.

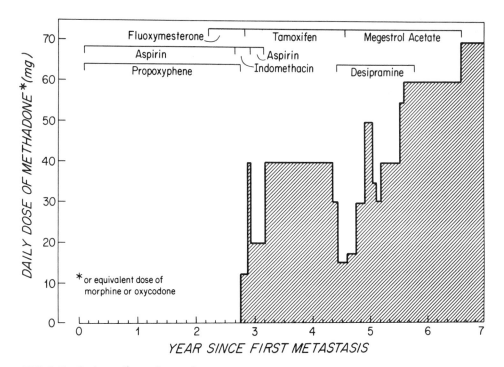

FIG. 1-5.   Prolonged use of narcotics

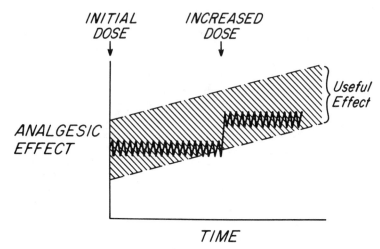

FIG. 1-6. Tolerance (After Vere DW: Pharmacology of morphine drugs used in terminal care. In Vere DW [ed]: Topics in Therapeutics 4, pp 75–83. Kent, England, Pitman Medical Publishing, 1978)

Physical dependence is a common phenomenon when opiates are taken regularly; it parallels the development of tolerance. Some degree of physical dependence can be detected after a few weeks or less of regular narcotic use. Withdrawal of the narcotic (or administration of a narcotic antagonist) produces a characteristic constellation of symptoms and signs: irritability, insomnia, tremor, lacrimation, rhinorrhea, yawning, perspiration, piloerection, chills, flushing, abdominal cramps, and muscle aches and spasm.

Contrary to the expectation of many health-care workers who have dealt with narcotic addicts, the usual opiate withdrawal among cancer patients, even among those who have been on high doses of analgesics, provokes only mild discomfort. The outpatient may not even bother to notify the physician, whereas an inpatient with this syndrome may pass unnoticed except for minor changes in the vital signs and a few nonspecific complaints that may not be recognized as representing withdrawal. Withdrawal in cancer patients (and presumably other patients who are not psychologically dependent) is usually not like the turbulent "going cold turkey," dramatically portrayed in movies about narcotics abusers.

Insofar as withdrawal can cause discomfort, physical dependence is easily managed by warning patients not to stop opiates suddenly and by tapering chronic analgesic regimens slowly rather than precipitously. Gradual withdrawal can often be accomplished over a few days and is easily accepted if pain does not emerge. Physical dependence does not prevent appropriate periodic attempts at downward adjustment of medication dosage.

Psychological dependence—a craving for the drug and for the pleasant feeling associated with its use, a preoccupation with securing its supply, or related compulsive patterns of drug-seeking and abuse, which deviate from accepted medical and social patterns—is hardly ever observed among chronic cancer-pain patients. In the hospital setting where most health-care workers learn about drug dependence, narcotic "addicts" make up the vast majority of patients who are recognized as undergoing withdrawal, and these patients show prominent physical symptoms and signs, along with striking drug-seeking behavior. Cancer patients who taper off medications will generally have little or no withdrawal symptoms and will be unlikely to complain, since they are not psychologically dependent. Lamerton, an experienced hospice physician comments:

> If for some reason the pain goes away . . . then the morphine can be tailed off and stopped. I have never known this process to present difficulties. Addiction is a myth.[50]

Statistics are lacking on the incidence of psychological dependence among cancer patients or in a general medical population to which narcotics are administered, but the following points deserve note:

1. Psychological dependence is a rarity among cancer patients. They seem to take just the amount of medication they need, often less, rather than escalating the dose. Indeed, undermedication and reluctance to use narcotics are common clinical problems, not drug-craving. Patients generally do not report a "high" from the medication, and they do not desire to continue analgesic use when their pain resolves. They taper the dose when pain improves.*

2. Withholding adequate doses of narcotics does not prevent psychological dependence. Indeed, one theory holds that insufficient analgesia may provoke psychological dependence, whereas prophylactic administration of proper doses of narcotics will interrupt the psychological link between pain, drug-taking, and the relief of distress, and thus will deter the development of a conditioned state of dependence. Thus, even the patient with a prognosis of prolonged survival should not be denied narcotics when these drugs are required for pain control.

3. After prolonged ingestion of large amounts of narcotics, medical patients (and substance abusers) may uneventfully stop the use of these drugs.[48,92] Neither lengthy narcotic treatment nor the prescription of higher doses of these drugs necessarily leads to the development of psychological dependence.

    The pattern of chronic recidivistic abuse of narcotics may represent an unusual or atypical response to these drugs. For instance, among 451 men who were chosen as a random sample of veterans ending their tour in Vietnam, 43% had used narcotics, 29% had used them regularly, and 20% had been dependent at some time, but only about 10% were drug dependent on returning to the United States.[76] Eight to 12 months later, 10% of this sample reported some narcotics use since returning, but only 2% noted current use, while 0.7% were addicted. In a sample of 490 men, drawn from the 10.5% of veterans who had positive urine tests for drugs upon returning to the United States, 89% were dependent on narcotics when they ended their tour, but only 8% were using narcotics when interviewed 8 to 12 months later. Thus, another author concluded that the "repeated self-administration of heroin does not invariably lead to compulsive daily use."[67]

---

*Kanner and Foley examined narcotic drug use in a cancer pain clinic.[48] Out of an original group of 103 patients who were referred, two patients took more medication than prescribed and overdosed themselves. Both patients were described as having chronic, non-malignant pain and a history of drug abuse. In reviewing many papers on narcotic addiction, the authors concluded that a "normal nervous constitution" is infrequent in an addict population, and that psychological dependence and substance abuse are rarely associated with legitimate opiate use for cancer pain. In the most worrisome study cited, 27% of white addicts and 1% of black addicts reported having first received narcotics from a physician to the point of addiction in the course of treatment for an illness.

4. Obviously, psychological dependence can occur. The "addictive personality" is not immune to cancer. Drug abuse, however, is usually not difficult to recognize, and does not itself necessarily pose a major problem for the physician who, still wishing to prescribe regular analgesic use for cancer pain, will simply need to supervise medication more closely. Patients who develop drug dependence are likely to be "problem patients," regardless of their use of narcotics.

5. Fears of tolerance and dependence are ubiquitous. Indeed, concerns about addiction are frequent in patients taking nonaddictive medications. Successful narcotic treatment of pain requires vigorous effort on the part of the physician to clarify misconceptions about tolerance and addiction with everyone involved in the patient's care. It is terribly cruel to suggest that cancer patients are abusing drugs when they need and deserve good painkillers to lead a decent life. Physicians should be alert to mindless antidrug sentiment among health-care professionals, patients, family members, and themselves.

> When Dr N came she begged, 'Let them inject me as often as necessary,' and she imitated the action of a nurse thrusting in the needle.
> 'Ha, ha, you are going to become a real drug-addict!' said N in a bantering tone. 'I can supply you with morphia at very interesting rates.' His expression hardened and he coldly said in my direction, 'There are two points upon which a self-respecting doctor does not compromise—drugs and abortion.'
>
> [Simone de Beauvoir, writing about her mother's terminal illness in a memoir ironically entitled *A Very Easy Death*[21]]

Judging Dosage and Timing of Narcotics

In the management of pain with narcotics, respect individual differences. Pharmacological research has documented wide variations in bioavailability, distribution, and clearance of these agents, and many psychological and social factors influence the appreciation and expression of pain and the efficacy of treatment.

Objective Measures

There are no objective clinical measures of analgesia. Miosis is frequently evident in properly medicated patients and in overmedicated patients, but pupillary size or response has not been demonstrated to be useful in assessing analgesic effect. Blood levels of narcotics, insofar as they have been studied, have not proved helpful[12]; they may correlate poorly with drug levels at the site or sites of analgesic action, somewhere in the central nervous system (CNS).

Subjective Measures

The reports of the patient and family are the basis for adjusting dosage and timing. The patient's account of pain is usually quite straightforward and clear, and the clinician will have little doubt about how the medication is working. Careful questioning, however, as described below, may be needed for optimal adjustment of medication.

When medication is begun, patients report that the pain becomes better or more tolerable. When the ideal dose is being approached, the pain is "no bother" or "fine" or present only when aggravated. At an ideal dosage, the patient reports no pain or has only mild discomfort when pain is provoked. Similarly, patients will describe various degrees of pain relief or toxicity (drowsiness or confusion) in relation to the timing of the dose (see Fig. 1-2). The complete obliteration of pain in a fully alert patient is a regularly achieved, wondrous action of these old "miracle" drugs.

Occasionally patients are unable to report pain accurately. Neuropsychiatric conditions may impair the patient's ability to describe symptoms, as may fear, depression, and chronic pain itself. Personal and cultural variations in the perception and reporting of pain may complicate the clinician's job. Even the patient who seems a "good historian" may need to learn to attend to particular sensations and situations. Coming to an understanding of how each patient experiences and expresses pain is a challenging and endlessly fascinating clinical task.

Some patients use words that suggest severe pain, yet do not appear to be very uncomfortable. The family's and health-care workers' observations of restlessness, facial expression, distractability, and sleeplessness may be helpful indications of the intensity of pain.

The Pain History

The following dimensions of pain, familiar to the physician from the earliest stages of clinical training, are reviewed with suggestions for their application to advanced cancer patients:

1. *Location*—Various sites of pain should be carefully distinguished. New sites often require new diagnostic efforts. Rather than using global descriptions of pain control, the success of treatment at each site should be reviewed, and separate approaches to pain at these various locations can be considered. Charting symptoms on body diagrams may be helpful, especially when a team of health-care workers is involved in the monitoring of pain and the adjustment of medication.

2. *Intensity* may initially be difficult to communicate, but each patient can develop with his or her physician a mutually understood vocabulary to grade the severity of pain. Pain can be judged in relationship to behavioral consequences:

   Can you concentrate on other activities?

   Can you sleep?

   Can you enjoy a meal (or conversation or listening to music)?

   The present discomfort may also be compared with previous experiences:

   How does it compare with that broken arm you had? With childbirth? With the day after surgery when you tried to get out of bed?

   Some patients can grade their pain on an imaginary scale:

   If zero represented no pain at all, and 10 were the worst imaginable pain, how would you rate this discomfort? How was it before you had any treatment? How is it a few hours after you take the medicine?

3. The *quality* of the pain has diagnostic implications, but also is a marvelous mirror of the patient's personality and emotional state: the flamboyant, colorful, vague discomfort of the hysteric; the overly detailed, impersonal ruminations of the obsessive; the persecutory overtones in the suspicious, paranoid personality; or the long-suffering masochist who seems both to reject help and demand sympathy.

4. *Chronology*—The *frequency, onset, and duration* of pain may need to be recorded by the clock and should be related to daily events and the time at which the medication is taken. The periods immediately before and after the narcotic dose are

critical for noting trough (undermedicated) and peak (overmedicated) effects. Paroxysmal or shooting pains, as discussed below, may respond better to anticonvulsants than to the usual analgesics.

5. *Aggravating and alleviating factors* include activity, position, and mood. Treatment success can be gauged by the degree of comfortable activity allowed the patient: resting, moving in bed, moving from bed to chair, ambulating with assistance, walking without assistance, carrying out normal indoor activities, and so on. Can the patient be distracted? Do heat, rest, massage, and various adjunctive measures help? How does the social situation influence pain?

6. *Associated symptoms*—Concurrent fear, anxiety, and depression are often amenable to treatment, and their relief will improve pain.

7. *Attributions*—Important clues to psychosocial management are provided by the patient's notions of what causes the pain, how it should be treated, how the medication effects well-being, what the pain means in terms of prognosis, and so on. As discussed at length in Chapter 5 (Feeling Secure), these attributions may not be stated forthrightly unless sought by the physician.

8. *Adaptation*—The physician needs to determine how the patient is coping with the pain:

> *How do you get along with this pain?*
>
> *How does it affect you?*
>
> *How do you tolerate it?*

Ethnic Styles

Cultural differences in dealing with pain are also worth noting.[103,104] For some patients and families, for instance, suffering is an accepted feature of the world, and the appearance of distress is met with a host of responses that make the problem understandable, shared, and perhaps more tolerable. For others, suffering is an entirely alien phenomenon, an affront to anticipated achievement and invulnerability, a defeat, or even a shame. Cultural stereotypes are hazardous when applied automatically to an individual, yet a study of cultural differences reminds the clinician of the various ways that individuals and families may respond to pain. Also, physicians may tend to be intolerant or to misinterpret or react inappropriately to ethnic styles that are unfamiliar and different from their own.

Jews are commonly perceived as skeptical, pessimistic, or worried. They seem sensitive to pain and are readily willing to express discomfort. Jewish patients feel that a sick person is entitled to complain and get help, and they may seem to demand sympathy from their families. Their descriptions of pain may be highly detailed and may suggest their own pathophysiologic explanations for the discomfort. They often seek foremost an intellectual grasp on the illness, on the cause and meaning of suffering. They are more concerned about getting rid of the underlying disease, the source of pain, than about achieving prompt symptom control. The hospital may be seen as an impersonal place; home is often preferred.

Italians seem to have a dramatic response to pain, and they often provoke anxiety in others. They may present with family members who are also visibly upset and who convey anxiety. They seem highly expressive of a discomfort that is often diffusely felt rather than localized—the total body pain or "I hurt all over" syndrome. These patients seem totally caught up in the immediate experience, and they seek not to discover the meaning of the symptom or to review the course of the illness, but to obtain prompt physical relief. They ask for sympathy, not worry. They often prefer home; the hospital seems alien. Like the fabled Frenchmen in E. M. Forster's story about a coach whose horses suddenly run wild, Italians recover their spirits quickly after the catastrophe (unlike the Englishmen in the carriage who were unruffled during the crisis but felt bad long afterwards, unable to enjoy food and companionship).[34] Similar generalizations have been made about Hispanics.

The Irish are commonly described as stoical. They are reluctant to present symptoms to the physician, perhaps waiting until the discomfort or worry has gotten almost out of hand. The family seems to tell the patient not to worry about the symptom, although the patient may eventually be "forced" to come in by a relative. Symptoms are minimized, and pain reports may seem to drift into dreamy stories and diversions. The patient's tendency to avoid acknowledging the symptom's seriousness may either fool the physician into not taking the complaint seriously or may inadvertently communicate a submerged terror, a sense that something frightening is being concealed.

The "WASP" (white Anglo–Saxon Protestant) or "older American" is described as future-oriented. Pain is not so much a problem of the moment as a worry about what will happen next week or month. Pain descriptions sometimes seem devoid of emotional content, yet laden with practical concerns about functioning properly and getting the problem fixed. Maintaining a "stiff upper lip," WASPs devalue the expression of discomfort and especially any amplification of distress. These patients report on pain rather than complaining about it. They feel that some pain is inevitable and should be tolerated, but that excessive suffering is unnecessary and should be reversed. When their bodies are not working well, they tend to withdraw from family and social contact rather than seeking support or sympathy. A well-equipped hospital is a good place to go for rational management of pain problems. This ethnic style characterizes, at least partly, most acculturated Americans, regardless of their ethnic background, particularly persons of higher educational and socioeconomic status. The dominant values of a busy hospital ward often reflect this style.

Goals of Treatment

The physician's realistic confidence that he or she can effectively control pain will convey a useful optimism and hopefulness to the patient. Prompt relief of severe pain (and its attendant anxiety) can be readily achieved, although optimal pain control may require lengthy adjustments of medication.

Patients can almost immediately become rather comfortable at rest and can generally obtain a good night of sleep as soon as careful supervision of medications is begun in the hospital. One or 2 days of adjustment may be necessary to achieve such comfort at home, where less intense supervision of treatment is available.

Complete comfort during periods of aggravation of the pain (*e.g.*, during exacerbation of colic or during activities that stress a bony metastasis) is less readily achieved. When pain is best during bed rest, the treatment can be calibrated similarly as with a patient with congestive heart failure—by the degree of comfortable activity permitted. After comfort at rest and the ability to sleep are secured, moderate mobility and a return to many normal activities should be sought. Finally, full mobility and resumption of activities are the goals, although many medical conditions may make such restoration of function impossible. The physician helps the patient and family by setting and sharing realistic expectations for the degree of attainable relief, emphasizing satisfaction with what has been achieved and seeking tolerance, compensations, and adjustment when activities cannot be restored.

The Clinical Pharmacology of Chronic Narcotic Usage[41–43,52]

Most pharmacological studies of narcotics deal with acute, time-limited pain (such as postoperative pain), rather than with chronic pain and its associated profound psychophysiologic and social consequences. Pharmacological studies usually compare the effects of single doses of drugs rather than examining the effects of repeated, long-term administration of these agents. Extrapolations of such studies of acute pain to the use of narcotics in the chronic treatment of chronic pain may be hazardous. A cautious, empirical approach is necessary.

Some writers on chronic pain have failed to distinguish between the management of patients whose painful illnesses appear to have a well-defined "organic" or "objective" basis—malignant disease and a variety of chronic or progressive conditions such as sickle cell anemia, angina pectoris, tic douloureux, postherpetic neuralgia, and migraine headaches—as opposed to those patients in whom psychiatric, behavioral, or "functional" factors are preeminent.*

No narcotic agent has been shown to be superior in its ability to control pain. All narcotics seem to have similar side-effects when used in an appropriate fashion to achieve similar analgesic effects. Limited data on the *duration* of action and relative oral and parenteral *potency* of the various narcotics (Table 1-3) lead one, at times, to favor certain drugs for convenience and for minimizing fluctuations in analgesic effect. Studies on the heterogeneity of opiate receptors provide hope of developing selective pharmacologic agents for the analgesic, autonomic, sedating, euphoric, behavior-rewarding, respiratory-depressant, and other components of opiate action, but presently provide little guidance for the clinician.[18,73]

The available pharmacological information on narcotics does not lead us to any but the most commonsensical principles regarding when to be concerned about drug absorption (orally or parenterally) or the effects of age, weight, or hepatic and renal function on drug metabolism. Hepatic biotransformation is the major route of morphine elimination.[83] Comparisons of chronic oral, sublingual, rectal, and parenteral (continuous and intermittent subcutaneous, intramuscular, and intravenous) regimens are generally lacking. The rationale of avoiding partial agonists is discussed later in this chapter. There is no information to favor a particular narcotic agent for its efficacy in "somatic" versus "affective" pain, for its anxiolytic effects, or for its use at various sites of pain (*e.g.*, viscera or bone).

Except for the use of acetaminophen and aspirin with codeine, there is a paucity of good data on the effect of combining narcotics or adding other analgesics such as anti-inflammatory agents or "adjuvants" (cocaine, alcohol, amphetamines, and bel-

---

*In this latter category is chronic "benign" pain (or the "learned pain syndrome" or the "pain prone patient"[24]), a topic about which there has been a great deal of recent writing.[31,85] The typical patient with this disorder has had a long-standing problem with bodily distress. The discomfort or disability may be difficult to explain on a physical basis, and may seem dramatized or exaggerated. Many observers have noted that passivity, secondary gain, and conditioned or learned behaviors influence the course of this illness. Drug abuse is common, and patients often have undergone multiple unsuccessful and costly medical and surgical treatments. These patients are currently being referred to "pain clinics"—therapeutic communities which emphasize personal responsibility for pain and which provide behaviorally-oriented, multidisciplinary approaches to management. In these settings, chronic "goal-directed pain behavior" is believed to be subject to relearning. Generalizations about the nature and treatment of chronic benign pain should not be routinely applied to patients with cancer.

TABLE 1-3
Approximate Equivalent Doses of Narcotic Analgesics for Chronic Pain*
(with approximate dosage intervals)

	Parenteral	*Oral*
COMMONLY USED NARCOTICS	10 mg Morphine sulfate SC/IM (q3–4h)	= 30 mg (q3–4h)
	130 mg Codeine (q3–4h)	= 200 mg (q3–4h)
	10 mg Methadone SC/IM (q3–6h)	= 20 mg (q3–6h)
	1.5 mg Hydromorphone (Dilaudid) IM (q3–6h)	= 7.5 mg (q3–6h)
	10 mg Oxycodone (Percodan, Tylox)	= 30 mg (q3–6h)
GENERALLY NOT USEFUL FOR CHRONIC PAIN	60 mg Pentazocine (Talwin) IM (q2–3h)	= 180 mg (q2–4h)
	100 mg Meperidine (Demerol) IM (q2–3h)	= 300 mg (q2–4h)
"NEW NARCOTICS"	2 mg Levorphanol (Levo-Dromoran) SC/IM (q3–8h)	= 4 mg (q3–8h)

*Data from Houde, [40,41] Beaver,[6] Jaffe,[44] Saunders[80]

ladonna alkaloids). The clinician is challenged by a therapy that rests a good deal on empiric management, guided by common sense, clinical experience, and data on drug use in acute pain.

The Choice of Treatment

A few useful generalizations about the choice of treatment follow.

Route

Oral regimens are preferred for ease of administration and evenness of action (see Fig. 1-2). Injections offer a rapid onset of analgesia, but tend to produce a peak-and-trough effect—alternating periods of toxicity and inadequate pain relief. Lamerton reports that only one third of his dying patients ever required injections.[50]

Nonsteroidal Anti-inflammatory Drugs

Nonsteroidal anti-inflammatory drugs (salicylates, phenylbutazone, indomethacin, ibuprofen, etc.) are thought to be particularly useful for bone pain.[88,92,95] Occasionally, patients with bony disease who are receiving narcotics and are quite comfortable only at rest will be able to walk easily when an anti-inflammatory agent is added. Regardless of the cause of pain, these agents may be used alone, or they may be added to narcotic regimens, perhaps allowing for a reduction of the narcotic dose and its attendant toxicity.[39,63,64]

Among the many drugs in this class, none has been shown conclusively to excel in analgesic or anti-inflammatory action or to have lesser toxicity. Many of the newer agents have a long duration of action, and some may be slightly more effective or better tolerated than aspirin.[2,3] Because a marked variability among patients in the clinical response to a given drug has been noted, the physician may prescribe serial trials of several different agents.[81] At full doses, the clinical response to the drug should be evident within a week. A recent study of zomepirac (Zomax) prescribed for acute postoperative pain indicated that standard oral doses of this drug (which is no longer marketed) have an analgesic potency greater than morphine 8 mg SC.[32]

Indomethacin has proved effective when given as a suppository,[75] but aspirin is the only agent in this class that is commercially available in the United States for rectal administration.

Steroids

Steroids may be useful when tissue swelling is contributing to discomfort.[92] Classically, swelling occurs from a CNS mass, but also when other rigid enclosed spaces (such as the pelvis) are distended or when there is painful compression of nerves or distension of an organ (such as the liver). Begin with prednisone 10 mg po tid; depending on the response, taper or increase the dose. Steroids may also be useful in refractory bone pain and can help improve appetite and mood.[92]

Lack of Response

Patients who do not respond as expected to analgesics may not be absorbing drugs, or they just may require higher doses. Poor efficacy of analgesic drugs also commonly occurs when emotional distress is prominent. In such cases, concurrent measures are needed to address anxiety and depression. The rare patients who want more narcotics when they are drowsy from an earlier dose may need opiates for physical pain but probably are trying to use these drugs for their mood-altering action, a use that rarely proves satisfactory.

Mild-to-Moderate Pain[7,44]

Simple regimens are often adequate:

Acetaminophen (Tylenol) 650 mg po q3–4h up to about 3.0 g daily; also available as a liquid and in rectal suppositories

Aspirin 650 mg po q4h, which may be increased to 1300 mg po q4h; often best taken with meals or with antacids or in a buffered or enteric-coated form. Salsalate (Disalcid) is a salicylic acid preparation that may cause less gastrointestinal irritation and interference with platelet function than aspirin. A liquid preparation, choline salicylate (Arthropan 870 mg in 5 ml q3–4h) is occasionally useful. Rectal suppositories are also available

Propoxyphene compounds (Darvon, etc.) 1–4 tabs po q3–4h have little experimental justification for their use but seem appreciated by and effective for many patients

Codeine 30–120 mg po q3–4h; usually with aspirin or acetaminophen

Oxycodone compounds (Percodan, Percocet, Tylox) 1–4 tabs po q3–4h

Nonsteroidal anti-inflammatory drugs. These drugs can all cause gastric irritation (and hence are given initially with a meal or snack); sodium retention, nephrotoxicity, and platelet inhibition also occur

Indomethacin (Indocin) 25–50 mg po 3–4 times daily

Ibuprofen (Motrin) 300–400 mg po 3–6 times daily or 600 mg po 3–4 times daily

Naproxen (Naprosyn) 250–500 mg po twice a day or Anaprox 275 mg po 2–5 times daily

Piroxicam (Feldene) 20 mg po daily

Studies of oral analgesics indicate that 650 mg of aspirin or acetaminophen and 30 to 60 mg of codeine are roughly equianalgesic, and that codeine 65 mg or oxycodone 9 mg, when combined with 650 mg of aspirin, is superior to aspirin alone.[63,64] Additive effects have also been noted with aspirin and intramuscular morphine.[39]

Moderate-to-Severe Pain

Morphine

Morphine is a versatile drug for oral and parenteral use and is favored in most hospice programs for the oral treatment of moderate pain, regardless of the patient's expected remaining lifespan.[66,92] When treatment is switched from a parenteral regimen to oral use, the dose is doubled.

Morphine is now marketed in the United States as tablets, an elixir, suppositories, and an injectable solution. Elixirs can be prepared that conveniently deliver in 10 to 20 ml a dose of morphine that ranges from the equivalent of a single codeine pill to the equivalent of ten or more of the strongest narcotic analgesic tablets. Initial doses are usually 2.5 to 20.0 mg po q4h, combined with an antiemetic such as prochlorperazine (Compazine) or, if sedation is desirable, with a tranquilizer with antiemetic properties, such as chlorpromazine (Thorazine):

Morphine 2.5–120.0 mg (or more)
    plus
Compazine (as syrup) 5–10 mg
    or
Thorazine (syrup) 10–25 mg

QS to 10–20 ml, with honey water, cherry syrup, or other palatable solution
± 1.5 ml of 98% EtOH per 20 ml to prolong shelf life

An active hospice pharmacy might stock standard preparations of elixir of morphine in strengths of 2.0, 4.0, and 20.0 mg per 1.0 ml from which commonly required dosages can be prepared.

A patient who previously took a weak narcotic will probably start at the 10-mg dose of morphine. (See Table 1-3 for guidelines.) If the first one or two doses are not effective, the strength can be promptly increased by 50% to 100%. Once initially acceptable pain control is achieved, the dosage is adjusted every 2 to 3 days until the optimal effect is reached. Since the full impact of a dose change is often not appreciated for a few days, the medication should not be adjusted more frequently unless the patient is grossly over- or undermedicated. The sequential doses are usually 2.5, 5, 10, 15, 20, 30, 40, 60, 90, and 120 mg; finer adjustments of doses may be required. Figure 1-7 describes the range of maximum doses of morphine in 490 terminal patients.

Rectal and sublingual administration may offer alternate effective routes, producing satisfactory plasma levels for 3 or more hours,[71] but rigorous studies are lacking. Rectal suppositories or dilute solutions administered by rectal syringe are preferred

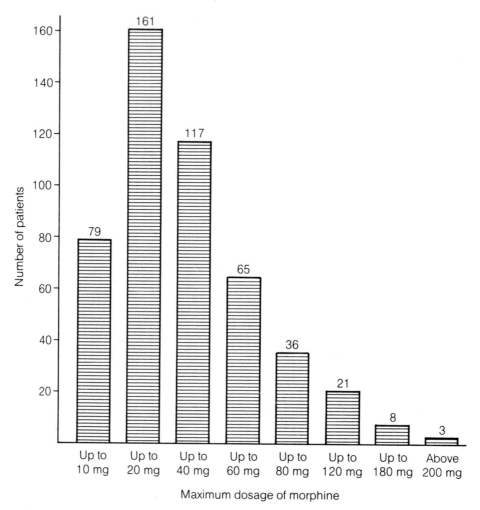

FIG. 1-7. Maximum dose of morphine in 490 terminal patients (Redrawn from Lamerton R: Care of the Dying, revised and expanded edition. New York, Penguin, 1980)

when emesis prevents oral intake. Lacking sublingual preparations, the sublingual route may be attempted with morphine solutions held in the mouth for 10 minutes.

Brompton cocktail, consisting of cocaine, alcohol, a phenothiazine, and either morphine or heroin, has recently received wide attention, but has no apparent advantage over morphine with a phenothiazine.[60] Cocaine may be useful as a local anaesthetic, but has no demonstrated long-term efficacy when combined with oral narcotics.[93] The inclusion of alcohol in an elixir should be considered if the patient finds it tasty or pleasant, but alcohol is often best enjoyed in its usual socially prescribed forms. Alcohol may sting an injured mouth, throat, or upper gastrointestinal tract and may aggravate pain in some patients, particularly those with lymphomas. The addition of 1.5 ml of 98% ethanol to each 20 ml of morphine elixir prolongs the mixture's shelf life by inhibiting microbial growth.[60]

Rate-controlled drug-delivery systems[36]—oral, transdermal, parenteral, and local—may have a valuable role for patients who cannot be well-managed on morphine elixir. Controlled-release morphine sulphate tablets, recently commercially available in the United States, are reported to produce analgesia for about 6 to 12 hours and compare favorably with intramuscular morphine in postoperative patients.[28]

Morphine may be given intravenously by continuous infusion.[35] After surgery, patients on continuous intravenous morphine had less pain and better respiratory function and required lower total doses than comparable patients on regimens of intramuscular injections.[77] Continuous-infusion rates should be based on previous medication requirements. A low starting dose is 1.0 mg/h. Doses of 5 to 30 mg/h can be anticipated, but higher doses (95 and 144 mg/h) have been reported.[35] Comparisons of the analgesic potency of intravenous morphine with various other routes are lacking, and no extensive experience with this form of administration has been reported.

Portable infusion devices are becoming widely available. A recent report described continuous subcutaneous morphine infusion by a portable pump.[16] The subcutaneous route was felt to be safer for outpatient management than the intravenous route. In addition, machines have been devised that deliver boluses of intravenous narcotics upon patient demand.[37] This method appears to be safe and effective for postoperative and obstetric pain (and provides another example of how patient-controlled analgesia does not lead to narcotic abuse), but has not been well-studied for treating chronic pains. An intramuscular on-demand system has also been described.[38]

Epidural and intrathecal morphine injections have been popular procedures for pain relief in some centers.[102] Continuous intrathecal morphine administration has been reported to provide good analgesia without the side-effects of parenteral medication and with a surprising lack of development of tolerance.[68,74] Remarkably, profound analgesia can be achieved by this technique without affecting proprioceptive or motor pathways. Intrathecal or epidural morphine may be attractive for patients with "intractable" pain in the abdomen, pelvis, or lower extremities, especially when oral agents are poorly tolerated.

Other Narcotic Drugs

Heroin, which is available in Great Britain, is more potent for a given volume of injection than morphine. When high doses of parenteral narcotics are administered, the smaller volume of heroin is convenient and more comfortable. However, hydromorphone (Dilaudid) is even more potent for injection and is available in the United States. Heroin has no other advantage over morphine, and its legalization in the United States promises little benefit to patients.[47,51,60,65,89,91]

Methadone is also a versatile drug, available in oral (tablet and elixir) and parenteral forms. Anecdotal reports and data on methadone use for the maintenance and withdrawal of narcotic addicts suggest that the drug can be effective when given one to four times a day. Indeed, methadone has a long serum half-life, and plasma levels of the drug continue to rise over 4 days at a steady-state dose.[97] However, plasma levels have poor correlation with analgesic (and presumably toxic) effects.[12] Moreover, methadone's ability to prevent narcotic withdrawal should not be confused with its analgesic properties, nor should studies on narcotic abusers be readily applied to nonaddict populations. In chronic use for pain, the dosage and duration of action of methadone are similar to those of morphine.[9] Some patients may need to take this drug only every 6 or even 8 hours, but 4-hourly regimens are the general rule. Warnings must be heeded about toxicity from cumulative effects that develop after days or weeks of using the drug, especially in the debilitated or elderly patient.[26]

Hydromorphone (Dilaudid) is particularly useful for providing low-volume, high-potency injections. It is now available in a 10-mg/ml solution and is favored for patients who require very strong narcotic injections, especially if the shots are discomforting. For both oral and parenteral use, hydromorphone may be more readily available than morphine or methadone in the United States, but its duration of action is often bothersomely short. A rectal suppository is also marketed.

Levorphanol (Levo-Dromoran) is available in oral and parenteral forms. A long duration of action (6–8 h) has been claimed.

Suppositories

Suppositories may be preferable to injections when patients are vomiting or do not absorb oral medication:

Oxymorphone (Numorphan) 5 mg pr
Hydromorphone (Dilaudid) 3 mg pr
Morphine sulfate 5 mg, 10 mg, or 20 mg pr

These medications are not commonly stocked in drugstores. A cooperative pharmacist may prepare rectal suppositories (*e.g.,* morphine in cocoa butter).

Further Considerations in the Use of Analgesics

Constipation

Constipation is a common side-effect of narcotics. *Do not wait for constipation and impaction to develop.* Prescribe stool softeners or laxatives prophylactically, for example:

Docusate sodium (Colace) 100–200
   mg po 2–3 times daily, or another
   stool softener   hold if having frequent bowel
            and/or   movements
Bisacodyl (Dulcolax) 5 mg po 2–3
   times daily, or 10 mg pr qd

Prune juice, other fruit juices, and hydration may be helpful. A more vigorous bowel regimen is occasionally required, particularly in poorly hydrated patients.

Nausea

Nausea is also such a frequent side-effect that prophylactic antiemetics should be routinely given when the stronger narcotics are begun. Nausea is apparently less common at low doses of narcotics, and gradually increasing doses may not lead to the appearance of nausea. Bedridden patients also are reported to suffer less nausea and vomiting, presumably because they experience less vestibular stimulation. The following are good drugs for treating nausea initially, the latter being more sedating:

Prochlorperazine (Compazine) 5–10 mg po q6–8h
Chlorpromazine (Thorazine) 10 mg po q4–6h

Alternative routes and doses of these drugs and the use of other antiemetic agents are described in Chapter 2, Section A. If a stable dosage of narcotics has been achieved and nausea and vomiting are not present, an attempt can be made gradually to discontinue antiemetics.

Drowsiness

Pain relief with an unclouded sensorium and normal affect can almost always be achieved through careful adjustment of dosage and timing. However, drowsiness is reported to be common during the first 2 to 3 days after the dosage is increased. Patients who have suffered with insomnia because of pain may "catch up" on sleep when the narcotics have made them comfortable; they may sleep nearly continuously for a few days, but generally appear alert when fully aroused.

When patients are drowsy but still request analgesia, two diagnoses should be considered:

1. The drowsiness is not due to the narcotic. Consider other causes of somnolence that might not produce concomitant analgesia. The lack of miosis may help confirm the impression that narcotic effects are not prominent.
2. The complaint of pain is occurring independently of physical distress. For instance, the patient may be using the opiate as an anxiolytic and trying to obliterate consciousness rather than eradicate pain.

Nighttime Pain

Pain is often more prominent at night. A 25% to 100% increase in dose may be useful at bedtime and in the middle of the night. Drowsiness is acceptable at these times. Predictable periods of increased pain (*e.g.*, taking a trip for radiation treatment) should be managed similarly. During episodes of aggravated pain, higher doses are tolerated without evidence of toxicity.

Dosage

For the vast majority of patients with relatively stable pain, fixed dosage schedules are preferable to prn orders. The dose and timing need to be carefully tailored and monitored. Occasionally, prn orders to increase or decrease the fixed dose or interval are useful; many patients make such adjustments without professional coaching.

Four-hourly regimens are the rule. Older patients may experience greater duration of analgesia from morphine.[45] When pain relief does not last 4 hours, the dose may be too low, perhaps signalling the development of tolerance; increased drug dosage may be more convenient than increased frequency of the same dose.

Initially, patients should be aroused for their middle-of-the-night dose, rather than being allowed to awake in pain. After an appropriate narcotic regimen has been established, many patients can skip this middle-of-the-night dose without awaking or arising in pain, especially if the bedtime dose has been increased.

Effects on Respiratory Function

Respiratory depression is rarely a concern unless the patient has a severe respiratory impairment or is grossly or repeatedly overmedicated. Parenteral regimens hold the highest risk of respiratory toxicity, although poorly supervised chronic oral narcotic administration can also slowly lead to overdosing. Considering how rarely significant respiratory depression develops when drugs are used carefully,[62] this sign of severe narcotic toxicity receives far too much attention in the medical and nursing literature. When gross measures of respiratory function were assessed 4 hours after narcotics were administered, moderate or high doses (100 mg/day or more) of oral morphine sulfate did not produce ventilatory failure.[98] Subclinical or more subtle changes in respiration may develop but have not been adequately documented.

Cough suppression, produced by low doses of narcotics, is sometimes desirable. A diminished cough reflex is rarely problematic. Indeed, narcotics seem to cause subjective improvement in coughing without decreasing the frequency or productivity.[10]

In the infrequent situation in which respiratory depression is a concern with a terminally ill patient, pain control is usually a much higher priority than the preservation of optimal ventilation. Moreover, as discussed in Chapter 2, Section F (Dyspnea), narcotics are of value in reducing respiratory distress.

Very rarely a patient with chronic drowsiness or significant respiratory depression from narcotics might benefit from the following:

Methylphenidate (Ritalin) 5–10 mg po bid
Dextroamphetamine 5 mg po q8–12h

These stimulants may also potentiate narcotic analgesia. In a single-dose study, dextroamphetamine 5 mg IM with parenteral morphine produced relief of pain roughly equivalent to $1\frac{1}{2}$ times that of the morphine alone, while dextroamphetamine 10 mg IM doubled the effectiveness of the analgesic; both dosages improved self-reported sleepiness and objective measures of alertness.[33] The long-term usefulness of stimulants for advanced cancer patients with pain or other symptoms has not been studied. The anorectic effects of these drugs may be undesirable, while their mood-elevating effects can be valuable.

Dry Mouth

Dry mouth is a side-effect of narcotics and of the phenothiazines commonly prescribed with narcotics. It is also a side-effect of other drugs (e.g., tricyclic antidepressants) and commonly occurs in the debilitated patient who is dehydrated or breathing through the mouth. Treatment is discussed in Chapter 2, Section E.

Hypotension

Narcotics may produce or aggravate hypotension or orthostatic hypotension, especially in dehydrated patients. Patients and families may need to be warned about lightheadedness and fainting when the patient sits up or stands.

Neuropsychiatric Effects

Pronounced dysphoria, agitation, hallucinations, and toxic psychosis from narcotics are reportedly produced much more frequently by partial agonists (see below). Anecdotal reports suggest that dysphoria may be alleviated by switching to a different subclass of narcotics (e.g., from a partial agonist to a relatively pure agonist, or from morphine to methadone).

Minor neuropsychiatric and neurologic symptoms—exaggerated myoclonus when falling asleep, strange dreams or states described as being "half awake and half asleep," or a sense of shakiness without gross tremor—are common with narcotic usage. Kaiko noted a very high incidence of CNS excitatory effects—nervousness, tremors, twitches, multifocal myoclonus, and seizures—in patients receiving meperidine, especially with chronic use and when mild renal failure was present.[46] These effects correlated with the accumulation of a metabolite of meperidine. Naloxone fails to reverse the actions of this metabolite and may even exacerbate them.

Other Side Effects

Urinary retention is an occasional side-effect of opiates. Beware of prostatism. Other side-effects of narcotics are worth keeping in mind, but are rarely important with advanced cancer patients (see Further Side-Effects of Narcotics).

FURTHER SIDE-EFFECTS OF NARCOTICS

Lowered seizure threshold
Bronchospasm (especially in asthmatics)
Increased biliary tract sphincter tone
Bradycardia
Syndrome of inappropriate antidiuretic hormone

Combination Therapy

Partial agonists (or agonist–antagonists), particularly pentazocine (Talwin), but perhaps also codeine, butorphanol (Stadol), nalbuphine (Nubain), and others, may actually *reduce* pain relief when combined with other narcotics. The combining of any two narcotics is rarely appropriate. If attempted, combination therapy should be handled cautiously, since the drug interaction is unpredictable. The concurrent use of narcotic or narcoticlike antitussive medications with opiate analgesics is senseless.

Increasing Doses

Gradually increasing doses are commonly required during the first few weeks and months of narcotic use, even when the disease is relatively stable. Tolerance often presents as the reemergence of pain just before the next narcotic dose is due to be administered. Otherwise, any escalation in the required dose should suggest a change in the underlying disease.

Attempting to Lower Doses

In all patients who are experiencing good pain control, gradual lowering of the dose should be attempted periodically. Dosage should be tapered after any additional treatment (*e.g.,* nonsteroidal anti-inflammatory drugs or radiotherapy) has reduced pain. When evidence of drowsiness or clouded sensorium from narcotics is detected, the medication usually needs to be reduced.

Stopping Narcotics

Patients should be warned about suddenly stopping narcotics or rapidly tapering dosage, lest they experience physiologic withdrawal symptoms.

Switching Medication

When patients are switching between oral and parenteral preparations or between various narcotic analgesics, Table 1-3 is useful. Few physicians are familiar with the data on equianalgesic dosages of narcotics. Hence, *prescribing errors are common.* A patient with uncontrolled pain on one drug will often be changed to ineffective treatment *via* another route or with another drug.

In general, switching can best be managed by calculating the total daily dose of the new drug, which would provide an effect comparable to the total daily dose of the current drug. The total dose of the new medication is then divided into an appropriate number of individual doses, based on the approximate dosage intervals. The author has found Table 1-3 relatively accurate for chronic analgesic use, but the data should be viewed as "approximate" for many reasons, including inevitable individual variations in absorption and sensitivity and possible variable cross-tolerance to narcotics.

Self-Administration
Alert patients can administer their own medication. Even mildly confused patients who need supervision can usually clearly indicate when additional medication is required.

Potential for Poisoning
Narcotics are highly poisonous and, along with other medications that are often kept closely at hand by the patient or family, should be placed out of the reach of children.

Masking of Symptoms
Patients on narcotics require frequent assessment for signs of illness that may be masked by the drugs. When narcotics are being used regularly, many of the complications of cancer and its treatment will not be clearly heralded by pain. Patients may unwittingly develop or aggravate decubiti or fail to notice other instances of tissue damage.

Phenothiazines and Other Sedatives
Despite their widespread use in conjunction with opiates, the phenothiazines have not been clearly shown to be effective analgesics or potentiators of narcotics.[59] A possible exception is methotrimeprazine (Levoprome), which is available only in parenteral form but can be considered for pain control in the rare patient who cannot tolerate narcotics. Also, hydroxyzine (Vistaril, Atarax), a nonphenothiazine antihistamine with antiemetic properties, appears to have an analgesic effect; 100 mg IM is roughly equal to morphine sulfate 8 mg IM, and additive effects were noted when hydroxyzine and morphine were used together.[8] Long-term oral administration of hydroxyzine in conjunction with narcotics has not been studied.

The phenothiazines and other sedating drugs (including alcohol) can be extremely helpful in relieving the tension and anxiety that often complicate advanced cancer and other serious illnesses. The reports that these drugs are effective for controlling pain may reflect their sedating properties rather than any intrinsic analgesic effect. Similarly, other psychotropic drugs, especially antidepressants, should be considered for patients in pain whenever emotional suffering is prominent.

ADDITIONAL MEASURES FOR PAIN CONTROL

The analgesic drug regimens described earlier in this chapter are regularly effective and well-tolerated, but a host of additional pain treatments, outlined in Table 1-4, should be considered periodically, especially when (1) analgesia does not seem optimal, (2) side-effects of drugs are troublesome, or (3) prolonged use of medication is anticipated and a "definitive" pain-relieving procedure is preferred. Many of these additional measures have already been noted or are described in subsequent chapters: all of the usual oncological methods (surgery, radiation, chemotherapy) to shrink the tumor, especially radiation therapy in the late stages of cancer as a treatment for bone

TABLE 1-4.
Additional Measures for Pain Control in Terminal Illness*

Treatment for the painful process
　Chemotherapy
　Radiation
　Surgery
　Antibiotics
　Steroids

Local anesthetics
　Topical
　Injected

Interruption of pain pathways/counter-irritation
　Nerve blocks and other neurosurgical procedures
　Transcutaneous electrical stimulation
　Acupuncture

Pituitary ablation/alcohol injection (mechanism of its analgesic effect is unknown)

General anesthetics
　Nitrous oxide or short-acting parenteral agents (for dressing changes, other painful
　　procedures)

Behavioral techniques
　Hypnosis
　Relaxation, guided imagery, biofeedback

Heat, cold

Immobilization

Muscle relaxants, massage, and physical therapy

Additional drugs
　Antidepressants
　Anticonvulsants
　Sedatives/hypnotics/antipsychotics
　Steroids
　Stimulants

Consultation (to reconsider diagnosis and management)
　Oncology
　Psychiatry
　Neurology
　Neurosurgery
　Rehabilitation medicine

* After Foley[30] and Twycross[90]

pain and some visceral pain; steroids; behavioral techniques; and the use of psychotropic agents.

　Antidepressant medications deserve special mention. The diagnosis of depression and the use of antidepressants is reviewed in Chapter 6. Antidepressants have long been used for refractory and unusual pains. They are highly effective in relieving the pain commonly experienced by depressed patients,[99] and considerable experimental evidence suggests that they might have an analgesic effect in other situations.[54] Unfortunately, since uncomfortable side-effects occur frequently enough, especially in debilitated patients, antidepressants must be prescribed cautiously. Moreover, they are slow-acting drugs, so their efficacy is not easily demonstrated by stopping and restarting treatment (as can readily be done with stimulants, sedatives, steroids, nonsteroidal anti-inflammatory agents, and narcotics).

Local anaesthetics can be used in many parts of the body:

Oropharyngeal lesions
  Lidocaine (Xylocaine) 2% viscous solution, "swish" and spit out or swallow 15 ml q3h prn up to 120 ml/day
  Dyclonine (Dyclone) 1% gel i–ii gtt q4h to affected area

External otitis
  Auralgan otic solution (antipyrine and benzocaine) q1–2h prn

Superficial irritation of skin or mucous membranes
  Dibucaine (Nupercainal) 1% ointment to affected area prn

Irritation of bladder and urethra
  Phenazopyridine (Pyridium) 100–200 mg po tid

Local anaesthetics may also be used to test nerve blocks prior to the injection of alcohol. They are sometimes added to substances injected into body spaces (*e.g.*, pleura, joints) to reduce the pain associated with the procedure. Injections of local anaesthetics, sometimes combined with steroids, have been used to treat "trigger points" and persistent postsurgical scar pain.

Anticonvulsant drugs should be considered for paroxysmal pains (either spontaneous or triggered). They are also employed for a variety of peculiar sensations that respond poorly to analgesics.[86] Among the diagnostic terms used to describe such sensations are thalamic pain, deafferentiation pain, causalgia, and neuralgia. These pains have a delayed onset after tissue injury and may have bizarre qualities—lancinating, shooting, or burning—and may be associated with hyperesthesia, dysesthesia, or other neurologic findings. Both antidepressants and anticonvulsants—diphenylhydantoin, carbamazepine, and sodium valproate—may produce gratifying results. Anticonvulsant drug schedules are identical to those used for seizures; the medication is increased until symptoms resolve, toxicity ensues, or blood tests indicate that a high therapeutic serum level of the medication has been achieved.

Neurosurgical procedures[13,56] are popular in some medical centers for pain management. Many surgical procedures have been developed for chronic pain. Neurosurgery is often the last resort for patients in severe intractable pain; neurosurgeons less commonly consult on patients with more manageable problems. Not surprisingly, therapeutic results have often been disappointing. Furthermore, studies of these procedures are often difficult to interpret—the criteria for entry into the treatment group are vague, controlled series are rare, the placebo effect is overlooked, and rigorous methods of evaluation and long-term follow-up are generally lacking. Studies are needed of the usefulness of some relatively benign interventions—nerve blocks and spinal cord stimulation—that could be offered to cancer patients who are not desperate for help but simply seek a definitive procedure or wish to avoid medications. Peripheral nerve blocks are probably underutilized for chest wall pain; celiac plexus and sacral blocks are also feasible for some patients.

Pituitary ablation is a neuroendocrine technique that has been favored for hormone-responsive tumors of the breast and prostate, while alcohol injections (which may not completely ablate the pituitary) have been reported to relieve pain from a variety of malignancies. Other CNS ablative procedures should almost never be done. Some of the rare candidates for unilateral cordotomy, midline myelotomy, and sacral rhizotomy can now be referred for chronic epidural morphine infusion. Patients with head and neck tumors may occasionally benefit from ablative procedures on the 5th and 9th cranial nerves.

Behavioral techniques for adults, including hypnosis, relaxation, and imaging techniques, should probably be reserved for patients who are feeling relatively well at the moment, but who anticipate pain or wish to improve pain relief or to decrease analgesic use.

Hypnosis[5,69] and a host of psychotherapies that have goals such as relaxation, positive thinking, or directing one's attention away from the body's sensations may be beneficial for some patients, but convincing evidence has not been demonstrated of their general usefulness and long-term efficacy, and they have not been shown to have analgesic potency comparable to that of drug regimens. Laypersons may embrace nonpharmacologic techniques of pain management enthusiastically and uncritically, whereas physicians, having seen so many popular "snake oils" come and go, may tend to be skeptical. On the other hand, physicians regularly practice hypnosis in the informal and often unconscious use of "suggestion." Like the placebo effect, hypnotic suggestion is an ever-present factor in patients' experience of pain and may have beneficial as well as noxious effects. The physician who attends to suggestion and uses word, tone, and manner for the patient's benefit has access to a powerful analgesic technique.[25]

Enthusiasts of behavioral techniques have contributed to the unfortunate pressure on some patients to avoid useful analgesic drugs. Inappropriate attempts to overcome pain with these methods are to be condemned, especially their use for sudden, intense pains or for those patients who are undermedicated and could promptly and reliably be made comfortable with standard analgesics. The proliferation of behavioral methods, most of which seem safe in themselves, has not been accompanied by rigorous evaluation of their acceptability or effectiveness for a cross section of patients.

Acupuncture and *transcutaneous electrical stimulation* have not been rigorously studied for use in cancer pain but may be attractive and beneficial to some patients.

Consultation to reconsider the diagnosis and to suggest further management is an excellent technique for the stymied physician to improve pain control, learn about new analgesic techniques, or share frustration.

SELECTED REFERENCES

1. Angell M: The quality of mercy (Editorial). N Engl J Med 306:98–99, 1982
2. Anonymous: Prostaglandin-inhibitor analgesics. Med Lett Drugs Ther 23:75–76, 1981
3. Anonymous: Zomepirac sodium—A new oral analgesic. Med Lett Drugs Ther 23:1–3, 1981
4. Baines M: Principles of symptom control. London, St. Christopher's Hospice (mimeographed), no date (statistics for 1978)
5. Barber J, Gitelson J: Cancer pain: Psychological management using hypnosis. CA 30:130–136, 1980
6. Beaver WT: Management of cancer pain with parenteral medication. JAMA 244:2653–2657, 1980
7. Beaver WT: Mild analgesics: A review of their clinical pharmacology. Am J Med Sci 250:577–604, 1965; 251:576–599, 1966

8. Beaver WT, Friese G: Comparison of the analgesic effects of morphine, hydroxyzine, and their combination in patients with postoperative pain. In Bonica JJ, Albe-Fessard D: Advances in Pain Research and Therapy, vol 1. New York, Raven Press, 553–557, 1976

9. Beaver WT, Wallenstein SL, Houde RW, Rogers A: A clinical comparison of the analgesic effects of methadone and morphine administered intramuscularly, and of orally and parenterally administered methadone. Clin Pharmacol Ther 8:415–426, 1967

10. Beecher H: Measurement of Subjective Responses. New York, Oxford University Press, 1959

11. Beecher H: Relationship of significance of wound to pain experienced. JAMA 161:1609–1613, 1956

12. Berkowitz BA: The relationship of pharmacokinetics to pharmacological activity: Morphine, methadone, and naloxone. Clin Pharmacokinet 1:219–230, 1976

13. Black P: Management of cancer pain: An overview. Neurosurgery 5:507–518, 1979

14. Bonica JJ: Cancer pain. In Bonica JJ (ed): Pain, pp 335–362. New York, Raven Press, 1980

15. Bonica JJ: Important clinical aspects of acute and chronic pain. In Beers RF Jr, Bassett EG (eds): Mechanisms of Pain and Analgesic Compounds, pp 15–29. New York, Raven Press, 1979

16. Campbell CF, Mason JB, Weiler JM: Continuous subcutaneous infusion of morphine for the pain of terminal malignancy. Ann Intern Med 98:51–52, 1973

17. Cartwright A, Hockey L, Anderson JL: Life Before Death. London, Routledge & Kegan Paul, 1973

18. Chang K, Cuatrecasas P: Heterogeneity and properties of opiate receptors. Fed Proc 40:2729–2739, 1981

19. Charap AD: The knowledge, attitudes, and experience of medical personnel treating pain in the terminally ill. Mount Sinai J Med 45:561–580, 1978

20. Cohen FL: Postsurgical pain relief: Patients' status and nurses' medication choices. Pain 9:265–274, 1980

21. de Beauvoir S: A Very Easy Death. O'Brien P (trans). New York, Warner Paperback Library, 1973

22. Dickinson E: The Complete Poems of Emily Dickinson. Johnson TH (ed). Boston, Little, Brown & Co. no date

23. Egbert LD, Battit GE, Welch CE, Bartlett MK: Reduction of postoperative pain by encouragement and instruction of patients: A study of doctor–patient rapport. N Engl J Med 270:825–827, 1964

24. Engel GL: Psychogenic pain and the pain-prone patient. Am J Med 26:897–918, 1959

25. Erickson MH, Rossi RL, Rossi SI: Hypnotic Realities: The Induction of Clinical Hypnosis and Forms of Indirect Suggestion. New York, Irvington Publishers, 1976

26. Ettinger DS, Vitale PJ, Trump DL: Important clinical pharmacologic considerations in the use of methadone in cancer patients. Cancer Treat Rep 63:457–459, 1979

27. Evans FJ: The placebo response in pain reduction. In Bonica JJ (ed): Advances in Neurology, vol 4. New York, Raven Press, 1974

28. Fell D, Chmielewski A, Smith G: Postoperative analgesia with controlled release morphine sulfate: Comparison with intramuscular morphine. Br Med J 285:92–94, 1982

29. Foley KM: Pain syndromes in patients with cancer. In Bonica JJ, Ventafridda V (eds): Advances in Pain Research and Therapy, vol 2, pp 59–75. New York, Raven Press, 1979

30. Foley KM: The management of pain of malignant origin. In Tyler HR, Dawson DM (eds): Current Neurology, vol 2, pp 279–302. Boston, Houghton Mifflin, 1979

31. Fordyce WE: Behavioral Methods for Control of Chronic Pain and Illness. St Louis, CV Mosby, 1976

32. Forrest WH Jr: Orally administered zomepirac and parenterally administered morphine: Comparison for the treatment of postoperative pain. JAMA 244:2298–2302, 1980

33. Forrest WH, Brown BW Jr, Brown CR et al: Dextroamphetamine with morphine for the treatment of postoperative pain. N Engl J Med 296:712–715, 1977

34. Forster EM: Notes on the English character. In: Abinger Harvest. New York, Harcourt, Brace, Jovanovich, 1964

35. Fraser DG: Intravenous morphine infusion for chronic pain. Ann Intern Med 93:781–782, 1980

36. Goldman P: Drug therapy: Rate-controlled drug delivery. N Engl J Med 307:286–290, 1982
37. Graves DA, Foster TS, Batenhorst RL, Bennett RL, Baumann TJ: Patient controlled analgesia. Ann Intern Med 99:360–366, 1983
38. Harmer M, Slattery PJ, Rosen M, Vickers MD: Intramuscular on demand analgesia: Double blind controlled trial of pethidine, buprenorphine, morphine and meptazinol. Br J Med 286:680–683, 1983
39. Houde RW: Medical treatment of oncologic pain. In Bonica JJ, Procacci P, Pagni CA (eds): Recent Advances on Pain, pp 168–188. Springfield, IL, Charles C Thomas, 1974
40. Houde RW: Systemic analgesics and related drugs. In Bonica JJ, Ventafrida V (eds): Advances in Pain Research and Therapy, vol 2, pp 263–273. New York, Raven Press, 1979
41. Houde RW: The use and misuse of narcotics in the treatment of chronic pain. In Bonica JJ (ed): Advances in Neurology, vol 4, pp 527–536. New York, Raven Press, 1974
42. Houde RW, Wallenstein SL, Beaver WT: Clinical measurement of pain. In de Stevens G (ed): Analgetics. New York, Academic Press, 1963
43. Houde RW, Wallenstein SL, Beaver WT: Evaluation of analgesics in patients with cancer pain. In Lasagna L (ed): Encyclopedia of Pharmacology and Therapeutics, section 6: Clinical Pharmacology. Oxford, Pergamon Press, 1966
44. Jaffe JH, Martin WR: Opioid analgesics and antagonists. In Gilman AG, Goodman LS, Gilman A (eds): Goodman and Gilman's The Pharmacological Basis of Therapeutics, 6th ed. New York, Macmillan, 1980
45. Kaiko RF: Age and morphine analgesia in cancer patients with postoperative pain. Clin Pharmacol Ther 28:823–826, 1980
46. Kaiko RF, Foley KM, Grabinski PY, Heidrich G, Rogers AG et al: Central nervous system excitatory effects of meperidine in cancer patients. Ann Neurol 13:180–183, 1983
47. Kaiko RF, Wallenstein SL, Rogers AG, Garbinski PY, Houde RW: Analgesic and mood effects of heroin and morphine in cancer patients with postoperative pain. N Engl J Med 304:1301–1303, 1981
48. Kanner RM, Foley KM: Patterns of narcotic drug use in a cancer pain clinic. Ann NY Acad Sci 362:161–172, 1981
49. Lack S: Hospice—A concept of care in the final stage of life. Conn Med 43:367–372, 1979
50. Lamerton R: Care of the Dying. New York, Penguin, 1980 (revised and expanded edition)
51. Lasagna L: Heroin: A medical "me too" (Editorial). N Engl J Med 304:1539–1540, 1981
52. Lasagna L: The clinical evaluation of morphine and its substitutes as analgesics. Pharmacol Rev 16:47–83, 1964
53. Lasagna L, von Festinger JM, Beecher HK: Drug-induced mood changes in man. 1. Observations on healthy subjects, chronically ill patients, and "postaddicts." JAMA 157:1006–1020, 1955
54. Lee R, Spencer PSJ: Antidepressants and pain; A review of the pharmacological data supporting the use of certain tricyclics in chronic pain. J Int Med Res 5:146–156, 1977
55. LeShan L: The world of the patient in severe pain of long duration. J Chronic Dis 17:119–126, 1964
56. Long DM: Relief of cancer pain by surgical and nerve blocking procedures. JAMA 244:2759–2761, 1980
57. Marks RM, Sachar EJ: Undertreatment of medical inpatients with narcotic analgesics. Ann Intern Med 78:173–181, 1973
58. Maciewicz R: Central pain pathways. Mediguide to Pain 3(4):1–4, 1982
59. McGee JL, Alexander MR: Phenothiazine analgesia—Fact or fantasy? Am J Hosp Pharm 36:633–640, 1979
60. Melzack R, Mount BM, Gordon JM: The Brompton mixture versus morphine solution given orally: Effects on pain. Can Med Assoc J 120:433–438, 1979; also reprinted in Ajemian I, Mount MB (eds): The R.V.H. Manual on Palliative Hospice Care. New York, Arno, 1980
61. Melzack R, Ofeish JG, Mount BM: The Brompton Mixture: Effects on pain in cancer patients. Can Med Assoc J 113:123–129, 1976; also reprinted in Ajemian I, Mount MB (eds): The R.V.H. Manual on Palliative Hospice Care. New York, Arno, 1980
62. Miller RR: Clinical effects of parenteral narcotics in hospitalized medical patients. J Clin Pharmacol 20:163–171, 1980

63. Moertel CG, Ahmann DL, Taylor WF, Schwartau N: A comparative evaluation of marketed analgesic drugs. N Engl J Med 286:813–815, 1972
64. Moertel CG, Ahmann DL, Taylor WF, Schwartau N: Relief of pain by oral medications: A controlled trial of analgesic combinations. JAMA 229:55–59, 1974
65. Mount BM: Medical applications of heroin. Can Med Assoc J 120:405–407, 1979; also reprinted in Ajemian I, Mount BM (eds): The R.V.H. Manual on Palliative Hospice Care. New York, Arno, 1980
66. Mount BM, Ajemian I, Scott JF: Use of the Brompton Mixture in treating the chronic pain of malignant disease. Can Med Assoc J 113:122–124, 1976; also reprinted in Ajemian I, Mount BM (eds): The R.V.H. Manual on Palliative Hospice Care. New York, Arno, 1980
67. Newman RG: Sounding boards: The need to redefine addiction. N Engl J Med 308:1096–1098, 1983
68. Onofrio BM, Yaksh TL, Arnold PG: Continuous low-dose intrathecal morphine administration in the treatment of chronic pain of malignant origin. Mayo Clin Proc 36:316–320, 1981
69. Orne MT: Pain suppression by hypnosis and related phenomena. In Bonica JJ (ed): Advances in Neurology, vol 4. New York, Raven Press, 1974
70. Osler W: Maeterlinck on death. Spectator, November 4, 1911. Quoted in Harvey Cushing: The Life of Sir William Osler, vol II, pp 298–299. Oxford, Oxford University Press, 1923
71. Pannuti F, Rossi AP, Iafelice G, Marraro D et al: Control of chronic pain in very advanced cancer patients with morphine hydrochloride administered by oral, rectal and sublingual route. Clinical report and preliminary results on morphine pharmacokinetics. Pharmacol Res Commun 14(4):369–380, 1982
72. Parkes CM: Home or hospital? Terminal care as seen by surviving spouses. J R Coll Gen Pract 28:19–30, 1978
73. Pasternak GW: Opiate, enkephalin, and endorphin analgesia: Relations to a single subpopulation of opiate receptors. Neurology (NY) 31:311–313, 1981
74. Polletti CE, Cohen AM, Todd DP et al: Cancer pain relieved by long-term epidural morphine with permanent indwelling system for self-administration. J Neurosurg 33:381–384, 1981
75. Reasbeck PG, Rice ML, Reasbeck JC: Double-blind controlled trial of indomethacin as an adjunct to narcotic analgesia after major abdominal surgery. Lancet 2:113–118, 1982
76. Robins LN: The Vietnam drug user returns. Special action office monograph, Series A, No. 2. Washington, DC, US Government Printing Office, 1974
77. Rutter PC, Murphy F, Dudley HA: Morphine: Controlled trial of different methods of administration for postoperative pain relief. Br Med J 280:12–13, 1980
78. Saunders C: The Management of Terminal Disease. Chicago, Year Book Medical Publishers, 1978
79. Saunders C: The nature and management of pain in terminal malignant disease. Mimeographed transcript of a tape for the Medical Recording Service, 3rd edition. London, St Christopher's Hospice, 1975
80. Saunders C, Baines M: Living with Dying: The Management of Terminal Disease. New York, Oxford University Press, 1983
81. Simon LS, Mills JA: Nonsteroidal antiinflammatory drugs. N Engl J Med 302:1179–1183, 1237–1243, 1980
82. Smith OM, Semke CW, Beecher HW: Objective evidence of mental effects of heroin, morphine and placebo in normal subjects. J Pharmacol Exp Ther 136:33–38, 1962
83. Stanski DR, Greenblatt DS, Lowenstein E: Kinetics of intravenous and intramuscular morphine. Clin Pharmacol Ther 24:39–52, 1978
84. Staub E, Kellett DS: Increasing pain tolerance by information about adverse stimuli. J Pers Soc Psychol 21:198–203, 1972
85. Sternbach RA: Pain Patients: Traits and Treatments. New York, Academic Press, 1974
86. Swerdlow M: The treatment of "shooting" pain. Postgrad Med J 56:159–161, 1980
87. Tolstoy L: The death of Ivan Ilych. In Great Short Works of Leo Tolstoy, pp 243–302. New York, Harper & Row, 1967
88. Twycross RG: Bone pain in advanced cancer. In Vere DW (ed): Topics in Therapeutics 4. Kent, England, Pitman Medical Publishing, 1978

89. Twycross RG: Choice of strong analgesic in terminal cancer: Diamorphine or morphine? Pain 3:93–104, 1977

90. Twycross RG: Diseases of the central nervous system: Relief of terminal pain. Br Med J 347:212–214, 1975

91. Twycross RG: Morphine and diamorphine in the terminally ill patient. Acta Anaesth Scand (Suppl) 74:128–134, 1982

92. Twycross RG: Relief of pain. In Saunders CM (ed): The Management of Terminal Disease, pp 66–92. Chicago, Year Book Medical Publishers, 1978

93. Twycross RG: Value of cocaine in opiate-containing elixirs. Br Med J 2:1348, 1977

94. Twycross RG, Fairfield S: Pain in far-advanced cancer. Pain 14:303–310, 1982

95. Ventafridda V, Fochi C, DeConno D, Sganzerla E: Use of nonsteroidal anti-inflammatory drugs in the treatment of pain in cancer. Br J Clin Pharmacol (Suppl 2) 10:343s–346s, 1980

96. Vere DW: Pharmacology of morphine drugs used in terminal care. In Vere DW (ed): Topics in Therapeutics 4, pp 75–83. Kent, England, Pitman Medical Publishing, 1978

97. Verebely K, Volavka J, Mule S, Resnick R: Methadone in man: Pharmacokinetic and excretion studies in acute and chronic treatment. Clin Pharmacol Ther 18:180–190, 1975

98. Walsh TD, Baxter R, Bowman K, Leber R: High-dose morphine and respiratory function in chronic cancer pain (abstr). Pain (Suppl) 11:539, 1981

99. Ward NG, Bloom VL, Friedel RO: The effectiveness of tricyclic antidepressants in the treatment of coexisting pain and depression. Pain 7:331–341, 1979

100. Weis OF, Sriwatanakul K, Alloza JL, Weintraub M, Lasagna L: Attitudes of patients, housestaff, and nurses toward postoperative care. Anaesth Analg 62:70–74, 1983

101. Wikler A: Opioid Dependence: Mechanisms and Treatment. New York, Plenum Press, 1980

102. Yaksh TL: Spinal opiate analgesia: Characteristics and principles of action. Pain 11:293–346, 1981

103. Zborowski M: Cultural components in responses to pain. J Soc Issues 8:16–30, 1932

104. Zola IK: Culture and symptoms—An analysis of patients' presenting complaints. Am Soc Rev 31:615–630, 1966

The Management
of Common Symptoms

2

Introduction

Patients with advanced cancer experience a variety of disagreeable symptoms in addition to pain. Table 2-1 indicates the frequency of some of these symptoms as reported in several series of dying persons who were evaluated at home or in an inpatient hospice. A number of common complaints—itching, hiccoughs, and dry or sore mouth—were not included in these reports.

Whereas standard medical training and practice focus on identifying and curing or ameliorating the underlying causes of an illness, the physician who cares for patients with chronic diseases, such as advanced cancer, must be preoccupied with the control of symptoms—reducing the disagreeable manifestations of disease.[2,3] The hospice approach contributes valuable lessons to general medicine by bringing greater attention to the nature of patients' discomforts and to the pharmacologic and non-pharmacologic modalities for effectively relieving distress.

HOW TO USE THIS CHAPTER

In keeping with an emphasis on comfort measures, this chapter is organized primarily according to symptoms rather than diagnoses. A typical section discusses a group of symptoms, their pathophysiologic basis, a differential diagnosis, and an approach to management. Information is reviewed that is particularly helpful in the care of

TABLE 2-1
Common Symptoms in Terminal Ilness
(percentage of patients experiencing symptoms)

Author:	Lamerton[7]	Lack and Buckingham[6]	Ward[9]	Baines[1]	Gotay[5]
Type of program:	Hospice/ Homecare†	Hospice/ Homecare*	Homecare	Inpatient Hospice*	Hospice/ Homecare*
PAIN	75	67	62	66	73
Headache	6			6	
GI					
Nausea	13				
Vomiting	20		38		
Nausea and vomiting		79		41	51
Anorexia	32	65	61	62	
Dysphagia				16	
Jaundice				8	
Bowel problems					41
Diarrhea	6	90			41
Constipation	48	68		46	
RESPIRATORY					41
Cough	29	83	48	49	52
Dyspnea	29	74	52	41	
BLADDER PROBLEMS					29
Incontinence				20	
(±frequency)		86			
SKIN					
Pressure sores				22	
Fistula				2	
Bleeding				9	
FLUID					
Edema		88			
Edema and/or effusion				27	
NEUROPSYCHIATRIC					
Confusion or drowsiness		90		10	16
Insomnia	7	82		24	60
Anxiety		86			
Weakness		45		20	
Paralysis				5	
GENERAL					
Weight loss				60	
Cachexia				12	
Fatigue					84

*Symptoms on or around time of admission
†Symptoms while in program

patients with advanced cancer and that is often lacking or underemphasized in general medical training or general textbooks on medicine and oncology. This chapter is based on the popular symptom-control cookbooks,[1] which have made the hospice approach widely available, but it tries to avoid their common tendency to present complex clinical issues in a highly simplified form. However, only an extremely lengthy textbook could aspire to address the detailed assessment and management of the protean manifestations of advanced cancer and the toxicity of cancer treatments. The reader is presumed to have a solid background in internal medicine and in the use of a variety of drugs in the care of debilitated patients.

Drug dosages have been suggested for average-size adults with normal hepatic and renal function. Individual differences must be respected. Reduced dosages are commonly required for debilitated patients with dysfunction of several organs. Before using an unfamiliar drug, the physician is encouraged to consult a pharmacology textbook and the manufacturer's package insert for a review of indications, dosage, major toxicity, adverse reactions, contraindications, drug interactions, details of administration, and recent warnings or precautions.

Much of the material presented in Chapter 2 is available in standard textbooks on medicine, pharmacology, oncology, and hospice care, as listed under General References, following this Introduction. Further documentation is offered under Selected References for each section.

GENERAL PRINCIPLES

The following general principles in symptom control should be noted:

1. *Take symptoms seriously.* Treat whatever hurts. In advanced cancer, the underlying problem often cannot be changed, but the symptoms can be palliated.

   Take seriously all symptoms, big and small. The wife of a dying patient who had been told that nothing could be done for his deafness described the simple prescription of a hearing aid as "a chance . . . a vote for life, not death."[8]

2. *Make the diagnosis.* A thorough medical evaluation is useful at all stages of illness and is the first step toward successful symptom control. Specific diagnoses may lead to specific treatments.

   At times, definitive diagnostic measures to delineate the cause of various symptoms are inappropriate in managing patients with advanced cancer. A carefully considered therapeutic trial to achieve comfort promptly may be more humane and sensible than waiting for clear indications for treatment. When treating "blindly" makes sense, however, it should be based on an informed opinion about the etiology of symptoms. The treatment regimen should be a thoughtful therapeutic trial, not a careless shotgun blast.

3. *Use simple measures before turning to the complex.* Simple steps are often sufficient. Reconsider the use of technologies that are discomforting or frightening and that may make the patient dependent on institutional care. Many of the standard measures of general medicine are unhealthy practices for the patient with advanced terminal illness. The parenteral line has become as much a part of the hospital admission procedure as a "johnny." Treat a dry mouth first with frequent sips of liquids, not with intravenous fluids.

   Easy methods are always virtuous, especially in the home, where elaborate regimens may overwhelm the family caretakers. Complicated methods are sometimes not worth the inconvenience they cause, and they can unnecessarily burden the home-care team. Gauge therapeutic efforts to the interest, willingness, and energy of the patient and family.

4. *Know your drugs.* Learn how to use a few therapeutic agents well. By concentrating on a select group of drugs, the clinician eventually becomes facile in optimizing treatment regimens and in rapidly establishing appropriate medication schedules for each individual.

   Beware of subtherapeutic doses; patients are often given too little of one drug, then switched to another drug without ever receiving an adequate trial of the original agent.

   Likewise, *beware of drug toxicity.* In the following sections on the symptoms of terminal illness, drug toxicity is a major consideration in differential diagnoses. Polypharmacy in elderly, debilitated, or malnourished patients with multiple organ failure is regularly associated with unanticipated drug effects, including over- and underdosing. Beware of drug interactions.

5. *Try hard and keep on trying.* Do not give up when first attempts fail. Persistence works. Everything learned while trying hard with one patient will help with subsequent patients.

   Do not wait for the definitive study on the treatment of a symptom; be empirical. Pick up tips from journals. Talk to specialists and old country doctors. Listen to patients' remedies.

   The very act of trying is evidence to the patient of your concern and hopefulness. The clinician's enthusiasm and persistence help the patient tolerate distress and can often make the difference between fair or satisfactory symptom control and excellent relief.

6. *Ample time is needed to do this work well.* More time is required for excellent symptom control than is generally allotted to physicians for a housecall or for an office or hospital visit. Nurses need more time than is generally allotted to a visiting nurse for a housecall or to a ward nurse for inpatient care. To provide good symptom control, arrange to have enough time, especially when techniques are first being learned.

7. *Adjust goals in order to enjoy the gratification of small improvements.* Because symptom control will not always prove to be excellent, be prepared to modify expectations for relief. Some of the hospice literature seems to suggest that every patient can be perfectly comfortable, that all symptoms can be totally alleviated, and that serenity can be the lot of all the dying. Strive for perfection, but be prepared for disappointment. A failure to suppress totally all symptoms is not a disgrace. Be pleased with doing some good—diminishing pain, increasing comfort, improving mobility, bringing momentary cheerfulness—rather than eradicating all symptoms.

8. *Treat the worry as well as the physical distress.* Ask what the symptom means to the patient and family. The worry about the personal meaning of the symptom can be more troubling than the physical discomfort and often may be quickly treated by appropriate reassurance (see Chap. 5, Feeling Secure).

9. *Help the patient and family accept "tolerable" symptoms.* Symptoms such as weight loss, weakness, fatigue, and anorexia are annoying or frustrating but are neither physically painful nor necessarily frightful portents. The patient and fam-

ily may take such symptoms very seriously. Redirect their concerns and educate them about the significance of these problems. Weight loss, for instance, need not be seen as a sign of treatment failure or impending doom. Similarly, in discussing weakness, one might say:

> The weakness isn't dangerous, but it is one of the most frustrating parts of having cancer. The treatment for it isn't very good. I'm going to give you these vitamins, which can help a little, but let's mainly try to see what we can do in spite of the weakness. It's something you can live with. You can still do many of the things you care about. . . . [Followed by a discussion about saving energy for important matters, planning extra rest during the day, identifying and emphasizing sedentary pleasures, finding aids to ambulation, and increasing home supports]

Beware also of elaborate measures to alleviate symptoms that are unlikely to respond to treatment; the disappointment over failure may be worse for the patient than the symptom itself.

10. *Anticipate and prevent symptoms.* Symptoms should be carefully anticipated and treated before they become intolerable, especially if keeping the patient at home is a goal. Patients will generally not stay at home if they are retching. Similarly, family members may only be able to stand the patient having 1 night of bad confusion and wandering before they demand institutional care. Do not wait for mild symptoms to become unbearable. Prepare the patient and family for predictable problems, showing them specific measures for getting help or for treatment.

11. *Know what treatment the patient is taking.* Compliance problems are common in the management of terminal illness, as in all areas of medicine. Patients and families will omit or modify the use of treatments that the physician considers essential or may add measures, some of which are useless or harmful. A careful review of the treatment regimen should be performed frequently. Families may also benefit from a variety of aids for remembering how to give medication properly. Routinely, a medication list which is intelligible to both professional and lay caretakers should be prepared, noting the name, color, purpose, and schedule for all drugs.

12. *When medications fail, think about the role of emotional distress.* Intractable complaints can express intractable despair. When symptoms do not respond to treatment that ought to have helped at least a little—when "nothing works"—the patient is often anxious, worried, depressed, or manipulative. Conversely, excellent symptom control rarely occurs when the patient has not achieved a relatively satisfactory frame of mind. Psychosocial support cures or alleviates many physical ailments.

13. *Multiple coexisting symptoms are the rule.* A problem-oriented approach, using a list of individual symptoms as well as diagnoses, is recommended for guiding clinical work.

14. *Provide comfort always; prolong life when appropriate.* Many well-intended therapeutic efforts that can be described as "palliative"—directed toward reducing symptoms of the disease itself—can prolong suffering rather than promote comfort. Tracheostomies, urinary and gastrointestinal diversionary procedures, and feeding devices can defer an untimely death but also may subject the patient to further discomforts and a more terrible dying. Avoid meddling, either by injudi-

ciously prescribing ineffective measures or by applying treatment aimed solely at prolonging life at a time when enhanced comfort is the appropriate therapeutic goal.

15. *Reassess constantly.*

REFERENCES FOR INTRODUCTION

1. Baines MS: Control of other symptoms. In Saunders CM (ed): The Management of Terminal Disease. Chicago, Year Book Medical Publishers, 1978
2. Cassell ES: The relief of suffering. Arch Intern Med 143:522–523, 1983
3. Cassell ES: The nature of suffering and the goals of medicine. N Engl J Med 306:639–645, 1982
4. Entralgo L: Doctor and Patient, Partidge F (trans). New York, McGraw-Hill, 1969
5. Gotay CC, Verhoof MJ, Lentjes DM: Symptom control in terminally ill patients receiving care at home. Presented at the Annual Meetings of the Royal College of Physicians and Surgeons of Canada, Calgary, Alberta, September, 1983 (and personal communication, CC Gotay)
6. Lack S, Buckingham RW: First American Hospice. New Haven, CT, Hospice, Inc, 1978
7. Lamerton R: Care of the Dying (revised and expanded ed). New York, Penguin, 1980
8. Lerner G: A Death of One's Own. New York, Simon & Schuster, 1978
9. Ward AM: Terminal care in malignant disease. Soc Sci Med 10:413–420, 1974

GENERAL REFERENCES FOR CHAPTER 2

1. Ajemian I, Mount BM: The R.V.H. Manual on Palliative Hospice Care. New York, Arno Press, 1980
2. Baines MJ: Control of other symptoms. In Saunders CM (ed): The Management of Terminal Disease. Chicago, Year Book Medical Publishers, 1978
3. Crowther AGO: Management of other common symptoms of the terminally ill. In Wilkes E (ed): The Dying Patient—The Medical Management of Incurable and Terminal Illness. Ridgewood, NJ, George A Bogden & Son, 1982
4. Dietz JH Jr: Rehabilitation Oncology. New York, John Wiley & Sons, 1981
5. Freitag JJ, Miller LW (eds): Manual of Medical Therapeutics, 23rd ed. Boston, Little, Brown & Co, 1980
6. Gilman AG, Goodman LS, Gilman A: Goodman's and Gilman's The Pharmacological Basis of Therapeutics, 6th ed. New York, Macmillan, 1980
7. Goroll AH, May LA, Mulley A: Primary Care Medicine. Philadelphia, JB Lippincott, 1981
8. Guyton AC: Textbook of Medical Physiology, 6th ed. Philadelphia, WB Saunders, 1981
9. Petersdorf RG, Adams RD, Braunwald E, Isselbacher KJ, Martin JD, Wilson JD (eds): Harrisons's Principles of Internal Medicine, 10th ed. New York, McGraw-Hill, 1983
10. McEvoy GK (ed): American Hospital Formulary Service Drug Information 84. Bethesda, MD, American Society of Hospital Pharmacists, 1984
11. Rubenstein E, Federman DD: Scientific American Medicine. New York, Scientific American, 1983
12. Schlang HA: Symptomatology of Metastatic Cancer. Garden City, NY, Medical Examination Publishing Co, 1981

A. Nausea and Vomiting

Nausea and vomiting are common troubling symptoms of cancer, sometimes appearing early in the course of the disease. They are also frequent sequelae of cancer chemotherapy and some forms of radiation therapy; patients often cannot or will not complete potentially useful, even curative, treatments because of such side-effects. About one third of terminally ill patients at St. Christopher's Hospice have a problem with vomiting.[3] The physician who is familiar with the pathophysiology of nausea and vomiting and with its pharmacologic control can substantially improve the well-being of patients suffering from these symptoms.

PATHOPHYSIOLOGY

There is little useful information on the pathophysiologic basis of nausea, which, like pain, is a subjective experience. The pathophysiology of vomiting, however, has been the subject of elegant studies.[4,5,7] This complex phenomenon has been shown to be controlled by the emetic center or integrative vomiting center (IVC) in the medulla oblongata (Table 2A-1). Retching, which commonly follows nausea and which may accompany vomiting, presumably has a similar neuroanatomic basis. The emetic center coordinates a complex set of actions of the gastrointestinal (GI) tract and of the respiratory and abdominal musculature, mediated by both somatic and visceral efferent nerves. Direct stimulation of this center by systemic emetogenic drugs or toxins has not been reported, but a number of drugs, particularly antihistamines, act directly on or near the emesis center to blunt its responsiveness to other stimuli. Pharmacologic blunting of the effector limb of the vomiting response has not been reported.

The emetic center receives input from at least four sources:

1. The *chemoreceptor trigger zone (CTZ)*, located in the medulla, is activated by chemical stimuli from the blood or cerebrospinal fluid (CSF). This center appears to mediate the response to a variety of drugs that cause vomiting—apomorphine, opiates, cardiac glycosides, and probably some chemotherapeutic agents. A number of antiemetic drugs appear to act directly on this site to block CTZ-induced vomiting. Experimentally, drugs acting on the CTZ are relatively ineffective in protecting against stimuli that impinge on the emetic center through other pathways.

2. *Peripheral input,* particularly from the GI tract and pharynx, is mediated through the autonomic nervous system (*i.e.,* vagal and, to a lesser extent, other cranial and sympathetic afferent nerves), acting directly on the emetic center. Early experiments demonstrated the emetic effect of GI irritants (*e.g.,* intragastric copper sulfate or traction on the intestines). Peripheral input is presumably responsible for the vomiting associated with abdominal and pharyngeal tumors and with many of the GI conditions caused by cancer and its treatment—biliary or intestinal obstruction, radiation enteritis, dumping, and so on. Peripheral input may mediate some chemotherapy-related emesis, presumably due to drug-induced intestinal irritation.

    Experimentally, neurosurgical interruption of the autonomic afferents can block vomiting from peripheral inputs. Pharmacologic blockade of these afferents has not been reported, but drugs that blunt the responsiveness of the emetic center are effective in inhibiting peripherally induced vomiting.

TABLE 2A-1
Pathophysiology of Vomiting

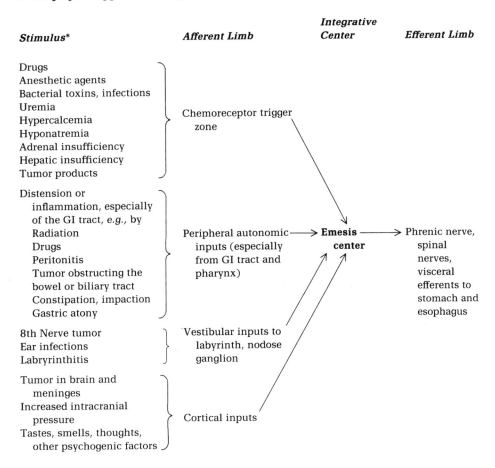

Stimulus*	Afferent Limb	Integrative Center	Efferent Limb
Drugs Anesthetic agents Bacterial toxins, infections Uremia Hypercalcemia Hyponatremia Adrenal insufficiency Hepatic insufficiency Tumor products	Chemoreceptor trigger zone		
Distension or inflammation, especially of the GI tract, *e.g.*, by Radiation Drugs Peritonitis Tumor obstructing the bowel or biliary tract Constipation, impaction Gastric atony	Peripheral autonomic inputs (especially from GI tract and pharynx)	**Emesis center**	Phrenic nerve, spinal nerves, visceral efferents to stomach and esophagus
8th Nerve tumor Ear infections Labryrinthitis	Vestibular inputs to labyrinth, nodose ganglion		
Tumor in brain and meninges Increased intracranial pressure Tastes, smells, thoughts, other psychogenic factors	Cortical inputs		

*Since reliable data on the site of action of many emetogenic stimuli are not available, groupings are theoretical.

3. *The vestibular apparatus* is responsible for the nausea and vomiting associated with motion sickness and ear disorders.[13,17,33,35] Vertigo may be an accompanying symptom. Some intracranial processes may also cause emesis by impinging on the vestibular tracts.

Stimulation of the vestibular apparatus (*e.g.*, head movement) seems to affect susceptibility to vomiting from stimuli that act on the emetic center through non-vestibular pathways (*e.g.*, apomorphine). The medications commonly used for motion sickness and vertigo apparently act near or directly on the emetic center, not on the inner ear or its neuronal pathways to the medulla.

4. Finally, *cortical centers* (including supramedullary centers in the hypothalamus and thalamus) impinge on the emetic center. Cerebral edema and some brain lesions may cause vomiting; other brain lesions may prevent it. An unusual form of sudden emesis without preceding nausea—projectile vomiting—is said to be pathognomonic of a cerebral lesion. Smells, tastes, and thoughts may provoke nausea and vomiting, whereas distraction from disagreeable associations can have some benefit in avoiding or controlling emesis of various etiologies.

CONDITIONED NAUSEA AND VOMITING

Patients who have vomited from chemotherapy may become nauseous or may start vomiting in the hours before the next course of treatment is to be started.[18,21] Such symptoms may be triggered by stimuli associated with the treatment—an ambulance ride, the smell from a cafeteria near the doctor's office, an alcohol swab used by a nurse, the sight of an intravenous bottle, or just the thought of a hospital examining room—or by the treatment itself, regardless of its actual emetogenic potential. Anticipatory nausea has been reported in 24% of patients receiving chemotherapy, beginning, on the average, 17 hours before treatment. Nine percent of patients note some anticipatory emesis beginning, on the average, 11 hours before treatment. Psychogenic emesis may develop after a single course of chemotherapy and presumably is induced by vomiting of other etiologies.

The psychological concept of "conditioned behavior" has provided a useful model for understanding this syndrome. The model suggests that once nausea or emesis has been provoked by any medical regimen—chemotherapy, analgesics, special diets, and so on—further treatments or events associated with that treatment may produce these symptoms, regardless of whether the initial stimulus for nausea and vomiting is present. Such conditioning might be prevented if the physician prophylactically administers effective antiemetics whenever important treatment is begun with agents that are likely to cause nausea or vomiting. If early signs of nausea are treated vigorously, and vomiting is prevented, the development of anticipatory or conditioned symptoms may be avoided.

A number of behavioral interventions have proved useful in managing conditioned nausea and vomiting.[19,26] Antiemetic drugs may also diminish or abolish these symptoms. Behavioral techniques have not been demonstrated to prevent or lessen vomiting due to unconditioned physical or psychological causes. Nevertheless, since stress or anxiety may play a role in the predisposition to nausea or vomiting, as well as in the development or learning of conditioned symptoms, relaxation techniques and anxiolytic therapy may be useful in the early course of any potentially emesis-provoking treatment.

EVALUATION

Table 2A-1 lists the common causes of nausea and vomiting. History-taking should delineate the situation in which the symptoms occur, particularly their relation to meals, abdominal pain, medication, emotional state, smells, and tastes. The quality of the emesis may give valuable clues to intestinal irritation and sites of obstruction (*e.g.*, hematemesis with a gastric ulcer or feculent vomitus with a low obstruction). Complaints referable to the GI tract should be sought. Impaction and obstipation are frequent causes of nausea and vomiting in the patient with advanced cancer. Concurrent neuropsychiatric symptoms suggest an intracranial mass. Cough-induced emesis is readily treated with antitussives.

Conditions that may provoke nausea and vomiting without a readily apparent diagnosis during the late stages of cancer include the following:

1. Adrenal insufficiency (Addison's disease) in patients who have received steroids or whose adrenal glands have been obliterated by surgery, radiation, and/or metastases
2. Brain tumors and cerebral edema
3. Meningeal carcinomatosis, which can be detected by attention to behavioral changes and cranial nerve signs
4. Conditioned or psychogenic vomiting, especially in patients who vomit in situations of anxiety
5. Multifactorial vomiting (*e.g.,* the patient with an intestinal tumor who has been made slightly nauseous by narcotics and develops emesis under the added stress of a respiratory tract infection, car travel, or an upsetting visit)

Laboratory studies may include determination of electrolytes (including calcium) and of renal and hepatic function. A flat plate of the abdomen may be helpful in identifying the site and cause of obstruction.

Both the patient's degree of distress from the symptom and the clinical sequelae of vomiting—fluid and electrolyte loss, malnutrition, erratic absorption of oral medication, and the risk of aspiration penumonia or of esophageal tear or rupture—should be gauged, especially when considering such disagreeable management measures as nasogastric intubation, intravenous therapy, or surgical treatment. Occasionally, for example, patients with partial bowel obstructions may be refractory to antiemetic medication, but their vomiting may be infrequent and well-tolerated. Other patients with frequent nausea or recurrent vomiting will be rapidly made miserable by their symptoms or may quickly become dehydrated.

MANAGEMENT

General Principles

Table 2A-2 reviews some of the specific treatments that may be useful when the cause of the nausea and vomiting are known. Unfortunately, nausea and vomiting often are produced by unclear or multiple mechanisms. Attempts to understand the underlying etiology of the symptoms are often unsuccessful, and the pathophysiology of symptoms may not point to a drug of choice. Also, treatment is often desirable before diagnostic efforts are completed. Hence, a sensible trial-and-error or empirical approach may be used, employing both pharmacologic and nonpharmacologic techniques.

Table 2A-3 describes nonpharmacologic general measures. A relaxed, pleasant environment should be sought, and the patient's general ease should be promoted. Avoidance of vestibular stimulation, especially automobile and elevator rides, should be attempted; bed or chair rest may be useful. Environmental stimuli causing nausea and vomiting (*e.g.,* disturbing foods and odors or stressful interpersonal encounters) should be identified and, if possible, eliminated. Fasting or a diet of small, bland, liquid meals should be prescribed.

Drug treatment should be started promptly. Antiemetic drugs are generally con-

TABLE 2A-2
Etiologic Considerations in Choosing Treatment for Nausea or Vomiting

Condition	*Management*
Intestinal obstruction [peripheral input] Esophageal	Local anesthetics
Gastric, high intestinal	Metoclopramide Nasogastric tube Steroids Rule out postgastrectomy obstruction, afferent loop syndrome
Small intestine and colonic	Rule out impaction Steroids Consider tolerating infrequent emesis
Gastric irritation [peripheral input]	Antacids Cimetidine, ranitidine Metoclopramide Sucralfate
Metabolic problems [CTZ-induced] Uremia Hepatic failure Hypercalcemia Hyponatremia Ketoacidosis	Treat underlying cause
CNS [cortical input] Increased intracranial pressure	Diuretics Steroids Raise head
Drug-induced [CTZ-induced] [peripheral input]	Stop or decrease drugs Give drug with meal or snack
Psychogenic [cortical input]	Emotional support Environmental adjustment Sedation Hypnosis, relaxation
Vestibular [vestibular input]	Rest, lie flat Avoid travel and sudden head motions

TABLE 2A-3
Nonpharmacologic Measures for Nausea and Vomiting

Fasting when vomiting is troublesome—"resting" the bowels
Rest; avoiding vestibular stimulation
Diet
        Begin with liquid or soft foods
        Small, light meals, eaten slowly
        Attractive foods, carefully chosen by patient*
        Bland diets, avoidance of sweet, greasy, or spicy foods or strong odors
        Trial of avoiding fatty and fried foods
        (See also discussion on nutrition and feeding in Chap. 2C)
Fluids to prevent dehydration—ice chips, small sips
Trial of alcohol before meals
Pleasant atmosphere and companionship for meals
Relaxation techniques, desensitization, and hypnosis
(Encourage use of antiemetics well before symptoms develop)

*Suggestions and cookbooks are available through the American Cancer Society and National Cancer Institute.

sidered to be most effective in preventing symptoms and least effective in controlling symptoms that have already become severe. Moreover, use of the drugs at the earliest signs of nausea may avert the development of conditioned symptoms.

Parenteral administration of antiemetics is occasionally necessary for the initial control of symptoms and for adequately assessing the response to a drug that may be poorly absorbed orally. If vomiting is severe and repeated, injections are advisable for prompt control of symptoms. Oral medications can generally be used when symptoms are mild or infrequent and when an initial bout of sustained or violent vomiting has responded to injections. Most orally administered drugs require 20 to 40 minutes after ingestion to achieve an effect, and reach a peak level in 1 to 2 hours. When nausea and vomiting are associated with a meal or other stimulus, patients should be instructed to take the medication at least $\frac{1}{2}$ hour before the precipitating event.

Common errors in the use of oral antiemetic agents include (1) use of subtherapeutic doses; (2) improper scheduling, particularly when prn or infrequent doses produce systemic drug levels that are inadequate for prophylaxis and control of symptoms; (3) failure to try agents with different sites of action; and (4) lack of attention to absorption (e.g., expecting a patient with severe bowel disease or repeated vomiting to achieve good systemic levels with an oral agent).

Rectal suppositories are a logical alternative to injections in the patient who cannot keep down or absorb oral medication. The absorption of medications from the rectum may be erratic, but patients often can achieve excellent control of emesis with suppositories.

Choice of Drugs

Studies of antiemetic drug use during cancer chemotherapy can only cautiously be applied to the control of emesis induced by the cancer itself or by its complication.[6,8,9,11,12,14-16,27,29] Similarly, studies based on the control of vomiting from motion sickness,[2,33-35] anesthesia,[17,24,25] or other clinical[30] or experimental conditions[4,5,31] cannot be automatically applied to patients with symptoms from various manifestations of advanced cancer.

In patients for whom a pathophysiologic basis for vomiting is known, an antiemetic drug may be chosen for its action on the CTZ or on the emesis center.[3,32] Hypothetically, the former group of drugs (the phenothiazines, the butyrophenones, or metoclopramide) would be ideal for managing vomiting from uremia or sensitivity to narcotics (mediated through the CTZ), whereas the latter group (H1-blocking antihistamines) might be chosen for hepatic distension, biliary obstruction, or carcinomatosis of the peritoneum (mediated through peripheral input). Systematic clinical data to support this logical approach in choosing antiemetics are lacking.

When a clear etiology for vomiting is not established, treatment is generally begun with a phenothiazine. This class of antiemetics has the best established record of usefulness, and toxicity is generally mild. High doses of one agent should be attempted before switching to other agents in this class or other classes. Alternatively, a butyrophenone may be employed.

For patients with adequate, but not excellent, symptom control on either a phenothiazine or butyrophenone, a switch between these two classes of neuroleptics or between two phenothiazines may be worthwhile, or metoclopramide may be tried. For distressed patients with a poor response to these first-line drugs, a second drug with a different postulated mechanism of action should be added to the neuroleptic (e.g., an antihistamine or metoclopramide). If symptoms improve on a two-drug regimen, slow withdrawal of the first drug can be attempted later.

The patient who fails to respond to such combination treatments often has a cause for vomiting that is poorly amenable to any pharmacologic manipulation (e.g., partial bowel obstruction). Expectations for relief must be lowered. However, the addition of other drugs may be attempted (see Miscellaneous Agents, below), and three agents may be tried simultaneously, while empirical trials of antacids or cimetidine may be considered.

Review of Specific Drugs[10]

Phenothiazines

Phenothiazines act primarily on the CTZ, although they may have some peripheral action. The antiemetic action of these drugs is not correlated with their antihistaminic or anticholinergic properties, but has been postulated to reflect their dopamine antagonistic action on the CTZ, an area rich in dopamine receptors.[22]

The various phenothiazines have not been rigorously compared in terms of their clinical efficacy and their relative toxicities in combating various forms of nausea and vomiting, nor are appropriate dosage ranges and schedules well described. Phenothiazines with a halogenated R-1 side chain—prochlorperazine (Compazine) and perphenazine (Trilafon)—have more antiemetic effect and cause less sedation and hypotension than do other agents in this class (e.g., chlorpromazine [Thorazine]) but also have more extrapyramidal effects. Experimental evidence in dogs favors perphenazine over prochlorperazine for preventing apomorphine-induced emesis.[31] Clinical data favor perphenazine and thiethylperazine (Torecan).[14-16,24,25] When sedation is desirable, chlorpromazine is the drug of choice in this class. Thioridazine (Mellaril) has no antiemetic effect.

Common side-effects are sedation, hypotension (usually postural), and extrapyramidal reactions such as parkinsonism and akathisia (motor restlessness). Increased prolactin levels from phenothiazines have an unclear import in cancer progression. Tardive dyskinesias usually occur after long-term use and can be a practical concern when these drugs are administered chronically to cancer patients with indolent courses.

Many phenothiazines are available as syrups and suppositories.

PHENOTHIAZINES

Prochlorperazine (Compazine)	5–20 mg po q4–8h 25 mg pr q6–12h 5–15 mg IM q4–6h
Chlorpromazine (Thorazine)	10–50 mg po q4–6h 25–100 mg pr q6–8h 25–50 mg IM q2–4h
Perphenazine (Trilafon)	2–8 mg po q6–8h (up to 24 mg qd) 5–10 mg IM q4–8h
Thiethylperazine (Torecan)	10 mg po, IM, or pr q4–8h

Butyrophenones

Butyrophenones also inhibit the CTZ. Haloperidol has proved useful for chemotherapy- and radiation-induced vomiting. Extrapyramidal reactions develop more frequently than with phenothiazines; sedation, paradoxical agitation, and akathisia are not uncommon. These drugs have less cardiac toxicity than the phenothiazines and are also generally less sedating and better tolerated by elderly or debilitated patients.

BUTYROPHENONES

Haloperidol (Haldol)	0.5–2.0 mg po or IM q4–8h
Droperidol (Inapsine)	2.5–10.0 mg IM q6–8h

Metoclopramide

Metoclopramide (Reglan) is a procainamide derivative with both peripheral (GI) and central (CTZ) antiemetic actions. It has recently been released in the United States for limited indications and has been employed in other countries for many GI conditions. Its general use for nausea and vomiting require further study.[1,28] Metoclopramide accelerates gastric emptying and increases pressure in the lower esophageal sphincter, making it a logical choice as an antiemetic for patients with atonic, small, or compressed stomachs, especially when accompanied by early satiety. Vomiting due to gastroparesis would presumably respond well to this drug, whereas symptoms of intestinal obstruction might be worsened.

About 10% of patients receiving the drug at usual doses will have CNS side-effects—sedation, dizziness, fainting, or, rarely, extrapyramidal reactions. Metoclopramide may affect the absorption of drugs; its concurrent use with other pharmacologic agents requires further evaluation.

When administered intravenously, usually in doses that are high (1–2 mg/kg), repeated (q2–3h), and expensive, metoclopramide has proved useful for some chemotherapy-induced emesis.[9] High doses for other causes of emesis have not been studied but deserve consideration.

Metoclopramide (Reglan)	10–20 mg po q6h or ac and hs
	10 mg IV q2–4h (up to 60 mg/day)

Antihistamines

Antihistamines, H$_1$-blockers, although related to phenothiazines, have minimal CTZ-blocking effect and appear to act on or near the emetic center. The anti–motion-sickness potency of various drugs in this class is not proportional to antihistaminic or anticholinergic properties, although both histaminic and muscarinic cholinergic receptors have been noted to be highly concentrated in the emetic center and vestibular center.[12] H$_1$-blockers have demonstrated usefulness, particularly when given before the onset of motion sickness and when effective blood levels are maintained during the period of emesis-inducing stimuli.

While antihistamines might logically be first-line drugs for any vomiting not mediated through the CTZ, they are often weakly effective. Clinical practice dictates that antihistamines be tried after phenothiazines and butyrophenones, except when they are the drug of choice for motion sickness and for vomiting associated with vestibular disorders. When a first-line drug fails, an antihistamine may be added, and excellent responses occasionally occur. Side-effects, including sedation and dry mouth, are generally mild.

ANTIHISTAMINES	
Cyclizine (Marezine)	50 mg po or IM q4–6h
	100 mg pr q4–6h
Dimenhydrinate (Dramamine)	50 mg po or IM q4–6h
	100 mg pr q8–12h
Diphenhydramine (Benadryl)	25–100 mg po q4–6h
	10–50 mg IV or IM q4–8h
Hydroxyzine (Vistaril, Atarax)	25–50 mg po or IM q4–8h
	120 mg pr bid
Promethazine (Phenergan)— [a phenothiazine with H$_1$-blocking action]	25–50 mg po, pr, or IM q4–6h

Anticholinergic Drugs

Anticholinergic drugs with predominantly CNS action can block peripherally induced emesis in experimental situations and have proved clinically useful for preventing motion sickness.[17,33,34] Transdermal scopolamine has recently been marketed and is reported to produce dry mouth less than previously marketed centrally acting anticholinergics.[2] The dermal route is ideal for patients having difficulty with oral medications, and such a drug is attractive as an adjunct to current first-line treatments. Unfortunately, anticholinergics seem to have little efficacy in blocking CTZ-mediated vomiting, and they have not been shown to have broad use as antiemetics.

ANTICHOLINERGIC DRUGS

Scopolamine (Transderm Scōp)	q3d
Scopolamine bromide	0.3–1.2 mg IM,
	usual dose 0.6 mg IM q6h

Miscellaneous Agents

Benzquinamide (Emete-con) is a parenteral agent that appears to depress the CTZ. Since it is structurally unrelated to the phenothiazines and antihistamines and is relatively nontoxic, it may be tried in a variety of settings, particularly for patients who are allergic to or develop dysphoria with phenothiazines.

Benzquinamide (Emete-con)	50 mg (0.5–1.0 mg/kg) IM, repeat in 1 h, then give q3–4h

---

Cannabinoids (tetrahydrocannabinol [THC], marijuana) are useful antiemetics for some persons receiving chemotherapy, especially younger patients and those who have had previous enjoyable experiences with such psychoactive drugs.[23] There is no good evidence that THC is useful for other causes of emesis. THC has not been widely available, although illicit marijuana is readily obtained by many patients. Absorption of the drug from smoking and ingestion is erratic. Improved appetite may be a useful side-effect of cannabinoids, but troublesome toxicity may include somnolence, dizziness, ataxia, dysphoria, dry mouth, and tachycardia. Synthetic analogues of THC (*e.g.,* nabilone) are being developed and tested.[11]

Tetrahydrocannabinol (THC)	10–20 mg po q3–4h

Trimethobenzamide (Tigan) is a relatively weak and possibly useless antiemetic with minimal side-effects.[15,24]

Trimethobenzamide (Tigan)	250 mg po q6–8h
	200 mg pr q6–8h

Steroids are reported to be useful in some cases of recurrent emesis.[6] They inhibit prostaglandin synthesis, a presumed mediator of the emetic reaction. High doses are used (*e.g.,* dexamethasone 4–20 mg po or IV q4–6h).

Sympathomimetic drugs (*e.g.,* dextroamphetamine [Dexedrine] 5–20 mg po or ephedrine 25–50 mg po) are effective in preventing motion sickness, especially when combined with scopolamine or promethazine.[34] Repeated doses and prolonged usage have not been studied in terms of antiemetic usefulness, ability to counteract the drowsiness induced by other antiemetics, or toxicity.

Sedative–hypnotics, such as barbiturates (*e.g.,* pentobarbital 50–150 mg po or IV), are sometimes added to phenothiazines to treat chemotherapy-induced emesis.[27] Barbiturates and benzodiazepines have generally not been shown to be effective antiemetic agents when given alone[15] or when added to standard agents,[20] although they are likely to have some value in managing anxiety-related symptoms. Antidepressants may be effective in conjunction with phenothiazines.[20]

Nonsteroidal anti-inflammatory drugs (*e.g.,* ibuprofen) often cause gastric upset and vomiting, but may also have some antiemetic properties.[30]

SELECTED REFERENCES

1. Albibi R, McCallum RW: Metoclopramide: Pharmacology and clinical application. Ann Intern Med 98:86–95, 1983
2. Anonymous: Transdermal scopolamine for motion sickness. Med Lett Drugs Ther 23:89–91, 1981
3. Baines MJ: Control of other symptoms. In Saunders CM (ed): The Management of Terminal Disease. Chicago, Year Book Medical Publishers, 1978
4. Borison HL, McCarthy LE: Neuropharmacologic mechanisms of emesis. In Laszlo J (ed): Antiemetics and Cancer Chemotherapy. Baltimore, Williams & Wilkins, 1983
5. Borison HL, Wang SC: Physiology and pharmacology of vomiting. Pharmacol Rev 5:193–230, 1953
6. Cassileth PA, Lusk ES, Torri S, DiNubile N, Gerson SL: Antiemetic efficacy of dexamethasone therapy in patients receiving chemotherapy. Arch Intern Med 143:1347–1349, 1983
7. Feldman M, Fordtran JS: Vomiting. In Sleisenger MH, Fordtran JS (eds): Gastrointestinal Disease: Pathophysiology, Diagnosis, Management, vol 1, pp 200–216. Philadephia, WB Saunders, 1978
8. Frytak S, Moertel C: Management of nausea and vomiting in the cancer patient. JAMA 245:393–396, 1981
9. Gralla RJ, Hri LM, Pisko SE et al: Antiemetic efficacy of high-dose metoclopramide: Randomized trials with placebo and prochlorperazine in patients with chemotherapy induced nausea and vomiting. N Engl J Med 305:905–909, 1981
10. Harris JG: Nausea, vomiting and cancer treatment. CA 28(4):194–201, 1978
11. Herman TS, Einhorn LT, Jones SE, Nagy C et al: Superiority of nabilone over prochlorperazine as an antiemetic in patients receiving cancer chemotherapy. N Engl J Med 300:1295–1297, 1979
12. Laszlo J (ed): Antiemetics and Cancer Chemotherapy. Baltimore, Williams & Wilkins, 1983

13. Mellencamp E, Wang RIH: The patient with nausea II: Motion sickness. Drug Ther 7:49–54, 1977
14. Moertel CG, Reitemeier RJ: Advanced Gastrointestinal Cancer—Clinical Management and Chemotherapy. NY, Harper & Row, 1969
15. Moertel CG, Reitemeier RJ: Controlled clinical studies of orally administered antiemetic drugs. Gastroenterology 57:262–268, 1969
16. Moertel CG, Reitemeier RJ, Gage RP: A controlled clinical evaluation of antiemetic drugs. JAMA 183:116–118, 1963
17. Money KE: Motion sickness. Physiol Rev 50:1–39, 1970
18. Morrow GR, Arseneau JC, Asbury RF, Bennett JM, Boros L: Anticipatory nausea and vomiting with chemotherapy. N Engl J Med 306:431–432, 1982
19. Morrow GR, Morrell C: Behavioral treatment of the anticipatory nausea and vomiting induced by cancer chemotherapy. N Engl J Med 307:1476–1480, 1982
20. Neidhart JA, Gagen M: Experimental antiemetic agents (other than cannabinoids and metoclopramide). In Laszlo J: Antiemetics and Cancer Chemotherapy. Baltimore, Williams & Wilkins, 1983
21. Nesse RM, Carli T, Curtis GC, Kleinman PD: Pretreatment nausea in cancer chemotherapy: A conditioned response? Psychosom Med 42:33–36, 1980
22. Peroutka SF, Snyder SH: Antiemetics: Neurotransmitter receptor binding predicts therapeutic actions. Lancet 1:658–659, 1982
23. Poster DS, Penta JS, Bruno S, Macdonald J: Delta 9 - tetrahydrocannabinol in clinical oncology. JAMA 24:2047–2051, 1981
24. Purkis IE: The action of thiethylperazine (Torecan): A new anti-emetic compared with perphenazine (Trilafon), trimethobenzamide (Tigan), and a placebo in the suppression of postanaesthetic nausea and vomiting. Can Anaesth Soc J 12:595–607, 1965
25. Purkis IE: The effectiveness of anti-emetic agents. Can Anaesth Soc J 10:539–549, 1963
26. Redd WH, Andresen GV, Minagawa RY: Hypnotic control of anticipatory emesis in patients receiving cancer chemotherapy. J Consult Clin Psychol 50:14–19, 1982
27. Sallan SE, Cronin CM: Nausea and vomiting. In Vincent TD Jr, Hellman S, Rosenberg S (eds). Cancer: Principles and Practice of Oncology, pp 1704–1707. Philadelphia, JB Lippincott, 1982
28. Schulze-Delrieu K: Drug therapy: Metoclopramide. N Engl J Med 305:28–33, 1981
29. Seigel LJ, Longo DL: The control of chemotherapy-induced emesis. Ann Intern Med 95:352–359, 1981
30. Stryker JA, Demers LM, Mortel R: Prophylactic ibuprofen administration during pelvic irradiation. J Radiat Oncol Biol Phys 5:2049–2052, 1979
31. Wang SC: Perphenazine, a potent and effective antiemetic. J Pharmacol Exp Ther 123:306–310, 1958
32. Weis OF, Weintraub M: New developments in the treatment of nausea and vomiting. Drug Ther 12:167–170, 1982
33. Wood CD, Graybiel A: Antimotion sickness and antiemetic drugs. Drugs 17:471–479, 1979
34. Wood CD, Graybiel A: Evaluation of sixteen anti-motion sickness drugs under controlled laboratory conditions. Aerospace Med 39:1341–1344, 1968
35. Wood CD, Graybiel A: Theory of antimotion sickness drug mechanisms. Aerospace Med 43:249–252, 1972

B. Hiccoughs

Chronic hiccoughs typically are associated with upper gastrointestinal disease and with other medical conditions affecting or adjacent to the diaphragm or phrenic nerve. In addition, a host of metabolic conditions (especially renal failure) and neurologic and psychological illnesses may be accompanied by hiccoughs.

Acute hiccoughs respond to a variety of home and bar remedies. Rapid ingestion of a large spoonful of dry granulated sugar is one effective treatment.[1] Alternative techniques available in the home include rebreathing into a paper bag or nasopharyngeal stimulation with a cotton swab or a nasogastric tube.

When simple remedies for acute hiccoughs fail,[2] phenothiazines (as listed under A. Nausea and Vomiting) are the treatment of choice. Intravenous chlorpromazine (Thorazine) 50 mg has proved a good agent; oral regimens may also be effective. Metclopramide 10 mg q6h by oral or parenteral route can also be tried. Minor tranquilizers (e.g., diazepam [Valium] IV or po) have also been used. After the hiccoughs resolve, drug treatment may be continued to prevent recurrence. Neurosurgical procedures have been used for rare refractory cases.

SELECTED REFERENCES

1. Engleman EJ, Lankton BL. Granulated sugar as treatment for hiccups in conscious patients. N Engl J Med 285:1489, 1971
2. Williams BWA, MacIntyre JMD: Management of intractable hiccup. Br Med J 2:501, 1977

C. Anorexia and Nutritional Care

INTRODUCTION

The relationship between nutrition and cancer has been widely cited in the popular press. A critical reading of studies on this topic, however, suggests few clinically useful nutritional strategies for patients with advanced disease.[12,20,29] In evaluating nutritional research and prescriptions, the reader should keep in mind that diet may have a different significance in specific stages of cancer: the predisposition to and initial development of neoplasms; tumor growth and spread; and the response of the tumor to treatment. Furthermore, the value of general nutrition should be distinguished from the roles of specific forms of protein, carbohydrates, and lipids, of food groups and fiber, of vitamins, minerals, additives, and contaminants, and of food preparation.

The important role of diet in the initial development of cancer will not be reviewed here. For established cancer, no dietary intervention has a clearly proved beneficial effect on tumor progression. A well-publicized regimen of high doses of vitamin C (10 g a day, given parenterally for the first week, then orally) is probably harmless, but has no convincingly demonstrated value.[9] Vitamin A and related retinoids also show promise, although toxicity may limit their usefulness.[6,31]

The poorly understood phenomena of cancer-related anorexia and cachexia are often naively attributed to malnutrition; yet the importance of nutrition in their etiology, sequelae, or treatment remains unclear.[11,24] Common sense and custom dictate that good nutrition helps a person to feel well and to fight off illness, that unintended weight loss is harmful, and that a cancer patient who eats properly can improve or prolong life by preventing or reversing cachexia. Scientific support for many of these notions, however, is lacking. Few studies of humans, or even animals, touch on these matters. Weight loss is clearly a worrisome sign in a patient with cancer and is one of the strongest prognostic indicators of poor outcome. Nutritional deficits are common.[10] Treatment of the weight loss itself, however, does not necessarily improve the patient's well-being or survival.[7,13,18,26,29] Insofar as studies are available, experimental evidence suggests that poorly nourished animals are *less likely* to get cancer than well-nourished animals and that their tumors grow more slowly. Furthermore, while forced feeding may lead to weight gain, the increase in tumor weight is proportionately greater than the increase in weight of the rest of the animal's body. Such worsening of the tumor has not been reported as a consequence of improved nutrition in humans, but vigorous nutritional support currently has little justification as a general cancer treatment, despite the regular association of cachexia with cancer death.

Nutritional counseling in advanced cancer, therefore, is primarily intended to enhance the comfort and pleasure of the patient whose food preference and tolerance is altered by the disease and its treatment. In addition, nutritional counseling alleviates the patient's and family's concerns about diet and weight loss. Also, a number of complications of terminal illness are treated, in part, by dietary methods, but are not discussed here as nutritional problems, namely:

1. Sodium and water retention
2. Increased or decreased serum osmolality, sodium, potassium, calcium, phosphate, magnesium, and glucose
2. Renal failure
4. Hepatic failure

PATHOPHYSIOLOGY[10,12,30]

Malnutrition has multiple causes (Table 2C-1). Of first concern for the physician are those treatable conditions of the gastrointestinal tract that discourage or prevent eating, especially subliminal nausea, stomatitis, xerostomia, and dysphagia. Second, potentially reversible conditions that cause maldigestion and malabsorption should be addressed. Third, psychological factors (depression, anxiety, and conditioned aversions) should be considered.

Anorexia is common in the absence of identifiable treatable factors. Anorexia may be a presenting sign of cancer and may be seen with relatively limited or localized disease.[11,24] It may sometimes be accompanied by nausea and vomiting. Its pathogenesis is poorly understood. Animals with cancer have been shown to have disturbances in the regulation of their feeding behavior, whereas both animals and humans with cancer have been shown to develop taste disorders. In general, patients with anorexia will show decreased sensitivity (or increased threshold) to tasting sweets, an increased sensitivity to bitterness, and aversion for various foods, particularly meat. These taste disturbances may be a consequence as well as a cause of malnutrition and do not necessarily respond to treatment of the tumor. Learned (conditioned) aversions may be induced by cancer treatments that cause nausea or vomiting[4,5] and probably develop in other settings. Disorders of smell, frank "taste blindness," and early satiety have also been described in cancer patients.[25,28]

Weight loss and *cachexia* may be partially explained by anorexia and difficulty in eating or absorbing food, but may develop despite seemingly adequate nutritional

TABLE 2C-1
Pathophysiology of Malnutrition in Advanced Cancer: Nutritional Disturbances and Their Etiologies

ANOREXIA
　　Primary or metastatic tumor
　　　　Local effects (*e.g.*, pelvic/abdominal tumors, hepatic metastases, compression of the
　　　　　　intestines)
　　　　Remote effects
　　　　　　Taste disorders
　　　　　　Food aversions
　　　　　　Early satiety
　　Treatment-related
　　　　Postsurgical small stomach or stasis
　　　　Drug-related, including chemotherapy
　　　　Radiation—local and systemic effects
　　Systemic illness
　　　　Infection
　　　　Hepatitis, pancreatitis
　　　　Endocrinopathies
　　Taste disorders
　　　　Drug-related (*e.g.*, metronidazole)
　　　　Remote effects of neoplasm and its treatment
　　　　Local disease (*e.g.*, stomatitis, nasopharyngeal tumor, radiation, surgery)
　　　　Associated with nausea and vomiting (see Chap. 2A)
　　　　Psychogenic
　　　　　　Depression
　　　　　　Anxiety
　　　　　　Conditioned aversions
　　Intolerance of institutional food

DIFFICULTY EATING (see Chap. 2E)
　　Head and neck tumors and their treatment
　　Xerostomia
　　Stomatitis
　　Loss of teeth, dental problems
　　Dysphagia, odynophagia

MALDIGESTION/MALABSORPTION
　　Pancreatic insufficiency
　　Bile salt deficiency
　　Hypersecretory states
　　　　Zollinger–Ellison syndrome
　　　　Pancreatic cholera (4)
　　Bowel infiltration
　　　　Diffuse (*e.g.*, lymphoma)
　　　　Local blockage
　　　　Fistula
　　Postsurgical
　　　　Esophageal surgery (with vagotomy, gastric stasis, diarrhea, steatorrhea)
　　　　Gastrectomy—dumping, achlorhydria, afferent loop syndrome (1,2)
　　　　Small intestine resections (2,3)
　　Postradiation
　　　　Enteritis (may occur as late sequela)
　　　　Fistula

TABLE 2C-1 *(continued)*

> Stenosis
> Obstruction
> ?Direct effect of malnutrition on the gut

PROTEIN-LOSING ENTEROPATHY

MALUTILIZATION

> "Cancer cachexia"
> Steroids—nitrogen wasting, hyperglycemia, calcium loss (4)

Specific nutritional deficiencies also develop, for example:
   1. Loss of intrinsic factor
   2. B_{12} deficiency
   3. Bile salt deficiency
   4. Electrolyte and water disorder

intake. Malutilization of nutritional supplies and widespread metabolic abnormalities have been demonstrated in cancer patients. The tumor can be shown to command excessive amounts of nutrients for its own needs. Organs without evidence of metastases exhibit abnormal metabolism, perhaps owing to remote effects of the tumor. Muscle wasting may be prominent. Cancer patients adapt poorly to starvation, showing high rates of protein breakdown. When they receive parenteral hyperalimentation, they are relatively inefficient in maintaining or increasing their lean body weight or in raising their serum albumin as compared with patients with uncomplicated starvation.

EVALUATION

Objective, practical measures of nutritional status are not readily available. Malnutrition is recognized by clinical evaluation[3,22]:

1. A history of grossly inadequate intake (with special attention to anorexia, vomiting, and unusual diets)
2. Weight loss
3. A physical examination that reveals muscle wasting, loss of subcutaneous fat, edema, cheilosis, or glossitis

   Laboratory findings suggesting malnourishment include a serum albumin of less than 3.5 mg/dl and anergy.

MANAGEMENT

Reasonable nutritional goals in terminal illness include the following:

1. Comfort, well-being, and pleasure in eating
2. Preventing gross malnutrition, supplementing deficient diets, maintaining weight when practical, and, rarely, slow rebuilding of body mass
3. Treating or preventing specific, symptomatic nutritional difficulties such as fat malabsorption or hyperkalemia

Vigorous nutritional support—aggressive techniques of enteral or parenteral hyperalimentation—should not be used to treat cancer or cancer-related anorexia/cachexia, but may have a limited role in managing specific nutritional problems and in preventing or reversing general malnutrition in a debilitated patient preparing for or undergoing strenuous treatment aimed at the neoplasm (e.g., a surgical procedure or a course of chemotherapy or radiation).

A clinical approach is suggested in the following sections.

General Measures to Treat Malnutrition

Identify and treat reversible factors contributing to difficulty in eating and to maldigestion/malabsorption (see Table 2C-1 and discussion below). Xerostomia, for instance, is a common condition that makes mastication difficult and depresses the appreciation of taste. Experimentally, exogenous and endogenous opiates stimulate food intake,[23] but narcotic analgesics may affect nutritional intake adversely by depressing the sense of smell[21] or causing nausea.

Identify and treat nausea and vomiting. Is there mild nausea, which might respond to antiemetics, antacids, or other measures?

Characterize anorexia, if present, and help the family prepare meals with the following considerations[1]:

Is there aversion to certain foods, particularly meats and chocolate?

Are there disturbing odors? What about tobacco?

Can the patient, by testing foods or just imagining foods, identify menus that might be appealing or distasteful? Consider, particularly, the attraction of sweet, spicy, bitter, bland, tart, or salty foods, of meat, fish, poultry, eggs, and milk and other dairy products. Bland foods and milk shakes, which so often are used as nutritional supplements, can be a poor choice of food for patients who want spicy, strongly flavored meals.

Consider seasonings such as lemon juice or mint. Patients with depressed appreciation of sweetness may enjoy additions of sweetness or flavorings to their diet. Patients with insensitivity to sour or salty tastes may prefer tart juices or foods flavored with lemon juice. Meat aversion may be managed by reliance on other protein sources—grains, legumes, milk, egg, and cheese. Cold, clear liquids are often favored, for example, fruit drinks (not tart juices) or carbonated beverages, as well as such foods as Popsicles or Jello. The addition of butter, gravy, cream, or other moisturizing agents may improve taste perception for drier foods. Switching frequently from one food to another while eating has been proposed as a measure to heighten taste appreciation.

Is there a preferred food temperature (e.g., hot, cold, or room temperature)?

Are there preferred textures (e.g., liquid, soft or blenderized, or solid)?

Can a colorful presentation of food enhance appetite?

Preferred meal size? Some patients can ingest larger total daily amounts if they take small, frequent feedings or if they slowly sip or nibble on high-calorie snacks throughout the day. The addition of metoclopramide (Reglan) may prevent gastric stasis in a small, compressed, or atonic stomach.

Are low-nutritional liquids or other substances producing satiety? The ingestion of large amounts of liquids with low caloric density may inhibit intake of more nutritionally valuable substances. The common encouragement to take fluids should be reevaluated.

Is there a diurnal variation in appetite, which might suggest preferred times for feeding? Thoughtfully timed meals or readily available meals can greatly enhance intake and pleasure.

Would the patient like alcohol? Does it help or hinder the appetite? Most patients with tissue irritation in the mouth or upper gastrointestinal (GI) tract find alcohol disagreeable; patients with lymphomas sometimes report aggravation of pain with this drug.[8] Others find that alcohol, especially before meals, stimulates the appetite and increases the pleasure of meals.

Zinc has been proposed as a treatment for some taste disorders, especially hypogeusia following radiation treatment[16,27] (e.g.,zinc sulfate 109.95 mg [25 mg elemental zinc] po qid with meal or snack). GI disturbances may occur with zinc. Pellagra may produce taste disorders, and niacin has also been proposed as a treatment for hypogeusia.[14] Niacin or niacinamide 100 mg qid should reverse subclinical pellagra within a few days.

Most of the measures noted above can be viewed as attempts to please the patient, to help with nutrition by paying careful attention to personal tastes which may be altered by cancer. Menu books or suggestions from a registered dietitian/nutritionist are often useful in developing a palatable and nutritious food plan tailored to individual needs. High-calorie, high-protein recipes may be offered and the patient may be assisted in experimenting with seasonings and flavorings.

In the hospital, patients and their families should have access to cooking facilities and should be encouraged to prepare foods as they prefer. Ideally, the patient will be able to obtain food whenever desired, including both hot and cold meals. If nutrition is important, hospital routines should not interrupt or interfere with eating.

Beware of the nutritional prescriptions that abound in the popular press and in lay gossip. Occasionally, patients adopt expensive, disagreeable, useless, or unhealthful nutritional "cures." More commonly, patients devise unpalatable diets or deprive themselves of favorite foods when casually advised to take in lots of potassium, eat dry toast and crackers, avoid alcohol, and so on. A plethora of well-meaning advice often overwhelms the patient and family while failing to address their specific needs.

Fatigue is a common cause of malnutrition. Who shops and prepares meals? What food is available to the patient without great effort?

General health measures—improved sleep and comfort, exercise, treatment of an infection, or transfusion for severe anemia—may yield excellent results in stimulating appetite.

Psychological Response to Nutritional Disorders

Identify the personal reactions of the patient and family to poor intake, weight loss, and cachexia. Many patients and families place very high significance on eating regularly and well, and they overrate the importance of nutrition for a person who is severely debilitated and will die soon regardless of intake. Family members may become very upset if a few meals are rejected, believing that the patient will starve or die quickly from inadequate nutrition. They may not appreciate that a patient can survive for long periods with little intake or that a liquid diet can provide adequate nutrition. In such situations, the family can be reassured of the diminished importance of eating, although counseling will not always alter deeply held beliefs. Acknowledge frustration and helplessness about feeding and note the good efforts and intentions of the family:

He is sick. The sickness makes him lose his appetite. We should try to feed him if he wants food or will take it, but we don't need to force him. He will still be sick if he eats.

He really does not want to eat. He can live for a long time, even if he hardly eats at all. People live for many months on a semistarvation diet.

Do not weigh the patient unless the information is useful. Documentation of weight loss only reinforces the patient's and family's concerns.

Guilt and blame are frequent features of family dynamics around feeding. Beware of meal times that focus on getting the patient to eat, perhaps depriving the patient and family of a cherished social gathering:

Her body controls her appetite, so she takes what she needs. You don't need to force her or trouble her with eating. But let her sit with you at meals and enjoy your company.

Many patients realize or learn to accept that anorexia and cachexia are disagreeable accompaniments of cancer, not major matters for concern. Like the weakness associated with cancer, these problems can be acknowledged as tolerable, but do not require treatment. Nutritional efforts should be gauged, in part, to how much the patient and family are bothered by anorexia/cachexia, how much effort they want to make to prevent malnutrition, and how the patient tolerates efforts to improve intake, including the prescription of food supplements that are often distasteful.

Appetite Stimulants

In rare instances, *consider appetite stimulants.* The best stimulant is a meal prepared to the patient's taste. Other measures may be considered:

Alcohol before meals
Prednisone 5–10 mg po tid

Steroids are frequently useful in far-advanced cancer for controlling pain, promoting general well-being, and improving appetite. Antidepressants work marvelously for depressed patients who are anorectic. Cyproheptadine (Periactin) may produce appetite stimulation as a side-effect, but has not been studied in anorectic cancer patients.

Nutritional Supplements

Commercial enteral nutritional supplements (Tables 2C-2 and 2C-3) may be considered when the patient has continued weight loss or muscle wasting or when oral intake is clearly inadequate despite attention to the matters noted above. They are also convenient for tube-feeding.

For patients taking oral feedings, special nutritional supplements rarely have much advantage over carefully prepared foods from the home kitchen. For instance, patients generally obtain more pleasure and calories from drinking Carnation Instant Breakfast or homemade milkshakes than from using canned liquid diets. The patient and family may be pleased that "something special" is being done or may attribute

TABLE 2C-2
Special Diets

Condition	Dietary Prescription (and Other Treatments)	Commercial Supplement*
Require meal replacement with soft or liquid foods	Blenderized diets Carnation Instant Breakfast, milk shakes, and other nutritional liquids	Liquid supplements— Precision Isotene, Ensure Plus, Sustacal, Meritene
Fat maldigestion	Medium chain triglycerides Supplemental vitamins A, D, K	Portagen, MCT oil
Pancreatic insufficiency	(See fat maldigestion) Cimetidine, pancreatic enzymes, B_{12} injections	Portagen, MCT oil
Enteral disease (short bowel, GI fistula, enteritis, inflammatory bowel, acute diarrhea, postsurgery)	"Elemental diet" Protein hydrolysate (iso-osmolar, lactose-free, low-fiber, low-fat, low-gluten) Avoid milk, milk-based products	Vivonex, Vivonex HN, Flexical, Precision LR
Salt retention	Sodium restriction	Isocal, Ensure Osmolite
Renal insufficiency	Salt and potassium restriction	Amin-Aid
Hepatic failure	Branched amino acids (vs. aromatic amino acids or methionine)	Hepatic Aid†
Lactose intolerance	Avoid lactose Lactose added to milk products	Ensure Plus, Isocal, Sustacal Liquid

*Not an exhaustive listing of commercially available preparations
†Efficacy is questionable.

great nutritional potency to commercial dietary preparations, but high-calorie supplements are expensive and often seem monotonous and unpalatable. They tend to suppress the patient's appetite for preferred, more pleasing foods. Because acceptance of supplements parallels acceptance of a regular diet, commercial preparations rarely are successful in greatly changing tolerance to feedings.

In general, commercial supplements should be used as additional sources of nutrition rather than as replacements for enjoyable foods. An exception to this rule is the patient who cannot prepare foods and for whom canned feedings are convenient. Also, patients who, owing to vomiting or dysphagia, can take in only small volumes of oral feedings may benefit from the concentrated calories available in supplemental feedings. High-caloric density, however, can be achieved with noncommercial diets or by the addition of commercial supplements to regular food. Dietitians may offer a

TABLE 2C-3
Dietary Supplements

Dietary Prescription	*Commercial Supplement**
High-fat diet	Lipomul
	MCT oil
High-carbohydrate diet	Polycose
High-protein diet	Citrotein (low-fat, low-residue, gluten-free)
	Casec

*Not an exhaustive listing of commercial preparations

"taste tray" of commercial supplements, allowing the patient to identify preferred brands.

Inexpensive multivitamins are easily tolerated by most patients and are often greatly appreciated by the patient and family.

Tube-Feeding

The introduction of small-bore nasogastric catheters and enteral formulas has made *tube-feedings* so much more acceptable to patients and so much less likely to cause significant discomfort or side-effects that this nutritional method deserves brief mention, although it is rarely required in far-advanced cancer.[17]

A small-bore, flexible catheter (Dobhoff, Entriflex) should be passed through the nose into the stomach or upper small intestine. A continuous drip of isotonic solutions at half strength or of hypertonic solutions at quarter strength (diluted with water) is generally begun at 50 ml/hr. Every day, the infusion rate is increased 25 ml/hr (to 100–125 ml/hr) or the concentration is increased (quarter to half to three-quarter to full strength), as long as complications do not arise (*i.e.*, diarrhea and cramps, reflux or aspiration) or until the required nutrition (usually 1000–2500 calories/day) is delivered.

The head of the bed should be elevated 30° to prevent reflux and aspiration. The bags of supplement should hang for no longer than 6 hours, and the administration set should be changed daily. Initially, the tube is aspirated every 4 hours to check for a large residual. Medications can be delivered through the tube but should be flushed through.

If the patient accepts a feeding catheter, blocked tubes or extruded tubes are major annoyances accompanying this treatment. The tube should be well secured.

Hyperalimentation

Hyperalimentation, particularly total parenteral nutrition, insofar as it has been studied among cancer patients, is not a life-prolonging or antitumor treatment. Aggressive enteral or parenteral nutritional support may help sustain life through a course of cancer therapy and thus may be considered an adjunct to surgery, chemotherapy, or radiation for malnourished patients, although its value is not clearly established.[7] Specific conditions (*e.g.*, radiation enteritis) may be indications for parenteral hyperalimentation. Similarly, patients who seem to be suffering from uncomplicated starvation (*e.g.*, due to irremediable swallowing disorders or high intestinal obstruction) are often felt to benefit from enteral nutrition and hydration (*via* nasogastric tubes or catheters placed elsewhere in the GI tract).

Enteral and parenteral total or supplemental alimentation are feasible at home, although parenteral regimens generally must be begun in the hospital, allowing for initial monitoring and training of the home-care team.[15] Commercial formulas are available for a variety of nutritional needs (*e.g.*, renal failure [Amin-Aid] and maldigestion of fats [Portagen]) (see Table 2C-2). The effectiveness of branched-chain amino acid solutions for hepatic encephalopathy (HepatAmine, Hepatic-Aid, Travasorb-Hepatic) has been questioned.[2]

ON DEATH FROM NUTRITIONAL DEFICIENCY

Decisions about the provision of nutrition for patients who are near death often reflect strong emotional influences, as well as uncertainty about the medical significance of food deprivation (or of dehydration, as discussed in Section J). The following points are helpful in making a decision.

Starvation is a word with powerful symbolic meaning, and it suggests withholding, neglect, punishment, and suffering. Fasting may have more positive connotations. Semistarvation is often a more accurate medical term to describe the nutritional status of patients with feeding difficulties. As with so many physical problems, the patient's and family's reaction to nutritional deprivation may be greatly influenced by the personal meaning attached to the experience, and thus the attitude and teaching of the medical staff can be a major determinant of how laypersons respond to this condition.

Prolonged fasting in healthy, alert adults is not necessarily described as disagreeable.[19] A brief initial stage of food craving is often followed, within a few days, by a long phase in which hunger is mild or absent. General well-being is otherwise relatively well maintained. The distress over starvation reported by concentration camp victims and other political prisoners, by persons lost at sea, and by dieters reflects the personal meaning of their situation as surely as does the euphoria, ecstasy or transcendental calm reported by religious fasters or the purification and cleansing reported by persons who fast for health reasons.

The medical consequences of nutritional deprivation in a debilitated patient who is nearing death are difficult to judge. Starvation in otherwise healthy, nonobese persons progresses rather slowly to death. Hunger strikers in Belfast lived $1\frac{1}{2}$ to 2 months, and many persons have fasted for periods of 3 weeks or longer without adverse consequences.[19] Fasting for weight reduction in obese patients has extended for months and, in at least one case, longer than a year.[32]

Based primarily on studies of healthy fasters, the following conditions are likely to develop during total starvation over a period of a week to a month: weight loss, bradycardia, hypotension (especially postural hypotension), lethargy, irritability, hyperuricemia, and ketosis. In general, deficiencies of minerals (including trace minerals) or vitamins are not evident. The major medical complications of prolonged semistarvation among obese patients on liquid-protein diets have been rare instances of ventricular arrhythmias and sudden death.

The important clinical question for the physician is how this particular patient—usually one who is debilitated, anorectic, or not fully alert, and who might not even enjoy much well-being if hyperalimented—feels when unable to eat. In contrast to the regular problem of thirst due to dehydration, very little suffering can usually be attributed to food deprivation, especially in the presence of anorexia. Occasionally patients are troubled by food craving, the loss of pleasure in eating, concern about not eating properly, weight loss (which is distressing because it changes one's appearance and is an outward sign of the illness), weakness, or postural hypotension. Such concerns tend to be diminished in many of the patients with advanced debility for whom tube-feedings are considered. In contrast, patients who are enjoying general well-being but are unable to ingest food (e.g., owing to an untreatable head-and-neck tumor or esophageal obstruction) or to absorb adequate nutrients are more likely to benefit from nutritional therapies. Even in such cases, the use of feeding tubes deserves careful scrutiny and rigorous studies. Feeding tubes may not reduce the distress and morbidity of aspiration and often seem merely to prolong suffering or to subject patients to new problems that are more distressing than would have been faced had aggressive nutritional support been foregone.

Members of the Nutritional Support Unit at Massachusetts General Hospital (MGH) and of the Nutrition Service of MGH and the MGH–Chelsea Memorial Health Center have provided useful information—lectures and written material—on this topic and have offered helpful comments on this section.

SELECTED REFERENCES

1. Aker SN: Oral feedings in the cancer patient. Cancer 43:2103–2107, 1979
2. Anonymous: Branched chain amino acids for the treatment of hepatic encephalopathy. Med Lett Drugs Ther 25:72, 1983
3. Baker JP, Detsky AS, Wesson DE et al: Nutritional assessment: A comparison of clinical judgment and objective measurements. N Engl J Med 306:969–972, 1982
4. Bernstein IL: Learned taste aversions in children receiving chemotherapy. Science 200:1302–1303, 1978
5. Bernstein IL, Webster M, Bernstein J: Food aversions in children receiving chemotherapy for cancer. Cancer 50:2961–2963, 1982
6. Bollag W: Vitamin A and retinoids: From nutrition to pharmacotherapy in dermatology and oncology. Lancet I:860–863, 1983
7. Brennan MR: Total parenteral nutrition in the cancer patient. N Engl J Med 305:375–382, 1981
8. Brewin TB: Alcohol intolerance in neoplastic disease. Br Med J 2:437–441, 1966
9. Cameron E, Pauling L: Megadoses of vitamin C as an adjunct in the treatment of cancer. Your Patient and Cancer pp 39–46, May 1982
10. Costa G, Donaldson SS: Current concepts in cancer: Effects of cancer and cancer treatment on the nutrition of the host. N Engl J Med 300:1471–1473, 1979
11. De Wys WD: Anorexia as a general effect of cancer. Cancer 43:2013–2019, 1979
12. De Wys WD: Nutritional care of the cancer patient. JAMA 244:374–376, 1980
13. De Wys WD, Kubota TT: Enteral and parenteral nutrition in the care of the cancer patient. JAMA 246:1725–1727, 1981
14. Green RF: Subclinical pellagra and idiopathic hypogeusia (letter). JAMA 218:1303, 1971
15. Grundfest S, Steiger E: Home parental nutrition. JAMA 244:1701–1703, 1980

16. Henkin RI: Prevention and treatment of hypogeusia due to head and neck irradiation (Questions and Answers). JAMA 220:870–871, 1972
17. Heymsfield SB, Bethel RA, Ansley JD, Nixon DW, Rudman D: Enteral hyperalimentation: An alternative to central venous hyperalimentation. Ann Intern Med 90:63–71, 1979
18. Karlberg, HI, Fisher JE: Hyperalimentation in cancer. West J Med 136:390–397, 1982
19. Kerndt PR, Naughton JL, Driscoll CE, Loxterkamp DA: Fasting, the history, pathophysiology and complications. West J Med 137:379–399, 1982
20. Kisner DL, Brennan MF. Malnutrition and nutritional support in cancer management. In Wiernik PH (ed): Supportive Care of the Cancer Patient. Mount Kisco, NY, Futura Publishing, 1983
21. Macht DI, Macht MB: Comparison of effect of cobra venom and opiates on olfactory sense (abstr). Am J Physiol 129:411–412, 1940
22. Michel L, Serrano A, Malt RA: Nutritional support of hospitalized patients. N Engl J Med 304:1147–1152, 1981
23. Morley JE, Levine AS: The central control of appetite. Lancet 1:398–401, 1983
24. Morrison SD: Origins of anorexia in neoplastic disease. Am J Clin Nutr 31:1104–1107, 1978
25. Nielsen SS, Theologides A, Vickers ZM: Influence of food odors on food aversions and preferences in patients with cancer. Am J Clin Nutr 33:2253–2261, 1980
26. Nixon DW, Lawson DH, Kutner M et al: Hyperalimentation of the cancer patient with protein–calorie undernutrition. Cancer Res 41:2038–2045, 1981
27. Russell RM, Cox ME, Solomons N: Zinc and the special senses. Ann Intern Med 99:227–239, 1983
28. Schiffman S: Taste and smell in disease. N Engl J Med 308:1275–1279, 1337–1343, 1983
29. Shils ME: Nutrition and neoplasia. In Goodheart RS, Shils ME (eds): Modern Nutrition in Health and Disease. Philadelphia, Lea & Febiger, 1980
30. Shils ME: Nutritional problems induced by cancer. Med Clin North Am 63:1009–1025, 1979
31. Sporn MB: Retinoids and suppression of carcinogenesis. Hosp Pract 18:83–98, 1983
32. Stewart WK, Fleming LW: Features of a successful therapeutic fast of 382 days' duration. Postgrad Med J 49:203–209, 1973

D. Constipation, Diarrhea, and Other Gastrointestinal Problems

CONSTIPATION

Advanced cancer patients frequently suffer the painful consequences of improperly managed bowels. The prevention of constipation becomes a regular concern for the physician.

Presentation

Mild constipation leads patients to complain of abdominal fullness, painful or hard stools, straining, rectal urgency, or a sense of incomplete defecation, and to develop troubling hemorrhoids. Some patients, of course, complain of infrequent stools but have no associated symptoms, and may merely require reassurance that only occasional bowel movements are necessary for good health. Other patients, however, not noticing a lack of normal bowel movements or not expecting to have regular stools when they are eating poorly, present with severe constipation.

Patients who are taking narcotics, including those who are relatively active and well-nourished, may stop having bowel movements and yet have no troublesome symptoms for a week or more until they develop a painful impaction. Impaction may be heralded by complaints of rectal pain and hard stools, but patients with impaired alertness or lack of normal sensation in the perineum often present with loose, frequent stools caused by seepage around a hard fecal mass in the rectum. The physician should be alert to the diagnosis of impaction and should not hesitate to perform a rectal examination when suspicious symptoms develop.

Obstipation can be mistaken for a catastrophic or terminal event: an acute abdomen, intestinal obstruction, or intractable vomiting. "Resuscitation by enema" is Richard Lamerton's term for a simple therapeutic intervention that rescues many debilitated patients from a premature death.

Pathophysiology

Among the common factors contributing to constipation in debilitated patients are weakness in straining, inattention to the urge to defecate, difficulty getting to the toilet, physical inactivity, poor fluid intake, and the use of opiates and other constipating drugs (*e.g.,* aluminum and calcium antacids, iron, tricyclics, or phenothiazines).

Conditions affecting the innervation of the bowel, especially the defecation reflex, may present as constipation. Constipated patients should be queried about concurrent bladder symptoms, and the physical examination should include attention to rectal tone and to lower extremity strength, sensation, and reflexes. Other diagnostic considerations include mechanical causes of constipation (tumor, stricture, volvulus) and metabolic processes (hypercalcemia, hypokalemia, and hypothyroidism). Constipation is also a common complaint in depression.

Management

Whenever a patient is taking opiates or undergoes prolonged bed rest with poor fluid intake, constipation should be anticipated and treated prophylactically. The patient and family need to be advised that such laxatives as dioctyl sodium succinate, Senokot, and bisacodyl may not produce immediate effects but can be beneficial if taken regularly. Medication is often best prescribed with instructions that it be taken daily *unless loose stools develop.* In general, the dosage should be titrated upward until satisfactorily soft bowel movements are produced at least every 3 days. The patient and family may benefit from being advised that bowel movements should continue regardless of diminished or absent oral intake.

Constipated patients should be encouraged to maintain a high fluid intake and, when feasible, to increase their activity level. An increase in dietary roughage (*e.g.,* bran or unprocessed wheat) or the use of psyllium preparations (*e.g.,* Metamucil) is occasionally helpful but is often found unpalatable. Moreover, the value of such roughage in a dehydrated or already seriously constipated patient is questionable. On the other hand, many severely ill patients can take prune juice or other fruit juices with laxative properties.

Senna, bisacodyl, and similar bowel stimulants are the mainstays of the prophylactic management and treatment of mild constipation. Dioctyl sodium sulfosuccinate, a stool softener, may be helpful when added to these mild cathartics, perhaps given in a drug combination (*e.g.,* Pericolace 1–4 times daily). In cases of severe constipation or when a preventive regimen with the above drugs fails, saline cathartics (milk of magnesia or magnesium citrate), castor oil, lactulose, and/or rectal suppositories should be tried. Also potentially useful is a new osmotic agent, Golytely—a balanced electrolyte solution with polyethylene glycol—which was developed for colon cleansing and which produces a profound diarrhea without inducing fluid or electrolyte disturbances; patients must be able to drink large amounts of the fluid.[1] Finally, enemas and manual disimpaction may be required. Topical anesthetics may ease the discomfort inflicted on patients by disimpaction, especially if hemorrhoids or proctitis have developed; premedication with systemic analgesics and sedatives should be considered.

A brief report of the successful use of oral naloxone for two patients with chronic idiopathic constipation raises the question of whether such an agent might counteract the constipation associated with opiate use without blocking systemic analgesia.[3] Currently, agents such as Senokot are satisfactory for controlling narcotic-induced constipation.

Weak patients should be assisted in getting to the bathroom once a day, or a bedside commode or bedpan should be prescribed. Patients whose mental status or rectal sensation is severely impaired may benefit from a bowel regimen that includes the following:

Regular laxative use to keep stools soft and avoid impaction
Being placed on the toilet, commode, or bedpan at least once a day
Daily stimulation of the defecation reflex with suppositories

---

MANAGEMENT OF CONSTIPATION

Senokot 1 tab or packet po 1–4 times daily to prevent constipation; hold if loose stools develop
    Alternative—Bisacodyl (Dulcolax) 5 mg po 1–3 times daily

Dioctyl sodium succinate (Colace, Doxinate) 200–600 mg po qd as tablets or syrup in 2–3 divided doses
    Alternative—Docusate calcium (Surfak) 240 mg po 1–2 times daily

Milk of magnesia 30 ml po hs prn no bowel movement in 2–3 days
    Alternatives:
        Magnesium citrate 200 ml po prn
        Castor oil 15–60 ml po prn
        Bisacodyl suppository 10 mg pr prn
        Glycerin suppository pr prn

Occasionally useful:
    Lactulose (Cephulac) 15–30 ml po 1–6 times daily—this is the agent of choice when concurrently treating hepatic failure
    Mineral oil 15 ml po hs—beware of aspiration
    Bulk-forming agents (*e.g.*, psyllium [Metamucil])
    Golytely solution (polyethylene glycol and electrolyte solution) 8 oz po repeated every 15 min or as tolerated over 3–4 hr until 1000 ml is taken or diarrhea ensues
    Enemas—tap water, saline, soapsuds, sodium phosphate (Fleet), oil

Neurogenic constipation (*e.g.*, in paraplegics):
    Bethanecol 10 mg po tid
    Neostigmine bromide 25 mg po tid

DIARRHEA

The troublesome sequelae of diarrhea include fluid and electrolyte loss, fecal incontinence or soiling, and the development of severe perianal irritation.

Pathophysiology

A number of diarrheal illnesses are associated with cancer and its treatment: postsurgical conditions such as the postgastrectomy syndromes, postvagotomy diarrhea, and short bowel syndromes; radiation- and drug-induced colitis; enteroenteric fistulas; steatorrhea and other maldigestive or malabsorptive states from deficiencies of pancreatic enzymes or bile salts; diarrhea associated with drugs, especially antibiotics, and with immunosuppression; secreting villous adenomas, carcinoid tumors, Zollinger–Ellison syndrome, the pancreatic cholera (or watery diarrhea) syndrome, and medullary carcinoma of the thyroid; and fecal impaction.

In the terminal phases of cancer, patients are subject to all the common causes of acute and chronic diarrhea, including infectious, toxic, and functional etiologies. Anxiety may lead to diarrhea or rectal urgency. Compromise of the colon and rectum from local tumor (including partial obstruction) and the late sequelae of surgery and radiation (e.g., strictures) may occasionally produce loose bowel movements. Incontinence from neurologic lesions may be mistaken for diarrhea. Diarrhea presenting late in the course of advanced cancer commonly results from drug toxicity (from laxatives, antacids, or antibiotics) or fecal impaction. A rectal examination is required for evaluation of this symptom.

Management

Medications should be adjusted so as not to aggravate the diarrhea. Alcohol and caffeine should generally be avoided. Hydration can be maintained with fluids containing sugar and electrolytes. High potassium intake may also be advisable. Protective and emollient ointments (e.g., zinc oxide, A and D ointment) can be applied to irritated perineal skin. Open wounds in the area may require protective dressings. In rare instances, watery diarrhea can be conveniently managed for brief periods with a rectal tube.

Over-the-counter absorbent medications containing kaolin, pectin, or bismuth are rarely helpful. Many patients are already receiving narcotics, which are the most effective antidiarrheal agents; the dose can be cautiously increased. If narcotics have not been prescribed, the drugs of choice are the meperidine congeners: diphenoxylate (Lomotil), and loperamide (Lomodium). These medications have minimal systemic effects at usual doses; higher doses can be tried with caution, but systemic effects can be anticipated. Lomotil contains small amounts of atropine, which may cause toxicity when dosage is increased. Problems from the combined use of narcotic analgesics and antidiarrheal meperidine congeners have not been reported but might be expected (e.g., agonist–partial agonist interactions and cross-tolerance).

Anticholinergic drugs (e.g., propantheline [Probanthine] 15 mg po 3–4 times daily) are occasionally useful for the "irritable bowel syndrome" and abdominal cramps, but may have troublesome side-effects (e.g., atonic bladder, dry mouth, drowsiness, and other central nervous system [CNS] disturbances). They can be tried for refractory diarrhea.

MANAGEMENT OF DIARRHEA

Diphenoxylate with atropine (Lomotil) 2.5 mg po 1–2 tabs q4h (initially up to 20 mg daily)
Loperamide (Lomodium) 2 mg po 1–2 tabs q4h (initially up to 16 mg daily)
Alternatives:
    Tincture of opium 0.5–1.0 ml po q4h
    Paregoric 4 ml po q4h
    Codeine 15–30 mg po q4h
    Morphine 5 mg po q4h

MANAGEMENT OF STEATORRHEA FROM PANCREATIC INSUFFICIENCY

Pancreatin or pancrealipase with meals and snacks
Medium-chain triglycerides
High-calorie diet rich in protein and carbohydrates
Oral replacement of fat-soluble vitamins; consider parenteral administration
Antacids or cimetidine to help prevent inactivation of enzymes by gastric acid
Standard antidiarrheal agents as needed

Steatorrhea from pancreatic insufficiency is managed with oral enzyme replacement and diet, whereas steatorrhea from diminished small bowel function (*e.g.*, secondary to resection or radiation) is managed by a dietary regimen alone (see Management of Steatorrhea from Pancreatic Insufficiency). Bile (choleretic) diarrhea, usually seen with small bowel resections of less than 100 cm, may respond to cholestyramine (12–16 g po daily, given with meals).

Secretory diarrhea of the Zollinger–Ellison syndrome has been palliated with cimetidine. The watery diarrhea syndrome and other diarrheal states with a presumably endocrine or paraneoplastic basis have responded to prednisone, indomethacin, lithium, and clonidine.[4,5]

FECAL INCONTINENCE[6]

Fecal incontinence, or soiling, requires prompt action. It is a common, often preventable cause for failure of home care.

The clinician first needs to determine the etiology of incontinence, reviewing the conditions discussed above under Constipation and Diarrhea, as well as the neurologic disorders reviewed in Section G under Urinary Incontinence. In the alert patient with normally formed bowel movements, a rectal examination will identify sphincteric disturbances and the majority of local conditions that cause fecal incontinence.

Second, a detailed review should be undertaken of general nursing measures to prevent incontinence and minimize its physical and psychosocial sequelae (see Table 2G-1 for an analogous approach to urinary incontinence). The distress of fecal incontinence can often be greatly ameliorated by control of the consistency and frequency of bowel movements, regular toileting, and the provision of appropriate protective devices. Feelings of shame and disgust may make this condition far more difficult for laypersons to manage than urinary incontinence. The treatment regimen often must be tailored to the personal tolerance of the patient and family, and outside help may be required.

INTESTINAL OBSTRUCTION

Intestinal obstruction is a common presenting symptom for cancers and is a frequent complication of advanced abdominal malignancies that have already received primary treatment, particularly metastatic colonic and ovarian cancers. In contrast to the acute abdominal emergencies that are common presentations for intestinal obstructions encountered in hospitals, blockage secondary to advanced cancer can be insidious in onset, intermittent, and not terribly debilitating. The standard treatments for bowel obstruction—"conservative management" (nasogastric suction and parenteral administration of fluid and electrolytes) or surgical repair (bypass and/or ostomy)— have an occasional role in far-advanced cancer, but simpler interventions, comfort measures or nontreatment are often appropriate and satisfactory.

Esophageal obstruction is discussed under Dysphagia in Section E. Mild obstruction below the esophagus is characterized by bouts of colicky abdominal pain and anorexia. Vigorous bowel contractions may be localized over the area of obstruction, accompanied by loud borborygmi or visible peristalsis. Abdominal distention and transient loose stools may ensue. These attacks will often resolve spontaneously. Patients may instinctively treat themselves by withholding food during the attack and by taking only fluids as the bout subsides. Mild analgesics or antispasmodics are rarely required. A vigorous bowel regimen to avoid hard stools is the only treatment regularly indicated at this stage; stool softeners such as dioctyl sulfosuccinate are preferred to cathartic agents, which may acutely increase painful peristalsis. A prolonged survival is not incompatible with intermittent partial obstruction.

More severe and prolonged obstruction may cause nausea and vomiting, hard stools, or a lack of bowel movements. In high intestinal obstruction, the onset of vomiting may signal the end of discomfort. Vomiting once or twice a day is often well tolerated by patients, and may be considered preferable to a nasogastric tube, restrictive diet, or surgery. Such patients may gladly eat favorite foods and enjoy large meals, even if vomiting regularly ensues. Adequate nutrition can often be maintained, since some fluid and food are absorbed, though hypokalemia may develop.

Antiemetics are often ineffective for intestinal obstruction, but metoclopramide, antihistamines, and other standard agents can be tried (see Section A). In severe lower obstruction, stool softeners are the mainstays of treatment. Steroids may be tried for both high and low obstruction.

Some patients, especially those with severe lower obstruction, will receive prompt and satisfying relief from nasogastric suction. While the necessary equipment can be provided in the home, the monitoring of this treatment and the parenteral replacement of fluid and electrolytes are difficult to manage outside an institution.

Radiation therapy is occasionally indicated for localized high obstruction. Surgery has a role in severe blockage throughout the GI tract (e.g., stents or dilation to relieve esophageal obstruction, and bypass or removal of obstructed bowel), especially when obstruction is the major manifestation of a metastatic cancer.

When intestinal obstruction causes severe symptoms in the terminal phase of cancer, particularly in those patients who are not candidates for the above measures, or who are eager to remain at home or to avoid intravenous lines and nasogastric tubes, the condition can be comfortably managed with medication. The usual analgesics and antiemetics should be employed, although the latter are rarely effective. Narcotics worsen any associated constipation and will usually only blunt severe, crampy abdominal pain unless given in doses high enough to cause moderate sedation. Thus, narcotics should be avoided in mild recurrent attacks, whereas they are used vigorously for severe and terminal obstruction. Diphenoxylate (Lomotil) is a favorite additional drug for crampy abdominal pain, while antispasmodics can also be tried, as described above under Diarrhea. When medication cannot be given orally, injections or rectal suppositories are indicated.

JAUNDICE AND HEPATIC ENCEPHALOPATHY

Two concomitants of biliary obstruction and hepatic failure—pruritus and hepatic encephalopathy—deserve attention even late in the course of a terminal illness. Pruritus is discussed in Section H of this chapter.

The appearance of jaundice is usually alarming to the patient and family. It may indeed signal a serious complication of advanced cancer, and herald the onset of new, troubling symptoms and a phase of rapid deterioration. On the other hand, some deeply jaundiced patients will enjoy prolonged survival, experiencing minimal or manageable distress from pruritus, drowsiness, anorexia, weakness, and so on. The natural course of various forms of jaundice in advanced cancer and the value of major therapeutic interventions have not been well studied.

Patients who would seem to benefit from interruption of the natural course of extrahepatic biliary obstruction (usually caused by carcinoma of the pancreas, biliary

---

MANAGEMENT OF HEPATIC ENCEPHALOPATHY

Attention to precipitating factors:
  GI hemorrhage, other protein loads
  Metabolic disorders—hypokalemia, alkalosis, uremia
  Constipation
  Infection
  Drugs—especially narcotics, sedative–hypnotics*
  Alcohol
  Dehydration
Dietary protein restriction
Multivitamins—in prolonged hepatic failure, consider parenteral administration of fat-soluble
    vitamins
Lactulose 1–4 tbsp (10–40 g) po 3–4 times daily beginning with 2 tbsp po tid; increase dose
    every 3–6 days until clinical improvement occurs or diarrhea becomes troublesome; antic-
    ipate 2–3 soft stools daily when appropriate dose achieved
  Lactulose enema 300 ml of 50% lactulose in 700 ml tap water
Neomycin 0.5–1.5 g po qid
  Neomycin 1–2 g in 100–200 ml NS pr 2–3 times daily as retention enema
Adjust doses of drugs metabolized by the liver

  *Drugs associated with intrahepatic cholestasis (e.g., phenothiazines) can generally be
used without concern for long-term toxicity.

---

tree, or periampullary area or by metastases to the porta hepatis) may undergo trans-cutaneous stent insertion for internal or external biliary drainage.[2] These procedures are regularly successful, although there are a significant number of complications—bile leak, pain, bleeding, fever, and sepsis. Also, drainage tubes frequently dislodge or become blocked, requiring replacement. Alternatively, peroral endoscopic sphincter-otomy or placement of a biliary drain or stent may be attempted. Radiation therapy can also be considered for both extrahepatic and intrahepatic obstruction.

Hepatic encephalopathy produces weakness, fatigue, and lethargy, proceeding to drowsiness, stupor, and a peaceful death. The major manifestations of hepatic failure can be ameliorated by reducing the accumulation of those products of intestinal pro-tein breakdown which the damaged liver is not able to adequately remove from the circulation (see Management of Hepatic Encephalopathy).

SELECTED REFERENCES

1. Davis GR, Santa Ana CA, Morawski SG, Fordtran JS: Development of a lavage solution asso-ciated with minimal water and electrolyte absorption or secretion. Gastroenterology 78:991–995, 1980
2. Kozarek RA, Sanowski RA: Nonsurgical management of extrahepatic obstructive jaundice. Ann Intern Med 96(part 1):743–745, 1982
3. Kreek MJ, Schaeffer RA, Hahn FEF, Fishman J: Naloxone, a specific opioid antagonist, reverses chronic idiopathic constipation. Lancet 1:261–262, 1983
4. McArthur KE, Anderson DS, Durbin TE, Orloff MJ, Dharmsathaporn K: Clonidine and lida-mine to inhibit watery diarrhea in a patient with lung cancer. Ann Intern Med 96:323–325, 1982
5. Pandol SJ, Korman LY, McCartny DM, Gardner JD: Beneficial effect of oral lithium carbonate in the treatment of pancreatic cholera syndrome. N Engl J Med 302:1403–1404, 1980
6. Smith RG: Fecal incontinence. J Am Geriatr Soc 31:694–697, 1983

E.   Mouth Problems and Dysphagia

MOUTH CARE

The physician who begins to pay careful attention to dryness or soreness of the mouth may be surprised by the frequency of such complaints in terminally ill patients. Sim-ple treatment can produce gratifying relief, often allowing a patient to eat or feel com-fortable again.[4] For the dehydrated patient, easily managed local measures for improv-ing a dry mouth may be preferable to such cumbersome and disagreeable methods as nasogastric tube-feedings or an intravenous line.

General mouth care may include the following measures:

Careful attention to oral hygiene, especially if the patient is neglecting self-care for any prolonged period. Brush and floss the teeth frequently or use gentler, nonabrasive "Toothettes" to remove debris.

Use a cleansing mouthwash (*e.g.,* sodium bicarbonate in water or one part fresh hydrogen peroxide added to equal parts of a favorite mouthwash and normal saline or water). Beware that many commercial mouthwashes contain alcohol which may irritate or dry out the oral cavity. Carbamide peroxide is available commercially as an 11% gel (Proxigel) or 10% solution (*e.g.*, Gly-Oxide) and acts to debride and soothe the mouth, as well as to provide weak antibacterial action.

Check the comfort and fitting of dentures, and remove them at night. Check for sores.

XEROSTOMIA

The evaluation and treatment of xerostomia is summarized in Tables 2E-1 and 2E-2.

Glycerin swabs are commonly used for dry mouth, but they provide very brief relief. Also, some experienced nurses believe these swabs promote drying and moniliasis.

STOMATITIS

The pathophysiology of stomatitis is outlined in Table 2E-3. General measures are noted in Table 2E-4. Topical pastes, anesthetics, and other agents may be useful for a variety of oral sores (see Table 2E-4). When applied before meals, these substances may allow comfortable feeding.

Specific Conditions

Monilia

Oral nystatin suspension (100,000 units/ml) is the drug of choice. Two to 3 ml is applied to each side of the mouth, then swallowed, four times a day. Higher doses (6 ml [600,000 units] qid) are occasionally required. Vaginal suppositories (Nystatin 100,000 units) have been used orally when swishing of the suspension is difficult. Treatment should be continued for 7 to 14 days or at least until a few days after signs of the infection resolve. Prophylactic or continuous treatment is occasionally indi-

---

TABLE 2E-1
Etiology of Xerostomia

Drugs, especially:
  Anticholinergics
  Phenothiazines
  Antihistamines
  Tricyclic antidepressants
  Opiates
Mouth-breathing
Dehydration, hypovolemia
Local radiotherapy
Connective tissue disease (Sjogren's syndrome)
Disorders of the salivary glands, including xerostomia of aging

---

TABLE 2E-2
Management of Xerostomia

Frequent lubrication	Small sips of liquids
	Regular chewing of ice chips
	Popsicles, ice cream, fruitades, sugarless drinks
	Irrigation with bulb syringe
Moisturizing agent	Mineral oil, preferably cold and flavored with lemon juice; beware aspiration
	Saliva substitutes by applicator or spray
Stimulate saliva	Sour or bitter cough drops
	Sugarless candy
	Sugarless chewing gum
Gentle cleansing	$\frac{1}{2}$ tsp baking soda and 1 tsp hydrogen peroxide in a glass of water
Dietary measures	Avoid dry foods, bread, meat, nuts; moisten foods and add sauces, butter, syrup, salad dressing, gravy
	Soften foods (puree) and avoid crisp food
	Avoid sweet foods, sugar
	Beware of tart, acidic, and spicy food
	Avoid extremes of temperature; cold food often preferred
	Avoid alcohol and tobacco
Other remedies	Pineapple chunks (soothing, lubricating)
	Melon
	Bethanecol (Urecholine) 10–20 mg po 3–4 times daily (or neostigmine, pyridostigmine)—stimulate salivation and counteract anticholinergic agents
	Spray bottle to administer liquids

TABLE 2E-3
Etiology of Stomatitis

Infection
   Monilia (secondary to diabetes, esophageal motor disorder, antibiotics, steroids, immunosuppression)
   Aphthous ulcers
   Herpes
Poor dental hygiene
   Improperly fitting dentures
   Caries, gingivitis
Avitaminosis (often presents with cheilosis [angular stomatitis] and sore tongue)
Blood dyscrasias
Drugs
   Methotrexate, other cytotoxic agents
   Aspirin
Radiation therapy

TABLE 2E-4
Topical Agents for Stomatitis

Local anesthetics
  Dyclonine (Dyclone) 1% gel or 0.5% and 1% solution—1–2 drops of the gel can be applied
    to oral sores every 2–4 h
  Xylocaine (Lidocaine) viscous 2% 15 ml po q3h prn, up to 8 doses a day, swish and swallow
    for brief pain relief (*e.g.,* before meals)
Milk of magnesia—beware of drying
Antacids—beware of drying; may be mixed with topical anesthetics
Kaopectate and diphenhydramine (Benadryl) elixir in equal parts; 15 ml po, swish and spit out
    before meals—beware of crusting
Honey
Corn syrup

cated when infections recur regularly; lower doses (*e.g.,* Nystatin 200,000 units bid) may be sufficient.

Clotrimazole (Mycelex) troches 10 mg four to five times a day have been effective experimentally in treating oral candidiasis and have recently become commercially available.

Ketoconazole (Nizoral) 200 mg po, used only once or twice a day, has been effective in chronic mucocutaneous candidiasis.[1] While it is not approved for routine oral candidiasis, some patients may find ketoconazole treatment more acceptable than the above measures.

Aphthous Ulcers

In addition to the topical agents listed in Table 2E-4, consider hydrocortisone lozenges 2.5 mg po four times a day.

OTHER ORAL PROBLEMS

Necrotic oral tumors and *osteonecrotic bone* should be cleansed regularly with hydrogen peroxide or diluted sodium hypochloride (modified Dakin's) solution.

Bad tastes may respond to pineapple chunks or strong flavorings in food (*e.g.,* peppermint) or candies (*e.g.,* sourballs).

Thick secretions may be loosened with meat tenderizer or papase.

Drooling may cause perioral irritation. Aluminum pastes protect the skin. Anticholinergic drugs (tincture of belladonna, atropine, or propantheline) can be used to reduce secretions.

DYSPHAGIA

The common causes of dysphagia are reviewed in Table 2E-5.

Repeated esophageal dilatation or intubation under fluoroscopic or fiberoptic endoscopic guidance is now possible for many patients with malignant or postradiation strictures and tracheoesophageal fistulas.[2,3]

TABLE 2E-5
Etiology of Dysphagia

Stomatitis
Xerostomia
Esophageal candidiasis
Neuromuscular dysfunction
    Local surgery, radiation
    Local nerve compression from tumor or nodes
    Cerebral metastases; meningeal carcinomatosis
Mechanical obstruction
    Intrinsic
        Local tumor
        Stricture
    Extrinsic
        Local tumor, nodes
Mucositis
Psychogenic

General measures consist primarily of dietary manipulation (usually a liquid or soft diet). Patients with obstruction or neuromuscular dysfunction should sit upright as they eat. Topical anesthetic agents, when swallowed, may relieve esophageal pain, as may antacids.

SELECTED REFERENCES

1. Anonymous: Ketoconazole (Nizoral): A new antifungal agent. Med Lett Drugs Ther 23:85–87, 1981
2. Atkinson M, Ferguson R: Fiberoptic endoscopic palliative intubation of inoperable oesophagogastric neoplasms. Br Med J 1:266–267, 1977
3. Boyce HW Jr: Approach to management of cancer of the esophagus. Hosp Pract 17:109–124, 1982
4. Castigliano SG: Oral care of the dying patient. In Kutscher AH, Schoenberg B, Carr AC (eds): The Terminal Patient. New York, Columbia University Press, 1973

F. Dyspnea, Cough, and Other Respiratory Symptoms

DYSPNEA

Pathophysiology

Dyspnea is an uncomfortable awareness of breathing, a sensation similar to pain. It serves as a stimulus for relieving respiratory insufficiency: getting fresh air, clearing the airway, removing constrictive clothing, or breathing rapidly and deeply. As in managing chronic cancer pain, the symptom should be viewed first as a warning of disease, a call to investigate and treat the underlying medical condition. Second, dyspnea is a discomfort that can be relieved regardless of its pathophysiologic basis.

Respiratory failure, particularly pneumonia, is a frequent cause of death among cancer patients, and dyspnea may also occur with a variety of other terminal conditions (*e.g.,* sepsis, cardiac failure, severe anemia, and hypovolemic shock). Some common diagnostic considerations in evaluating dyspnea are noted in Table 2F-1. The symptom is often multifactorial. For example, a lung cancer patient with chronic obstructive pulmonary disease undergoes a pneumonectomy, develops radiation fibrosis while being treated for recurrent tumor, then presents with a respiratory tract infection complicated by cachexia and muscle weakness, diminished alertness, and suppressed cough.

The symptom, dyspnea, should not be confused with physical signs such as tachypnea or hyperpnea. Fast or deep breathing, for example, as occurs during exercise, is not necessarily disagreeable. Patients with acidosis or high fever may develop tachypnea without air hunger or prominent symptoms of respiratory distress. Some comatose patients develop periods of tachypnea, but there is no reason to believe that they suffer dyspnea.

Similarly, dyspnea does not imply hypoxia or hypercarbia, nor does the perception of breathlessness have a simple correlation with airway obstruction or other measures of lung volumes or mechanics.[2] A number of conditions may produce prominent respiratory symptoms with little effect on gas exchange (*e.g.,* mechanical impairment of ventilation from a tight bandage across the chest, mild airway obstruction, small

---

TABLE 2F-1
Common Etiologies of Dyspnea in Terminal Illness

MUSCULOSKELETAL
    Chest wall weakness or impaired movement
    Diaphragmatic paralysis or impairment

PULMONARY
    Airway obstruction
        Bronchospasm, chronic obstructive pulmonary disease
        Tumor
    Lymphangitic spread of tumor
    Infection, including opportunistic infections
    Loss of functioning lung tissue from surgical resection, replacement by tumor, fibrosis
        (postirradiation, secondary to chemotherapy)
    Pleural effusion or scarring
    Pneumothorax

CARDIAC
    Pericardial effusion or tamponade
    Congestive heart failure (CHF)

VASCULAR
    Pulmonary embolus
    Superior vena cava syndrome

EXTRATHORACIC
    Anemia
    Central (neurogenic), including anxiety

pleural effusions, small intrathoracic tumors, and postsurgical or postirradiation scarring). Improvement in respiratory muscle performance (*e.g.*, from removal of a large pleural effusion) may have a profound effect on dyspnea without much change in gas exchange, lung volumes, or pulmonary mechanics (see Pleural Effusion in Section I).

Anxiety is so regularly a concomitant of dyspnea that it deserves special mention here. The patient may wonder:

Will I suddenly choke?

If I go to sleep, will I just stop breathing and die, or maybe wake up choking to death?

The family and other caretakers may similarly fear that the patient will suffocate or suddenly stop breathing or that the breathlessness will become insufferable. Successful home care for severely dyspneic patients requires that anxiety be kept at a manageable level and that panic be avoided. If calm, assured attention is not available to seriously dyspneic patients in the home, institutional care is usually preferable.

Management

The treatments for specific causes of dypsnea such as anemia, congestive heart failure (CHF), bronchospasm, or respiratory infections are not reviewed here. The general measures and nonspecific pharmacologic treatments for dyspnea are listed in Tables 2F-2 and 2F-3.

When specific etiologic treatment for dyspnea is ineffective or unavailable, *opiates* are excellent palliative agents for respiratory distress. The mechanism of

---

TABLE 2F-2
General Measures for Dyspnea

Reduce need for exertion
    "Compact care" (see Chap. 4)
    Ready availability of help
Positioning
    Pillows, adjustable beds and chairs
Improve air circulation
    Fans, open windows
Adjust humidity
    Steam kettle or humidifier for dry airway or thick secretions
Chest physical therapy
    Deep breathing, coughing
    Postural drainage
    Percussion and vibration
    Suctioning
Treat anxiety, give reassurance
    Sit with patient
    Educate on significance of symptoms
    Review and rehearse plans for exacerbated symptoms
    Identify situational and psychological components
    Relaxation techniques

TABLE 2F-3
Pharmacologic Treatment for Dyspnea

Drug Class	Agent and Dosage
Expectorants	Glycerol guaiacolate 5 ml po q4h
Mucolytic agents	Acetylcysteine (Mucomyst) 10% 2–20 ml 3–4 times a day *via* nebulizer
Narcotics	Codeine 30 mg po q3–4h
	Morphine sulfate
	5–10 mg po q4h
	2–5 mg SC or IV q4h
	(increase prn)
Sedatives	Diazepam (Valium) 2–10 mg po, IM, IV, prn
	Promethazine (Phenergan) 25–50 mg po q4–6h prn
	Chlorpromazine (Thorazine) 25–100 mg po q4–6h prn
Steroids	Prednisone 10–15 mg po tid
	Dexamethasone 1–4 mg po qid
Antimuscarinic agents (for excess secretions)	Atropine 0.4–1.0 mg po or SC q4–12h
Oxygen	

action of these drugs in reducing breathlessness is unclear. Opiates may alter the central perception of breathlessness, reduce ventilatory drive, or reduce oxygen consumption. Studies of patients with chronic lung disease suggest that acute improvement in both breathlessness and exercise tolerance may be anticipated from opiates without deterioration of blood gases.[5] Long-term studies of such treatment are not available, although a brief report on the use of dihydrocodeine over 2 weeks suggested some value of 30 mg po tid, but not of 60 mg po tid, and noted troublesome extrapulmonary side-effects from the drug but no significant respiratory compromise.[7]

The common injunction to avoid narcotics and sedatives in patients with asthma or respiratory failure (except when morphine is used for CHF) should be reconsidered within the context of terminal illness. Dyspnea can often be improved with low doses of narcotics, yet significant respiratory depression or sedation does not regularly occur with the doses required to produce satisfactory symptom relief. Moreover, in the unusual situation when carefully titrated narcotic doses lead to significant respiratory depression and to a possible hastening of the patient's demise, the urgency of relieving suffering often assumes precedence over the goal of prolonging life. Proper use of narcotics to ensure patient comfort should not be subverted by medicolegal preoccupations or by reaction to instances of careless or unethical administration of these drugs.

Sedatives are also used for breathlessness. Insofar as can be judged from observing sedative overdoses, barbiturates and alcohol are more potent respiratory depressants than benzodiazepines. Reliable clinical studies comparing the chronic respiratory effects of various sedatives with those of narcotics are lacking. For patients with moderately severe chronic lung disease, alcohol appears to be inferior to a mild narcotic in relieving dyspnea.[5] In one study of "pink puffers," 125 mg daily of promethazine, an antihistamine–phenothiazine, was effective in reducing dyspnea, while 25 mg of diazepam neither reduced breathlessness nor improved exercise tolerance, although it frequently caused drowsiness.[6] In a smaller study of severely disabled "pink puffers," diazepam 25 mg four times a day improved breathlessness and exercise tolerance without affecting blood gases.[4] In clinical practice, acutely dyspneic, terminally ill patients are more commonly treated with benzodiazepines than with sedating antihistamines or phenothiazines.

Glucocorticoids may be useful for improving chronic dyspnea in patients with bronchospasm or malignant involvement of the lung. The usefulness of steroids in asthma is well accepted; their role in patients with lymphangitic spread of tumor or with intrapulmonary metastases is not well-documented, but is supported by frequent anecdotes. Laryngeal stricture and the superior vena cava syndrome may also respond to steroids.

Oxygen therapy is often prescribed routinely for dyspneic patients. Chronic oxygen use cannot be justified in the absence of hypoxia or of a convincing symptomatic response to treatment. Oxygen should be prescribed at the lowest effective dose and should be administered through nasal prongs or a light, comfortable, plastic face mask. A nebulizer or humidifier attached to the delivery system will prevent drying of the respiratory tract. When indicated, oxygen therapy can be readily provided at home. The hazard of fire or explosion is small, but smoking and the use of flammable substances should be forbidden in the patient's room, and electrical outlets should be examined for defects.

Chest physical therapy in the last days of life can cause discomfort, exhaustion, and increased worry without improved well-being. It should be prescribed selectively.

COUGH[3]

Pathophysiology

The cough reflex, an explosive expiration, is generally incited by irritative phenomena within the respiratory tract (*e.g.,* infection, inflammation, tumor, and other foreign matter or toxic substances). Both lower and upper respiratory tract lesions may produce cough, as may extrinsic lesions impinging on the airway (*e.g.,* thoracic nodes or tumors of structures within the chest wall).

Cough, like pain, is a valuable warning signal of tissue irritation, and the cough reflex serves a useful purpose, forcefully expelling foreign material and secretions from the respiratory tract. The complications of a persistent cough, however, include new pain (in the chest or abdominal wall or respiratory tract), aggravation of existing pain, rib fractures, tussive syncope, headache, exhaustion, insomnia, anorexia, and vomiting. When cough develops, an appropriate evaluation of the symptom should be initiated, and insofar as possible, treatment should be aimed at the underlying cause. When the symptom is not helping clear the respiratory tract or when its benefits are outweighed by the aggravation and discomfort of recurrent coughing, antitussive medication should be prescribed.

Management

Treatment of cough ranges from highly specific and effective measures aimed at the irritative phenomena (*e.g.,* radiation to the tumor or nodes, antibiotics for infection) to a host of nonspecific measures, some of unproved or doubtful efficacy (Tables 2F-4 and 2F-5).

TABLE 2F-4
Management of Cough Due to Specific Diagnoses

Pathophysiology	*Treatment*
Tumor	Radiation, chemotherapy, surgery, steroids
Infection	Antibiotics
	Treat obstructive tumor
Bronchospasm	Treat irritation, infection
	Bronchodilators
	Adrenergic agents
	Theophylline
	Glucocorticoids
Aspiration (secondary to vomiting, tracheoesophageal fistula, difficulties with swallowing, and/or suppression of cough and gag reflexes)	Dietary manipulation
	Tube-feeding
	Antibiotics
	Steroids
CHF	Diuretics
	Cardiac glycosides
Pleural effusions	See Section I (Fluid Accumulation)

TABLE 2F-5
Nonspecific Cough Treatments

Loosen a moist cough	Hydration
	Humidity
	Pulmonary toilet, drainage, physical therapy
	Iodides (as expectorants)*
	Mucolytic agents (acetylcysteine)*
Dry up a cough	Sympathomimetic decongestants
	Antihistamines
	Atropinic agents
Soothe throat and upper airways	Reduce environmental irritants, especially smoke
	Cough syrups† ± ethanol
	Terpin hydrate
	Glyceryl guaiacolate
	Cough drops
	Local anesthetics (e.g., Lidocaine viscous)
Suppress cough	Increase dose of current narcotic drug
	Or begin dextromorphan 15–30 mg po q4h
	or Codeine 15–30 mg po q4h and increase dose prn
	or Morphine 5–10 mg po q4h and increase dose prn
	Benzonate (Tessalon) 100 mg po q4–6h
Sedate‡	Benzodiazepines, phenothiazines, alcohol

*Probably efficacious but difficult to use
†Questionable efficacy, probably harmless
‡Unclear value, worth consideration

The prescription of antibiotics for cough, sputum production, or pneumonia in the terminally ill deserves careful consideration. For the patient who has evidence of a bacterial respiratory tract infection, and who can appreciate a prolonged survival, a course of antibiotics can improve comfort and the quality of life. When the patient is moribund, cough suppressants and antipyretics may be appropriate treatment, and antibiotics may be withheld.

Inhibition of the cough reflex can occasionally be achieved with topical anesthetics, especially when an upper airway lesion is causing irritation. In general, however, cough suppression requires the use of centrally acting narcotic drugs or narcotic analogues. Careful research on the use of narcotics for chronic cough suggests that the drugs do not reduce the objective signs (frequency and productivity) of coughing, but rather alleviate the distress associated with the symptom, improving the subjective evaluation of the severity of the cough.[1] Opiates seem to be effective cough suppressants in lower doses than those required for pain relief, although commonly prescribed doses of codeine (12–15 mg po q4–6h) may be subtherapeutic. Presumably, patients who have developed tolerance to opiates may require higher doses for effective cough suppression. When the patient's drug regimen already includes an opiate in doses appropriate for analgesia, the prescription of a narcotic cough syrup (e.g., terpin hydrate with codeine or guaifenesin with hydrocodone) is unreasonable. Moreover, the effect of the interaction of the two opiates is unpredictable. Instead, such patients should try slightly higher doses of their previously prescribed narcotic. If a cough syrup is desirable, either for psychological reasons (e.g., a favorable association in the mind of the patient or family) or for possible therapeutic effect (which has little experimental justification), nonopiate syrups may be prescribed concurrently, or the previously prescribed narcotic may be compounded with such a syrup.

Antitussive medication is often required only at bedtime or on a prn basis. When narcotic analgesics are already being used, a higher dose may be prescribed at bedtime and prn cough.

The common practice of adding an H_1-blocking agent, usually the phenothiazine, promethazine (Phenergan), to a narcotic agent for the purpose of cough suppression probably derives from the use of this combination for the common cold. Antihistamines may be helpful for allergic upper respiratory tract symptoms or as sedatives. Their usefulness for other causes of cough is not documented. They tend to cause drying of the bronchial secretions, an effect that may be desirable or that may make expectoration difficult.

Benzonate (Tessalon), a nonnarcotic drug related to procaine, may have central (CNS) and peripheral (pulmonary) antitussive effects, and can be added to a narcotic regimen.

"DEATH RATTLE"

In the final days or hours before death, certain patients who are semicomatose or who have an ineffective or suppressed cough will develop noisy or gurgling respiration from pooled pharyngeal or pulmonary secretions. Treatment for this "death rattle" may improve the family's comfort. Positioning the patient on his or her side may be sufficient treatment.

Antimuscarinic drugs, usually given parenterally in low doses, will decrease secretions in the nose, mouth, pharynx, and bronchi and produce relaxation of bronchial smooth muscle:

Atropine 0.4–1.0 mg po, SC q4–12h
Scopolamine 0.6–0.4 mg po, SC q4–12h

Transderm Scōp, a preparation of scopolamine that is absorbed through the skin, is marketed for motion sickness but may have some usefulness in drying secretions.

HEMOPTYSIS

Mild hemoptysis is common with many of the conditions that produce cough or dyspnea. For the average terminally ill patient who coughs up small amounts of dark blood, hemoptysis usually remains mild and resolves spontaneously or recurs infrequently. Treatment includes measures directed at the underlying condition (*e.g.*, radiation to the tumor, antibiotics for infection).

More severe, sudden bleeding occurs occasionally among patients with tumors in the respiratory tract or pharynx or with coagulopathies. Exsanguination is a dreaded complication of cancer, although death follows quickly and painlessly. Significant hemoptysis or the prospect of exsanguination may be very difficult for the patient and family to manage at home. Vigorous sedation may be considered for frank bleeding.

SELECTED REFERENCES

1. Beecher HK: Measurement of Subjective Responses. New York, Oxford University Press, 1959
2. Burdon JGW, Juniper EF, Killian KJ, Hargreave FE, Campbell EJM: Perception of breathlessness in asthma. Am Rev Respir Dis 126:825–828, 1982
3. Irwin RS, Rosen MJ, Braman SS: Cough, a comprehensive review. Arch Intern Med 137:1186–1191, 1977
4. Mitchell-Heggs P, Murphy K, Minty K, Guz A, Patterson SC, Minty PSB, Rosser RM: Diazepam in the treatment of dyspnea in the "pink puffer" syndrome. Q J Med 49:9–20, 1980
5. Woodcock AA, Gross ER, Gellert A, Shah S, Johnson M, Geddes DM: Effects of dihydrocodeine, alcohol, and caffeine on breathlessness and exercise tolerance in patients with chronic obstructive lung disease and normal blood gases. N Engl J Med 305:1611–1616, 1981
6. Woodcock AA, Gross ER, Geddes DM: Drug treatment of breathlessness: Contrasting effects of diazepam and promethazine in pink puffers. Br Med J 283:343–346, 1981
7. Woodcock AA, Johnson MA, Geddes DM: Breathlessness, alcohol, and opiates (letter). N Engl J Med 306:1363–1364, 1982

G.   Urinary Tract Symptoms

Many of the conditions causing painful, difficult, or frequent urination in the advanced cancer patient are familiar to the general physician and are not reviewed here. This section focuses on urinary incontinence, a topic that touches on all the common problems of voiding, and concludes by describing an approach to renal failure and urinary tract obstruction in advanced cancer.

Two urinary symptoms deserve brief mention. First, polyuria—a symptom associated with hyperglycemia, hypercalcemia, diabetes insipidus, fluid loads, and diuretics—is mentioned as a reminder that an increased urinary output may occasionally provoke incontinence or be confused with dysuria. Second, hematuria caused by neoplastic involvement of the urinary tract often requires no treatment or can be managed with occasional transfusions. However, drainage and irrigation may prevent obstruction from blood clots. Additionally, lower tract bleeding may be controlled by fulguration and other local measures performed through the cystoscope and, occasionally, by radiation, while troublesome renal hemorrhage may occasionally be palliated by arterial embolization.[3]

INCONTINENCE AND RELATED VOIDING PROBLEMS

Incontinence can be a terribly embarrassing symptom, and patients occasionally conceal or minimize this complaint unless questioned carefully and sympathetically:

> *Does urine ever come unexpectedly without your being able to stop it?*
>
> *Do you ever lose your urine or wet yourself?*

The pungent odor of urine-soaked clothes and bedding may be intolerable to patients or persons near them. Ongoing incontinence may produce serious irritation of the skin, perineal mucosa, and nearby wounds.

Four pathophysiologic categories of voiding problems and urinary incontinence are described below.[6-8] In clinical practice, patients can usually be assigned to one of these categories or subcategories on the basis of the history and physical examination, the analysis and culture of a clean-voided urine specimen, and, at times, the measurement of postvoid residual. The history should include an assessment of previous voiding patterns, especially of prior obstructive symptoms, stress incontinence, infections, and catheterization. Physical examination can detect bladder distension, impaction, and sphincter dysfunction. A chart of voidings or incontinence (noting the presence of wet clothes or sheets every 2 hours) may be useful. Urodynamic studies and other diagnostic procedures are often impractical and unnecessary.

Regardless of the etiology of incontinence, a number of general treatment measures, described in Table 2G-1, can be employed.

Causes of Incontinence

Overflow Incontinence

Overflow incontinence results from bladder outlet obstruction (*e.g.*, from local tumor or its treatment) or from detrusor failure. The latter condition—a loss of normal bladder contractility—typically occurs when the autonomic reflex arc is affected by anticholinergic drugs (tricyclic antidepressants, phenothiazines, and the agents used for detrusor instability) or when afferent spinal innervation is disrupted by pelvic surgery, tumor, or neuropathy. Suprapubic discomfort, urgency, and a feeling of inability to void are common symptoms. Urination may occur frequently and in small volumes and may be uncontrollable. The bladder may be palpable or percussable. The postvoid residual is large, and massive retention may ensue. Because rapid decompression of a severely distended bladder may be associated with intravesical bleeding, a common practice is to remove urine in 500-ml aliquots no more often than once an hour. Also, a postobstructive diuresis should be anticipated.

TABLE 2G-1
General Measures for Urinary Incontinence

1. Reduce delays in getting to the bathroom. Assess mobility, particularly the patient's ability to get to the toilet. Improve the responsiveness of persons who assist the patient in voiding. Consider use of a bedside commode, bedpan, or urinal, especially when assistance is not readily available.

2. Avoid fluid loads. For nocturnal incontinence, restrict fluids after the evening meal. Eliminate diuretics and dietary ingredients (such as coffee, tea, and alcohol) that aggravate incontinence. Consider evaluation for polyuric states.

3. Avoid medications that diminish alertness.

4. For patients who can cooperate, consider establishing a voiding regimen. For instance, if the incontinence chart indicates uncontrolled voiding at intervals of 2 hours or longer, prompt the patient to urinate regularly every 2 hours.

5. Male patients may use condom drainage or, rarely, penile clamps. If the voiding problem is intermittent (*e.g.*, nocturnal or only while ambulatory), these measures may be better tolerated if used only during periods either of high risk for incontinence or of low tolerance by the patient or family for wetting.

6. Consider incontinence sheets, pads, and pants; waterproof sheets and mattress protectors; and extra help for laundry and changing clothes. These measures can usually provide satisfactory control of skin irritation and urine odor.

7. Institute measures for perineal skin care (Section H, Skin Problems).

8. Intermittent or indwelling catherization should be considered to relieve pain, to prevent severe bladder distention or local tissue irritation, and to manage persistent incontinence that is personally or socially unacceptable. Chronic indwelling catheters, however, may be uncomfortable and occasionally cause serious, even fatal, complications.

9. In rare patients with prolonged anticipated survival and troublesome incontinence, especially those who have difficulty retaining or tolerating an indwelling catheter, consider a suprapubic cystostomy or an ileal loop ostomy.

MANAGEMENT OF OVERFLOW INCONTINENCE

Some patients merely need to be encouraged to void every 2–4 hours. Perineal or lower abdominal stimulation (Credé maneuver) may be helpful.

Stop or decrease anticholinergic drugs.

Intravesical pressure can be raised by muscarinic drugs that stimulate the detrusor. These drugs are generally not employed when bladder outlet obstruction is present. They are relatively ineffective and potentially quite toxic:

Bethanecol (Urecholine, Myotonachol) 10–50 mg po 3–4 times a day beginning with low doses and increasing gradually

---

Stress Incontinence

Stress incontinence (or low-pressure incontinence) occurs when bladder outlet resistance is low. Usual causes are pelvic relaxation and incompetence of the bladder sphincter resulting from tumor, local inflammation, and the complications of pelvic surgery and radiation. Voiding may occur without adequate warning when the patient coughs, laughs, or sneezes, or the patient may intermittently be unable to hold urine while attempting to reach the bathroom. Urine volumes are low or normal, and the postvoid residual is small.

MANAGEMENT OF STRESS INCONTINENCE

Program of regular voiding—void before leaving house.
Kegel exercises to strengthen pelvic musculature.
Women with pelvic relaxation may benefit from a pessary.
Men may use a penile clamp.
Alpha-adrenergic agents increase bladder outlet resistance:
    Ephedrine 25 mg po tid
    Phenylpropanolamine (Propadrine) 25 mg po 3–4 times a day—usually prescribed in combination with an antihistamine as Ornade SA bid
Tricyclic antidepressants also have alpha-adrenergic action:
    Imipramine 10–150 mg po qd—often effective in low doses (25–75 mg po qd)

Detrusor Instability

Detrusor instability (also called reflex, uninhibited, or urge incontinence) occurs in the following situations:

The bladder is irritated (e.g., from infection, radiation, chemotherapy, stones, or local tumor), or the voiding reflexes are otherwise impaired (e.g., from urethritis, urethral strictures, or local tumor)

A neurogenic (or spastic) bladder has resulted from loss of normal spinal cord inhibition of voiding (e.g., from a spinal cord lesion or from the loss of input from higher centers, as in dementia)

Patients with intact spinal cords—the first subcategory above—note an urgent (and sometime frequent) need to void and may be incontinent whenever a commode is not readily available. Dysuria may be prominent. Fecal impaction is a common, readily reversible cause of this form of incontinence. Patients with a reflex neuropathic bladder, on the other hand, do not experience urgency or an awareness of voiding. Cord compression (as discussed in Section L, Weakness and Fatigue) is one cause of urinary incontinence that may require emergency treatment. In both subcategories, the postvoid residual is small.

MANAGEMENT OF DETRUSOR INSTABILITY

Treat infections and irritants.

Local anesthetics suppress irritative phenomena:
    Pyridium 100–200 mg po tid

Anticholinergic drugs and smooth muscle relaxants may allow the bladder to hold larger amounts of urine before contracting. These drugs inhibit the detrusor, reduce intravesical pressure, and decrease bladder contractility. Since side-effects are common, dosage should be increased gradually:

Propantheline bromide (Probanthine) 7.5–30 mg po 3–4 times a day
Oxybutynin (Ditropan) 5 mg po 2–4 times a day

Tricyclic antidepressants have anticholinergic effects as well as an alpha-adrenergic action, which helps control the sphincter:
Imipramine 10–150 mg po qd—often effective in low doses (25–75 mg po qd)

Incompletely studied but potentially useful approaches include beta-adrenergic inhibition with baclofen or hydramtrazine and the use of calcium channel blockers such as nifedipine.

Uninhibited incontinence is often amenable to therapy without a catheter. Neurogenic bladders may be incited to contract by regularly scheduled perineal or lower abdominal stimulation (Credé maneuvers). Anticholinergic agents may still be prescribed to control frequency.

Continuous Incontinence

Continuous incontinence is characterized by regular dribbling of urine through a fistula (ureterovaginal or vesicovaginal) that has developed as a complication of surgery, radiation, or tumor. Incontinence pads are the major modality of treatment, sometimes aided by placement of an indwelling catheter or by urinary-diversion procedures. Dressings are described in Section H, Skin Problems.

THE USE OF INDWELLING CATHETERS[5]

Indications

The decision to use an indwelling urinary catheter is profitably discussed with the patient and family. Some patients have had previous experiences with catheters, and may recall significant physical discomfort from the device or find the apparatus extremely humiliating. Other patients will be grateful when the embarrassment or discomfort of wetting is ended. The patient's ambulation and travel outside the home may be inhibited by the catheter, but should not be prevented.

Important medical indications for chronic catheterization include painful bladder distension, maceration of skin or breakdown of the perineal skin, and contamination or aggravation of wounds from persistent urinary leakage. If the patient is oblivious to pain or local skin problems and is unlikely to suffer from their progression, catheterization may still be considered for the family's or caretakers' convenience and comfort. The risks of long-term catheterization need to be considered, but deserve little concern in the patient who is severely debilitated or nearing death.

For chronic control of incontinence, clean intermittent catheterization is medically preferable to an indwelling catheter, but is rarely practical for advanced cancer patients in the home, unless only infrequent drainage is required. An indwelling catheter with a closed drainage system is easily managed by most families and by many patients living alone.

Catheter Management

1. Silicon catheters may be preferable, since they seem to form less concretions.
2. The catheter should be inserted under aseptic conditions, preferably by specially trained personnel.

3. The catheter should be changed only if it becomes heavily encrusted or if partial or complete blockage develops. Many catheters can remain in place for over a month.
4. The system should be kept closed, except for when the bottom of the bag is drained or when obstruction necessitates irrigation under strict aseptic technique.
5. Downhill, unobstructed flow of urine should be maintained at all times by keeping the collecting bag below the bladder. Clamping of the system in order to obtain a urine specimen is unnecessary and potentially hazardous. The bag should not be allowed to fill up. The bag is best kept attached to the bed when the patient is lying down. A leg bag can be provided if the patient is ambulatory.
6. To prevent tension or dislodgement, the drainage system should be carefully taped to the patient's thigh or lower abdomen.
7. Urine specimens for laboratory studies should be obtained by cleansing the surface of a section of the catheter with an iodine disinfectant and then aspirating the urine with a 21-gauge sterile syringe.
8. The development of significant bacteriuria or of low-grade pyuria may be a harbinger of a serious infection and suggests the need for careful monitoring of the patient's condition. Bacteriuria, however, should be ignored unless the patient develops symptoms or signs of a urinary tract infection. Symptomatic infections are treated with systemic antibiotics. Reinfection with resistant strains of bacteria is likely to occur. Some infections will not respond to treatment unless the catheter is removed.
9. When recurrent symptomatic infections occur, consider removing the catheter. Prophylactic administration of antibiotics has not been demonstrated to be useful in long-term catheterization, but can be attempted (e.g., Trimethoprim 160 mg/sulfamethoxazole 800 mg [Bactrim, Septra] $\frac{1}{2}$ tab po bid). Urinary antiseptics (e.g., methenamine mandelate [Mandelamine]) are ineffective for catheterized patients.[4]

A number of inconvenient, useless, or potentially harmful regimens have been proposed for the care of indwelling catheters. Routine changes of the catheter have no definite value. Careful cleaning, dressing, or application of antibacterial substances to the catheter or urethral meatus have not been shown to prevent infections. Prophylactic use of antibiotics for a few days after catheter insertion has been recommended but not adequately studied. Other measures that have unproved value or are probably harmful include irrigation, routine use of urinary antiseptics (e.g., bladder instillations or oral hexamine mandelate, hexamine hippurate, or ascorbic acid), routine use of antibiotics, frequent urine cultures, and treatment of documented instances of significant bacteriuria in the absence of symptoms.

RENAL FAILURE AND URINARY TRACT OBSTRUCTION

Renal failure in the late stages of advanced cancer is usually due to hypovolemia or to ureteral or bladder outlet obstruction. Rarer causes include infiltrative tumor, radiation damage, acute tubular necrosis, hepatorenal syndrome, myeloma kidney, uric acid or xanthine nephropathy, hypercalcemia, disseminated intravascular coagulation, pyelonephritis, and damage from chemotherapeutic agents (methotrexate, platinum, streptozotocin) or other drugs (especially antibiotics). Common cancer-related renal conditions that may not cause significant azotemia include amyloidosis, renal vein thrombosis, and the nephrotic syndrome.[1]

Renal failure usually leads slowly, and with only moderate distress, to a uremic death. The management of dehydration, pruritus, hiccoughs, and nausea are discussed in other sections of this chapter. Unless renal function is stable or deteriorating very slowly, the usual dietary measures for renal failure (salt and protein restriction) are rarely appropriate or helpful. Similarly, treatments with phosphate-binding gels, bicarbonate, or hypouricemic agents are usually unnecessary.

Bladder outlet obstruction can be managed with a Foley catheter or suprapubic cystostomy, as discussed above. The management of ureteral obstruction deserves brief discussion here.[2] This condition is associated with metastatic tumors, especially of the pelvis, as well as with hematuria, pyuria, nephrolithiasis, sloughed renal papillae, and scarring from cancer treatments. Ureteral obstruction may be asymptomatic or may cause flank pain, hematuria, uremia, or oliguria. When obstruction is associated with pyuria, fever, or other signs of infection, it should be viewed as an acutely life-threatening problem.

A new diagnosis of ureteral obstruction should not be sought in the late stages of terminal illness when a slow death from uremia is acceptable, when invasive studies or procedures are shunned, or when a prompt demise from another complication is anticipated. Some patients with advanced cancer, however, can anticipate benefit from unilateral procedures to correct obstruction, especially if the relatively simple technique of percutaneous nephrostomy is available. Other surgical techniques, particularly retrograde catheterization of the ureters with the placement of internal stents, may occasionally be appropriate.

SELECTED REFERENCES

1. Fer MF, Mckinney TD, Richardson RL et al: Cancer and the kidney: Renal complications of neoplasms. Am J Med 71:704–718, 1981
2. Gutman FD, Boxer RJ: The pathophysiology and management of urinary tract obstruction. In Rieselbach RE, Garnick MB (eds): Cancer and the Kidney, pp. 594–624. Philadelphia, Lea & Febiger, 1982
3. Lodish JR, Boxer RJ: Urinary tract hemorrhage. In Rieselbach RE, Garnick MB (eds): Cancer and the Kidney, pp. 625–661. Philadelphia, Lea & Febiger, 1982
4. Vainrub B, Busher DM: Lack of effect of methenamine in suppression of, or prophylaxis against chronic urinary infection. Antimicrob Agents Chemother 12:625–629, 1977
5. Warren JW, Muncie HL Jr, Bergquist EJ, Hoopes JM: Sequelae and management of urinary infection in the patient requiring chronic catheterization. J Urol 125:1–8, 1981
6. Wheatley JK: Bladder incontinence. Postgrad Med 71:75–82, 1982
7. Williams ME: A critical evaluation of the assessment technology for urinary incontinence in older persons. J Am Geriatr Soc 31:657–664, 1983
8. Williams ME, Pannill FC: Urinary incontinence in the elderly: Physiology, pathophysiology, diagnosis, and treatment. Ann Intern Med 97:895–907, 1982

H. Skin Problems

i. Pruritus

Lymphomas, mycosis fungoides, polycythemia vera, and other myeloproliferative dis-orders may be associated with pruritus, even in early stages of the illness. Generalized itching is otherwise uncommon in late-stage cancer, except when specific skin con-ditions develop or as a complication of systemic processes such as cholestasis and uremia (Table 2H-1).

TABLE 2H-1
Common Causes of Pruritus

SKIN DISEASE
>   Xerosis
>   Urticaria
>   Atopic dermatitis
>   Infestations, bites
>   Infections—candida, pyoderma
>   Local irritation
>   Chemicals, soaps
>   Tape
>   Body fluids
>   Burns
>   Postherpetic
>   Fungating tumors
>   Mycosis fungoides
>   Wounds

SYSTEMIC DISEASE
>   Cholestasis
>   Uremia
>   Hematologic
>   Polycytemia vera
>   Lymphoma
>   Leukemia, myeloma
>   Mastocytosis
>   Iron deficiency
>   Endocrine
>   Diabetes
>   Thyroid disease
>   Carcinoid
>   Hypercalcemia
>   Parasitosis
>   Psychogenic
>   "Senile pruritus"
>   Drugs
>   Drug reactions and toxicity, including aspirin, opiates
>   Drug withdrawal

PATHOPHYSIOLOGY[1]

The pathophysiology of pruritus has not been well-elucidated. A variety of local cutaneous chemical mediators have been implicated; histamine may be involved in some pruritic conditions, and bile salts may play a role in the pruritus of cholestatic disease.

A unique neuroreceptor for itch has not been described. Pain and itch are transmitted along similar neural pathways, yet the two sensations clearly differ in their precipitants and their responses to drugs. The scratch response is specific to pruritic states.

MANAGEMENT[3]

Pruritus that is associated with *allergic phenomena* or *primary skin diseases* will often respond readily to specific topical measures or to removal of irritants. Antihistamines (H_1-blockers), local anesthetic agents, and topical and oral steroids can be quite useful (Tables 2H-2 and 2H-3). H_2-blocking antihistamines (*e.g.*, cimetidine) and serotonin blockers (*e.g.*, cryoheptadine) may also have a role in the management of pruritus associated with skin diseases. In addition, psychotropic drugs (phenothiazines and antidepressants) have been used for pruritus; many of these agents have antihistaminic or antiserotonergic effects.

Pruritus associated with *nonallergic systemic conditions* (*e.g.*, uremia or cholestasis) responds poorly to H_1-blocking antihistamines. An exception to this generalization may be the myeloproliferative diseases, in which pruritus has responded to both H_1- and H_2-blocking agents.

Antihistamines

Antihistamines are relatively nontoxic and, regardless of their anticipated efficacy, should be tried, along with the general measures noted below, for all pruritic conditions. The full therapeutic potential of these drugs is usually not realized because they are commonly prescribed at subtherapeutic doses.

TABLE 2H-2
Topical Agents for Pruritus

TOPICAL ANESTHETICS
   Phenol (0.5%–1.0%), usually with menthol 0.5% or camphor—its bacteriocidal action is
      occasionally useful
   Benzocaine—concern about sensitization with this or related agents is generally
      irrelevant in managing terminal illness
   Calamine lotion or other zinc-containing creams and lotions—since calamine tends to be
      drying, it is preferable for "wet" lesions

TOPICAL STEROIDS
   Lotions or creams
      Triamcinalone 0.025% tid
      Fluocinalone 0.1% tid
   Spray

TABLE 2H-3
Systemic Antipruritic Drugs

H₁-BLOCKING ANTIHISTAMINES
    Diphenhydramine (Benadryl) 25–100 mg q4–6h
    Tripelennamine (Pyribenzamine) 25–75 mg q4–6h
    Chlorphenireamine 2–16 mg q4–6h (also sustained-action tabs)
    Phenothiazines (see Anxiety) or Promethazine 25–50 mg q4–6h

SEROTONIN ANTAGONIST
    Cryoheptadine (Periactin) 4 mg 3–4 times a day

H₂-BLOCKING ANTIHISTAMINE
    Cimetidine (Tagamet) 200–400 mg qid
    Ranitidine (Zantac) 150 mg bid

SEDATIVES—BENZODIAZEPINES
    See Chap. 6, Coping with Loss

TRICYCLIC ANTIDEPRESSANTS
    See Chap. 6, Coping with Loss

NONSTEROIDAL ANTI-INFLAMMATORY AGENTS
    See Chap. 1, Pain Control

STEROIDS
    Prednisone 5–20 mg tid

All H_1-blocking agents may produce sedation and other central nervous system disturbances (*e.g.,* dizziness), dry mouth, and other atropinic symptoms, and occasional gastrointestinal disturbances (including nausea and anorexia). The choice of H_1-antihistaminic agents can be guided somewhat by preferred side-effects. Chlorpheniramine is relatively nonsedating, as is hydroxyzine (which also has analgesic properties), whereas diphenhydramine or tripelennamine more commonly cause drowsiness, a side-effect that may be desirable for nocturnal itching or for anxious patients. The profound antianxiety and antipsychotic actions of phenothiazines may be useful at times. Switching among various agents in this class of drugs will often be worthwhile, either for improving therapeutic response or for minimizing undesirable side-effects.

Anti-Inflammatory Agents

Nonsteroidal anti-inflammatory agents should be considered first-line treatment for pruritus that accompanies nonallergic systemic conditions, especially when pain and pruritus coexist (*e.g.,* from cutaneous metastases).[7] Aspirin and such agents as ibuprofen or indomethacin may be tried along with or after an adequate trial of H_1-blockers. The patient who responds poorly to a first trial of H_1-antihistamines and anti-inflammatory agents can be tried on other agents in these classes or on related drugs (*e.g.,* an antiserotonergic agent rather than an antihistaminic one, or ibuprofen rather than aspirin). Alternatively, systemic steroids may be considered (see Table 2H-3).

When these measures fail, an H_2-blocking agent, cimetidine, may be added. Cholestyramine, a bile-salt–binding agent, has proved useful in pruritus associated with cholestasis, but also seems helpful in uremia and has been used for pruritus associated with hematologic malignancies; however, it is usually difficult to ingest and is poorly tolerated.

The importance of emotional factors in the perception and response to itching should be especially considered when routine antipruritic treatments fail. The management of anxiety, boredom, and depression by pharmacologic and nonpharmacologic methods may provide dramatic relief of pruritus. A sedative–hypnotic, such as diazepam, is commonly useful for distressed patients, especially at bedtime.

The usefulness of opiates in treating pruritus is unclear. These agents may cause pruritus, but also may relieve some itching. They generally are ineffective, though not harmful, in pruritic skin conditions. Naloxone, the opiate antagonist, has an antipruritic effect when administered parenterally for experimental, histamine-induced pruritus.[2]

General Measures

1. Choose clothing for comfort.
2. Avoid drying of skin:
     Increase ambient humidity
     Avoid hot or frequent baths
     Use bath oils to preserve skin moisture
3. Treat dry skin with emollients and lubricants:
     Alpha Keri
     Eucerin
     Avoid drying, irritating soaps
4. Trim nails and avoid excoriation.
5. Avoid drugs and foods that provoke itching (*e.g.,* coffee and alcohol may cause vasodilation and induce pruritus).
6. Tepid baths may produce temporary relief.
7. Treat anxiety, boredom, and depression. Provide distraction.
8. Treat insomnia. Like pain, pruritus may be worse at night. Hypnotic drugs may allow sleep despite pruritus.

Disease-Specific Measures

Cholestasis
Cholestyramine is the treatment of choice for cholestasis:

Cholestyramine 12–16 g po qd in divided doses with meals, mixed with applesauce or pureed, tart fruit

A number of other treatments have been reported, including androgens (methyltestosterone 25 mg SL qd), ultraviolet phototherapy, and plasma perfusion.

Uremia
Hypercalcemia should be treated (as described in Section N). If pruritus persists despite normocalcemia, correction of hyperphosphatemia, if present, should be attempted. Cholestyramine may be useful. Also reported to be effective are ultraviolet phototherapy (which has produced remission after 8 biweekly treatments),[4] oral activated charcoal (6 g qd),[5] and parenteral lidocaine.

Hematologic

Consider a trial of H_1- and H_2-blocking agents. Plasma exchange helped one patient.[6]

Special Problems

Anogenital pruritus is frequently associated with piles, fissures, and other forms of proctitis, local yeast infections, parasitic diseases, localized primary skin disease (*e.g.*, psoriasis), and irritation associated with vaginal discharge, urinary, or fecal incontinence, or poor local hygiene. Perirectal abscess may lead to pruritus ani. Patients who use topical antihistamines or anesthetic agents or who are sensitive to soaps may develop allergic reactions in the anogenital region. Systemic pruritic conditions may cause localized itching, as may local tumor or irradiation.

Treatment includes removal of irritants, attention to the bowel regimen (use of bulk-forming or lubricant laxatives), sitz baths, suppositories containing topical analgesics or steroids, and the systemic measures noted above.

Pruritus vulvae may occur with atrophic vaginitis, vaginal infections (candida, trichomonas), local irritation (urinary incontinence, poor local hygiene, soaps, deodorants), local carcinoma, and radiation treatment, and as a manifestation of systemic pruritic conditions. Vaginal suppositories containing steroids or appropriate antimicrobial agents should be considered in addition to the measures noted above for generalized pruritus.

SELECTED REFERENCES

1. Anonymous: Itch (Editorial). Lancet 2:568–569, 1980
2. Bernstein JE, Swift RM, Soltar K, Lorincz A: Antipruritic effect of an opiate antagonist, naloxone hydrochloride. J Invest Dermatol 78:82–83, 1982
3. Gilchrest BA: Pruritus: Pathogenesis, therapy, and significance in systemic disease states. Arch Intern Med 142:101–105, 1982
4. Gilchrest BA, Rowe JW, Brown RS, Steinman TL, Arndt KA: Ultraviolet phototherapy of uremic pruritus. Ann Intern Med 91:17–21, 1979
5. Pederson JA, Matter BJ, Czerwinski AW, Llach F: Relief of idiopathic generalized pruritus in dialysis patients treated with activated oral charcoal. Ann Intern Med 93:446–448, 1980
6. Shaw D, Trotter JM, Calman KC: Plasma exchange to control sweats and pruritus. Br Med J 281:1959, 1980
7. Twycross RG: Pruritus and pain in en cuirass breast cancer. Lancet 2:696, 1981

ii. Pressure Sores

PATHOPHYSIOLOGY

Pressure sores or pressure ulcers (also called bedsores, decubitus ulcers, or decubiti) are commonly associated with advanced, debilitating disease. While ulcers will occasionally be caused by discrete, reversible trauma (*e.g.*, by pressure from the edge of a cast or a tight bandage), they usually occur when advanced cancer patients are unable to protect themselves from the daily trauma of lying, sitting, or moving on a bed or chair (*e.g.*, from pressure over bony prominences and from friction or shearing forces). Decubiti develop when one or more of the normal mechanisms for the protection and maintenance of the skin are blunted:

The appreciation of and response to pain and irritation of the skin is diminished owing to altered mental status, hypesthesia or analgesic agents.

Weight loss and dehydration lead to a decrease of the soft tissues, which normally absorb and distribute pressure on the body and which cushion deeper tissues and protect bony prominences.

The usual shifting of weight on various portions of the body is prevented by paralysis, weakness, stupor, or other causes of immobility.

Normal nutrition and repair of the skin is impaired by malnutrition, advanced age, edema, venous stasis, ischemia, anemia, or other systemic illness or drugs (especially steroids).

Direct tissue damage occurs from urine, stool, or sweat on the skin—an exposure to irritants that a healthy person would not allow.

CLINICAL PRESENTATION[2]

Ulcers can be produced experimentally with a single exposure to mild pressure over only 2 hours. Intermittent pressure is better tolerated than continuous pressure.

Clinically, relatively mild trauma to the skin will produce reversible pressure sores. Areas of blanching erythema are the earliest detectable lesions, and they may resolve spontaneously if further trauma is avoided. Prolonged mild pressure can lead to irreversible damage, usually first evident when initial erythematous lesions become nonblanching. Further signs of damage to deeper tissue layers include edema, blister formation, and punctuate hemorrhages. Later, the overlying skin will slough, revealing a reddish ulcer. Small, superficial ulcers may be associated with large, undermining injuries to the deep tissues, and thus may herald the development of extensive soft-tissue necrosis. Over a few days or weeks, a waxy, yellow eschar or a gray–black area of necrosis may appear. Ulceration may extend into the subcutaneous fat or deep fascia. Complications include abscess formation, sinus tracts, osteomyelitis, and septic arthritis. Secondary infections are frequently polymicrobial, often including *Bacteroides fragilis.*

Once decubiti appear, progression and multiplication of lesions is the rule unless vigorous measures are taken to guard the skin and to heal existing lesions. Moreover, when the patient is positioned so as to avoid pressure on existing sores, new areas of the body become subject to prolonged pressure and skin breakdown.

Necrotic tumor masses occasionally present similarly to decubiti. Raised verrucous margins are typical of malignant ulcers. A biopsy can be used to identify malignancy, although both types of ulcers are often treated in an identical manner in the terminal phases of illness.

MANAGEMENT

Some patients may have little pain or distress from extensive decubiti. Surprisingly, very large, deep, gruesome wounds may be well tolerated, usually because of the same factors that led to the development of the ulcer. When such sores are not bothersome and reflect the advanced malnutrition and immobility seen *in extremis,* the family and staff need not busy themselves over difficult treatments that may be both futile and of no benefit to the patient.

> *He is so sick now that he can't even protect his skin by turning away from this sore. It looks awful, but doesn't seem to be bothering him.*

In general, however, the earliest evidence of pressure sores is cause for alarm. Vigorous treatment and instigation of preventive measures can often save the advanced cancer patient from serious discomfort or disability. *The avoidance of further pressure on the bedsores is the foremost goal of treatment.* Clean wounds (*i.e.,* nonnecrotic, noninfected ulcers) will usually heal when ongoing trauma is simply prevented.

Prevention of Pressure Sores and Management of Early Lesions (Erythema and Closed Blisters)

Inspection
The skin should be inspected a few times a day, especially during bathing or turning. The heels, sacrum, ischium, and greater trochanters deserve careful attention. Patients who are being turned side-to-side will commonly develop sores on lateral surfaces (shoulders, hips, ankles) or where limbs touch each other (medial knee or ankle).

Hygiene
The skin should be kept clean and dry. If moisture or irritation develops in any area (*e.g.,* perineal or intertriginous regions), the skin should be washed and carefully dried as required, usually two or three times a day. Otherwise, baths may be needed daily or only a few times a week.

Contact of urine and feces with the skin should be prevented. Soilage should be cleaned promptly.

Dry skin should be treated with moisturizing agents, (*e.g.,* Eucerin). Lotions or creams may be massaged into the skin. Talcum powder should be applied only to dry skin, since moist powder will increase friction on the skin.

Frequent Turning and Positioning
Once problems with decubiti develop, the patient should be moved in bed at least every 2 hours. Insofar as possible, the patient should be encouraged to shift his or her weight frequently. Direct pressure on existing wounds should not be allowed, while prolonged, intense pressure on any portion of the body should be minimized. By using pillows, blankets, and cushions, the weight of the body should be distributed over the largest possible surface.

Specifically, most patients will lie on a flat bed and be turned side-to-side (or to whichever positions prevent pressure on damaged areas) every 2 hours. Ideally, the patient should alternate between two positions on each side: half-way turned and fully turned (or tilted slightly face down). Some patients can also lie flat on the stomach.

Sitting up does not allow distribution of weight over a large surface and may predispose to pressure sores. For the patient with decubiti who can rest in a chair, periods of sitting up should be shorter than 2 hours. This position should be avoided if it causes pressure on existing sores.

Avoid Trauma and Corrosive Damage

The following should be avoided:

Sliding in bed, especially when moved

Rubbing skin dry—sensitive skin should be patted dry

Rough, starchy, wrinkled, or damp sheets

Tightly fitting bedclothes—use porous, absorbent materials that allow air circulation

Harsh soaps, including contact with strong laundry soaps used on sheets

Irritation from jewelry, buttons, snaps, food crumbs, dressing, and, especially, tape

Excess heat, particularly from lamps and similar devices used to dry wounds

Patient's long nails

Irritation from urine, stools, draining wounds, etc.

Guards

Sheepskin guards can be applied to heels and elbows. Blankets or sheepskin pads are placed between the legs when the patient lies on the side.

Bedding, Mattresses, and Cushions

Special bed surfaces (*e.g.,* sheepskin) can be less traumatic to the skin than sheets, especially rough hospital sheets.

Special mattresses or cushions that help distribute weight should be used on beds and chairs: air- or fluid-filled flotation mattresses, alternating-pressure mattresses, and foam mattresses (*e.g.,* "egg-crate mattresses").

Well-constructed "doughnuts" or cushions may be used to redistribute pressure. Commercial foam cutouts are often ineffective, since they do not employ enough cushioning. Foam should be 4 inches thick or more.

Systemic Measures

Systemic measures include the following:

Promote nutrition, and consider dietary supplementation with multivitamins, vitamin C, zinc, and magnesium.

Avoid steroids.

Treat pain, spasticity, and other causes of immobility, but also try to minimize the use of agents that diminish awareness of pain.

Treat infection, anemia, and other illnesses contributing to skin breakdown.

Additional Measures

Gentle massage

Bed cradles to promote ventilation

Treatment of Open Wounds

In addition to the measures described above, many regimens and agents have been proposed and used successfully (though not in controlled trials) for open pressure sores. Straightforward means to minimize pressure and to maintain local hygiene are far more important than the choice of topical agents (*e.g.,* antiseptics, enzyme preparations, stimulants to granulation, drying agents, or antibiotics). The favorite regimen of the attending nurse or family is often chosen, as long as it does not seem harmful, since it will be applied with enthusiasm and confidence.

Wounds should be carefully measured if progress in healing is to be gauged accurately.

General principles of treatment include the following.

Débride Necrotic Tissue
Devitalized tissue inhibits repair and promotes infection.

For superficially necrotic ulcers, apply wet-to-dry dressings. Deep wounds require loosely packed gauze and may benefit from irrigation. Fine mesh gauze can be soaked with normal saline or half-strength povidone iodine (Betadine) and changed four times a day. Once débridement is accomplished, wet-to-dry dressings will hinder healing and should be discontinued. Enzyme preparations (Elase, Travase) or dextranomer beads (Debrisan)[3] may enhance débridement and healing.

Sharp dissection is required for extensive necrosis or for thick eschars, especially if the eschar is associated with evidence of deeper necrosis or infection (e.g., erythema, tenderness, and fluctuance). Deep surgical débridement and a variety of surgical procedures that are used regularly in paraplegics and similarly rehabilitatable patients have little role in the management of the terminally ill cancer patient.

Local Hygiene
Wash with a mild surgical soap or apply a disinfectant three times a day (e.g., hexachlorophene [Phisohex], chlorhexidene [Hibitane], or half-strength povidone iodine [Betadine].

Clean, well-healing wounds can generally be left open to air. Clean, dry dressings may be applied when necessary to protect the wound. When the removal of dressings is painful, consider petroleum–gauze dressings.

Dry dressings, however, promote scab formation, and scabs may inhibit epithelialization. Healing of clean wounds may be further promoted by maintaining a moist wound surface with pectin–gelatin (e.g., Stomahesive, Duoderm) or vapor-permeable film dressings (e.g., OP-Site, Tegaderm).[1] The latter dressings are transparent, allowing for easy monitoring of the wound.

When the wound needs to be protected from urine, feces, or other drainage, these moist occlusive dressings, or barrier films, and less expensive plastic guards (e.g., Saran Wrap enclosed with tape) should be considered.

Dry Out Very Moist, Macerated Lesions
The following may be used to dry wounds:

Frequent washing and careful drying.

Ultraviolet light, heat lamps, standard lights or hair dryers—the risk of causing a burn is greater than the potential benefit when these measures are used by inexperienced persons or are not carefully supervised.

Drying agents (e.g., topical Maalox).

Topical Antibiotics
Topical, nonabsorbable antibiotics (e.g., Sulfadene) may have a role in preventing serious infection or treating mild local infections, but are generally not required.

Eradicate Local Infection

The presence of infection (cellulitis or deeper infections) should be determined by bedside clinical assessment, not by bacterial cultures. Many wounds are contaminated by bacteria and may yield high colony counts when cultured, but show little sign of tissue infection. The choice of antimicrobial agents may be guided by reports of the antibiotic sensitivity of the bacteria cultured from the wound.

Ultraviolet Light

Ultraviolet light, which may be bacteriocidal and may stimulate skin repair, has been shown in a well-controlled study to speed the healing of pressure sores that are less than 5 mm deep.[4] In contrast to the usual casual application of light treatments to pressure sores, this study followed a strict protocol, including skin testing to individualize doses, careful screening of surrounding skin, and the provocation of a strong inflammatory reaction with twice-weekly therapy.

SELECTED REFERENCES

1. Anonymous: Transparent wound dressings. Med Lett Drugs Ther 25:103–104, 1983
2. Reuler JB, Cooney TG: The pressure sore: Pathophysiology and principles of management. Ann Intern Med 94:661–666, 1981
3. Sawyer PN, Dowback G, Sophie Z, Feller J, Cohen I: A preliminary report of the efficacy of Debrisan (dextranomer) in the debridement of cutaneous ulcers. Surgery 85:201–204, 1979
4. Wills EE, Anderson TW, Beattie BL et al: A randomized placebo-controlled trial of ultraviolet light in the treatment of superficial pressure sores. J Am Geriatrics Soc 31:131–133, 1983

iii. Fungating Tumors and Ulcerating Wounds

Of all the manifestations of advanced cancer, fungating tumors and malignant ulcerating wounds can be among the most troubling and discouraging for the patient and family and for health-care providers. Such lesions may produce gross deformities, unsightly sores, or intolerable odors, and may plague the patient with drainage and bleeding. While the disheartening appearance of these growths is not always amenable to treatment, the odor, drainage, infection, and attendant discomfort can often be satisfactorily managed.[3]

> Radiation therapy can control many of the disagreeable manifestations of fungating tumors and malignant ulcers. Surgical techniques for wound management include débridement or palliative excision, amputation of the affected part, and vascular ligation to control bleeding. A toilet mastectomy may occasionally be indicated for troubling chest wounds from breast cancer. Chemotherapy, including topical chemotherapy, can also be considered.

ODOR

Odors generally result from bacterial growth in moist, necrotic tissues. The odor may be extinguished by cleaning and drying out the wound and by eradicating the bacteria.

Regular cleansing with soap and water or saline may be sufficient to clean wounds, but the following antiseptic agents are often useful:

Povidone iodine (Betadine) is a relatively mild, nonstinging and effective disinfectant and is available in a variety of forms, including 2% and 10% solutions and 2% aerosol spray, vaginal gel, and mouthwash.

Diluted sodium hypochlorite solution (modified Dakin's solution), used at half-strength (0.25%), is a favored disinfectant for dissolving necrotic tissues. The solution may be applied in soaked gauze. Because it can be irritating to the skin and will dissolve blood clots and delay clotting, it should not be used on clean, healing, or bleeding wounds. The solution must be freshly prepared.

Chlorhexidene gluconate—4% emulsion (Hibiclens) or 1% aqueous solution (Hibitane)—may be better tolerated at sensitive skin sites than the agents described above and is negligibly absorbed. It has been favored for vulvar lesions. Like hexachlorophene (and unlike iodine-containing agents), it produces a sustained antibacterial action, especially with repeated use.

Hydrogen peroxide is a frequently misused antiseptic. Since its effectiveness deteriorates quickly, it must be delivered from a fresh bottle. Even then, its antibacterial action is brief.

Systemic toxicity from topical agents applied to wounds or mucous membranes has been reported with multiple substances, including hexachlorophene, iodine-containing antiseptics, and boric acid. None of the commercial antiseptic solutions are reliably bacteriocidal for all organisms; gram-negative organisms, particularly *Pseudomonas*, may be resistant. Acetic acid may, at times, be chosen as an antiseptic because of its effectiveness against *Pseudomonas aeruginosa*.

Necrotic wounds can be cleansed and superficially débrided by frequent packing with moist gauze (see Section Hii, Pressure Sores). Moist and draining lesions can be dried by using wet-to-dry gauze dressings; the addition of modified Burow's solution (one Domeboro packet or tablet in 1 pint of water) may facilitate drying. Cleaning, drying, and scabbing may be facilitated with caustic agents (*e.g.,* acetic acid, silver nitrate, or potassium permanganate).

When scrupulous wound management and topical antiseptics fail to control odor, antibiotic agents are useful. Fungating wounds are typically populated by multiple organisms; cultures (which should include attention to anaerobes) are often little help in selecting treatment. Metronidazole (Flagyl) 250 mg po tid is an agent effective against anaerobic bacteria that often cause bad odor.[1] A course of chloramphenicol might also be tried. Topical antibiotic agents and sprays are rarely effective, although the addition of unabsorbed sulfa drugs—silver sulfadiazine (Silvadene), which seems to penetrate eschars, or mafenide acetate (Sulfamylon Cream)—may be considered. Anecdotal reports suggest that topical yogurt may be soothing and effective; presumably the lactobacilli compete favorably with the odor-producing bacteria.

A persistent odor can be made more tolerable by the following methods:

Prevent dispersion. Odors may be contained by placing an ostomy bag or similar odor-proof device or an odor-absorbent dressing over the wound. The addition of charcoal tablets or an ostomy deodorant (*e.g.,* Banish 2, M-9) to the ostomy bag may also help prevent dispersion of the odor. Charcoal (available for fish tanks or as briquettes for barbecues) may also absorb disagreeable odors when placed near the bedside. A nurse experienced with ostomies can suggest how to apply skin-barrier preparations and similar dressings.

Cover up the odor with other smells. Deodorant pads and sprays and solid air fresheners are occasionally useful. The addition of oil of orange or oil of peppermint to the dressings may also cover up disagreeable smells.

Improve air circulation near the patient. Fans, air conditioners, and other methods for promoting air circulation can lessen the intensity of bad odors.

BLEEDING

Radiation, arterial ligation, and cryosurgery have been employed to control excess bleeding.

Oozing may be managed with astringent and drying agents as described above. Pressure dressings should be applied. (For further help, see Management of Bleeding.)

MANAGEMENT OF BLEEDING

Topical, absorbable hemostatics—gelatin sponges (Gelfoam)—may be left on the wound indefinitely. Oxidized cellulose gauze (Oxycel, Surgicel) can also be used for immediate control of hemorrhage, but will inhibit epithelialization of the wound.

Thrombin powder can also be applied topically and can be used in conjunction with Gelfoam.

Gauze soaked in epinephrine 1:1000 may reduce capillary bleeding.

Silver nitrate sticks can be used for small bleeding points.

DRAINAGE AND FISTULAS

Two major hazards of drainage are the irritation of adjoining normal skin and the contamination of nearby wounds. Techniques for protecting adjacent skin (as described in Section Hii, Pressure Sores) include the careful use of dressings or ostomy bags on the wound, and the application of ointments (*e.g.,* A&D cream), standard dressings, or special barrier preparations (barrier films and sprays, pectin-based dressings, or vapor-permeable film dressings) to areas affected by the drainage. Silicone adhesive spray or similar sticky sprays or applications can ensure adherence of tape or dressings to the skin.

Measures suitable for drying moist wounds are discussed above under Odor. Small fistulas can often be dressed like small wounds; purulent drainage should be cultured and may respond to appropriate antibiotics. Larger, feculent, or copiously draining fistulas can be treated like ostomies; the preparation of appropriate dressings may be best handled in consultation with an enterostomal therapy nurse.[2]

> Diversion procedures are occasionally appropriate palliative measures for enterocutaneous fistulas or rectovaginal and rectovesical fistulas. Vesicovaginal and vesicocutaneous fistulas are generally managed with conservative measures, especially careful cleansing and dressing.

SELECTED REFERENCES

1. Doll DC, Doll KJ: Malodorous tumors and metronidazole. Ann Intern Med 94:139–140, 1981
2. Dunavant MK: Wound and fistula management. In Broadwell DC, Jackson BS (eds): Principles of Ostomy Care, pp 658–686. St Louis, CV Mosby, 1982
3. Wood DK: The draining malignant ulceration: Palliative management in advanced cancer. JAMA 224:820–822, 1980

I. Fluid Accumulation—Edema and Effusions

ETIOLOGY

Peripheral or dependent edema may have multiple etiologies in the patient with advanced cancer: lack of the normal muscular activity that facilitates venous and lymphatic return of fluids from the periphery to the central circulation; hypoalbuminemia (which is typically due to malnutrition and the metabolic effects of the tumor, but may also be associated with such conditions as malabsorption, infection, hepatic failure, and protein loss from drainage or exudation of protein-rich fluids); venous or lymphatic obstruction; and all the common (and not necessarily malignant) causes, such as peripheral venous disease and the sodium-retaining states associated with cardiac, renal, or hepatic failure.

The same systemic factors and similar local processes can contribute to fluid retention in the pleural, pericardial, or peritoneal cavities, although an effusion in these spaces frequently signals the presence of tumor or tumor products that alter tissue permeability or drainage.

Prolonged survival is not uncommon after the development of effusions or peripheral edema caused by malignant disease. Selected patients should be considered for vigorous measures to control fluid accumulation, including palliative uses of chemotherapy, radiation, and surgery. For example, satisfying improvement of malignant ascites has been noted with chemotherapy for ovarian carcinoma and with abdominal radiation for other groups of patients.

MANAGEMENT

General Measures[4,9]

Many patients with far-advanced disease will tolerate fluid accumulation with little or no discomfort and require no intervention for this condition. The following general measures may be useful when fluid accumulation produces disagreeable symptoms:

Restrict sodium intake to 2–5 g a day, and prescribe potassium salt substitutes.
Avoid drugs that contain sodium or that promote sodium retention (especially steroids, nonsteroidal anti-inflammatory agents, and some antibiotics).
Improve nutrition, especially protein intake.
If significant hyponatremia develops, institute moderate fluid restriction—2000 ml/day or less.
Increase bed rest.
Administer intravenous albumin or other plasma expanders—this stopgap measure is rarely appropriate, but can provide temporary relief in selected hypoalbuminemic patients.

Diuretics

Diuretics may alleviate fluid accumulation, even in situations where local tumor is producing exudative effusions or is blocking venous and lymphatic drainage. The value of symptomatic relief from fluid accumulation should be weighed against the risk that treatment will produce serious volume depletion and electrolyte abnormalities, especially when high doses of diuretics are employed.

Thiazides and furosemide are the first-choice diuretic agents. They should be begun at low doses and increased cautiously. Rapid fluid loss is generally hazardous and unnecessary. Patience is especially required in the management of ascites, a condition that usually responds only slowly to these drugs and in which overly vigorous diuresis is common and dangerous.

Secondary hyperaldosteronism is believed to be a factor in the perpetuation of many forms of fluid accumulation. Spironolactone, an aldosterone antagonist that is a weak diuretic when used alone, may provide profound benefit for some patients, especially when used in conjunction with the stronger agents. The addition of spironolactone will reduce potassium loss—an effect that is generally advantageous but may be perilous if renal failure predisposes to hyperkalemia. The potentially harmful endocrinologic effects of this steroid on tumor growth are rarely of practical concern.

SUGGESTED DIURETIC REGIMEN

Hydrochlorthiazide 25–50 mg po 1–2 times a day; begin with low doses and increase dose gradually

If no response to hydrochlorthiazide 100 mg po qd, add spironolactone 25 mg po 4id

    If no diuresis occurs or fluid loss is not maintained after 2–3 days, increase spironolactone to 50 mg po 4id, then 75 mg po 4id

For refractory fluid:

    Increase hydrochlorthiazide to 75–100 mg po bid, or

    Replace hydrochlorthiazide with furosemide (Lasix) 40 mg po bid and gradually increase dose to 80 mg po tid, as needed, with careful attention to electrolytes and renal function

Ethacrynic acid (Edecrin) is an alternative to furosemide

Triamterene and amiloride are potassium-sparing alternatives to spironolactone; they are not aldosterone antagonists

---

DEPENDENT EDEMA—ADDITIONAL MEASURES

Elevate edematous extremity as much as tolerated, using supports (*e.g.*, pillows) or slings

Compression:

    Elastic bandages or support stockings or sleeves

    Pneumatic intermittent compression

    When edema is maximally controlled, individually fitted elastic stockings and sleeves should be considered

Gentle exercise—isometric exercises are satisfactory

Attention to skin breakdown, injury, pressure sores, and signs of infection

Lanolin creams may soothe stretched skin

PLEURAL EFFUSIONS

Many patients with large pleural effusions are asymptomatic or only mildly symptomatic and require no intervention, while other patients with small effusions have troubling cough or dyspnea. Pleural effusions typically produce dyspnea by compromising chest-wall mechanics rather than by affecting gas exchange, lung volumes, or lung mechanisms.[3]

Symptomatic effusions will often respond to the general measures and diuretics described above for reducing fluid accumulation.[7] Antitussive agents may also be valuable. Hypoxia is rarely responsible for symptoms, although oxygen therapy occasionally produces subjective improvement. Thoracentesis can be considered when symptoms are marked (as well as when required for diagnostic studies). The pleural fluid should be drained as thoroughly as possible. If the determination of the etiology of the effusion might be useful for treatment, the fluid can be sent to the laboratory for cell count, cytology, and cell block, as well as measurement of protein and lactic dehydrogenase (LDH) levels. Thoracentesis is a senseless procedure for a patient who is not otherwise moribund or for whom brief relief of respiratory symptoms will not contribute significantly to well-being. As described in Section F, Dyspnea, a well-managed death from respiratory failure is not necessarily frightening nor associated with severe symptoms of dyspnea. Even without the use of narcotics or sedatives, patients may become drowsy, presumably from carbon dioxide retention, and may succumb gently to progressive stupor and coma.

In selected patients, the removal of a small amount of pleural fluid may produce dramatic relief of dyspnea. Symptomatic improvement from thoracentesis is typically brief, although an occasional patient may enjoy weeks of relief. If a significant symptomatic response is noted to the initial thoracentesis, repeated procedures can be performed in the home or office.

For those patients in whom a prolonged survival can be anticipated, especially those for whom the pleural effusion presents a life-threatening or disabling complication, more definitive therapeutic procedures can be considered. Prolonged palliation may be achieved by chest-tube drainage through a closed thoracotomy, followed by local instillation of sclerosing drugs or chemotherapeutic agents. Tetracycline is currently the sclerosing agent of choice; the concomitant instillation of Xylocaine may reduce the considerable discomfort often experienced with sclerosing procedures.[1] Radiation therapy to the mediastinum, hilum, or local tumor can also be considered, especially when examination of the pleural fluid reveals a transudate or a chylothorax indicative of lymphatic obstruction.

ASCITES

Paracentesis provides prompt relief from the discomfort and respiratory compromise of tense ascites, but the improvement is often mild and brief. Repeated paracentesis may cause protein loss, which further aggravates fluid retention. Happily, a large proportion of patients with ascites will enjoy good (but not prompt) results from moderate salt restriction and from resolute but cautious use of diuretics.[8]

Refractory, incapacitating ascites in a patient with a good long-term prognosis may be managed with a peritoneal–jugular venous (LaVeen) shunt, but complications from the procedure are numerous. Local instillation of chemotherapeutic agents has also been attempted.[6]

PERICARDIAL EFFUSION[10]

Pericardial effusions, especially when large or rapidly accumulating, may cause chest pain, cough, dyspnea, and a characteristic pattern of cardiovascular changes, including hypotension. Emergency pericardiocentesis produces prompt but usually short-lasting relief. The diagnosis and treatment of pericardial effusion should be pursued in those settings in which the patient and physician would consider either long-term drainage with an indwelling catheter or the use of other aggressive management techniques: surgical procedures (pericardial window or pericardiectomy), intracavitary instillation of chemotherapeutic or sclerosing agents,[2] local radiation therapy, or systemic chemotherapy.

LYMPHEDEMA

Lymphedema typically occurs as a consequence of radiation, surgery, thrombotic disease, or malignant infiltration of lymph nodes and lymphatics. Lymphedema of the upper extremity is a common postoperative complication of mastectomies, and its development long after surgery raises the question of whether cancer has recurred locally, although it often does not signify active disease.

The treatment of lymphedema is similar to that of peripheral edema, but the response to salt restriction and diuretics is poor.[5] Elevation, exercise, and compression are the mainstays of therapy for lymphedema of an extremity. Elastic bandages should be applied over the entire limb, beginning distally. A fitted sleeve or stocking can be applied when the lymphedema has substantially resolved. Manual or pneumatic massage may also be useful.

Because cellulitis is a frequent complication of lymphedema, the avoidance of injury and infection is a major concern in management. Patients with lymphedema of the arm should be instructed to use gloves while doing manual work that might lead to injury, and they should take special care to avoid skin damage from jewelry, burns, shaving, or nail trimming. Venupunctures and injections should not be performed in the affected limb. Scrupulous wound care is advised for even minor breaks in the skin, and patients are advised to contact their physician promptly if any signs of cellulitis develop.

Patients treated for head and neck tumors may also develop lymphedema. Some of the measures noted above can be adapted to the needs of these patients.

SELECTED REFERENCES

1. Anonymous: Treatment of malignant pleural and pericardial effusions. Med Lett Drugs Ther 23:59–60, 1981
2. Davis S, Sharma SM, Blumberg ED et al: Intrapericardial tetracyline for the management of cardiac tamponade secondary to malignant pericardial effusion. N Engl J Med 299:1113–1114, 1978
3. Estenne M, Yernault J, De Troyer A: Mechanism of relief of dyspnea after thoracentesis in patients with large pleural effusions. Am J Med 74:813–819, 1983
4. Flombaum C, Isaacs M, Scheiner E et al: Management of fluid retention in patients with advanced cancer. JAMA 245:611–614, 1981
5. Grabois M: Rehabilitation of the postmastectomy patient with lymphedema. CA 26:75–79, 1976
6. Howell SB, Pfeifle CL, Wung WE et al: Intraperitoneal cisplatin with systemic thiosulfate protection. Ann Intern Med 97:845–851, 1982
7. Leff A, Hopewell PC, Costello J: Pleural effusions from malignancy. Ann Intern Med 88:532–537, 1978
8. Moertel CG, Reitemeier RJ: Advanced Gastrointestinal Cancer: Clinical Management and Chemotherapy. New York, Harper & Row, 1969

9. Portlock CS, Goffinet DR: Manual of Clinical Problems in Oncology with Annotated Key References, pp 48–49, 272–275. Boston, Little, Brown & Co, 1980
10. Theologides A: Neoplastic cardiac tamponade. Semin Oncology 5:181–193, 1978

J. Is Dehydration Painful?

The decision to administer fluids to a dehydrated dying patient is often discussed primarily as an ethical issue, but sensible clinical choices should begin with a clear appreciation of the manifestations of water and electrolyte disorders and of the potential benefits of treatment. In this section, a series of common questions about dehydration in the terminally ill will be addressed: Does dehydration cause symptoms? Are these symptoms distressing to the patient? Is death from dehydration painful? Do fluid and electrolyte administration and other treatments help make dehydrated dying patients comfortable?

Dehydration—a loss of body water—is an imprecise term used to describe conditions with different etiologies and management.[16–18] Experimentally and clinically, two prototypical forms of dehydration have been described: sodium depletion and pure water loss.[21] As discussed more fully below, these conditions are characterized by loss of total body water and sodium. In the first case, the loss of salt is proportionately greater than the loss of water, whereas in the second case, sodium is relatively retained.

In general, research on fluid and electrolyte disorders has not been aimed at defining how dehydration of various degrees and duration is manifested symptomatically nor of how symptoms respond to treatment. Two small classic studies examine dehydration in normal subjects,[7,19,21] but the reports of healthy volunteers may be poor indications of the subjective responses of actual patients.[5] Systematic observations of patients are not available. Moreover, many reviews and studies of fluid and electrolyte disorders describe the symptoms of dehydration as manifestations of hyponatremia or hypernatremia, failing to address the possibility that water loss may produce symptoms independent of the serum sodium concentration (e.g., when isotonic dehydration develops). Likewise, the symptoms of hyponatremia or hypernatremia are often presented without distinguishing which findings occur in states of increased, normal, or decreased body water.[1–3,8,10,12,13,22,23]

HYPONATREMIC DEHYDRATION

One experimental form of water loss—hyponatremic dehydration—develops when subjects undergo salt and water depletion in a setting in which only water is restored. This condition can be produced experimentally and clinically when lost sweat or gastrointestinal (GI) secretions are replaced with salt-free fluids. Such patients have *pure salt or sodium depletion*. A similar pattern of clinical findings—perhaps best called *hyponatremic* or *hypotonic dehydration*—occurs when salt and water in body fluids are lost, but the loss of sodium is proportionately greater than the loss of fluid or the repletion of salt is inadequate.

Since salt is the principal cation of the extracellular fluid, hyponatremic dehydration leads predominantly to salt and fluid loss from the intravascular and interstitial compartments. Sodium depletion is thus sometimes called *volume depletion*—a term that is also imprecise, but that points to the prominence in this condition of signs of circulatory insufficiency.

Patients with pure salt depletion exhibit weight loss, poor skin turgor, dry mucous membranes, diminished sweat, and postural hypotension. Neuropsychiatric manifestations—weakness, apathy, lethargy, restlessness, confusion, delirium, stupor, and coma—also occur and may reflect primarily hyponatremia, since these symptoms are also seen in hyponatremia without volume depletion. Neuropsychiatric symptoms have been attributed to overhydration of brain cells and are similar to clinical findings in other hypo-osmolar states. Neuropsychiatric disorders occur especially when hyponatremia is severe or develops rapidly: a prompt lowering of serum sodium to 128 mmol/liter can produce symptoms, while a gradual lowering to 110 mmol/liter may go unnoticed. Subjects engaged in physical labor or undergoing relatively rapid onset of hyponatremia may complain of muscle cramps. Hyponatremia has also been reported to cause psychosis and localized neurologic findings such as aphasia, ataxia, and focal weakness.

Thirst may not be prominent in patients with hyponatremic dehydration, although marked volume loss is generally regarded as a stimulus to antidiuretic hormone (ADH) release and to thirst, as is apparent in the early signs of hypovolemic shock. McCance's experimental subjects did not regularly note thirst, perhaps reflecting the lack of severe dehydration in the study,[19] although McCance later postulated that a "curious loss of taste" associated with salt depletion is responsible for complaints expressed as "thirst."[20] Anorexia, nausea, and loss of taste have been noted in experimental and clinical subjects with hyponatremic dehydration. Occasionally reported symptoms include headache and vomiting (both of which are commonly seen with hyponatremia from water intoxication) and abdominal cramps. Vomiting is prominent in salt-depleted conditions such as diabetic ketoacidosis, Addison's disease, and heat exhaustion[14] and has been reported with diuretic-induced hyponatremia,[24] but anorexia, nausea and vomiting may be contributing causes rather than effects of dehydration. However, if hyponatremic dehydration produces these symptoms, a "vicious circle" of worsening salt depletion will occur.[18]

Azotemia, hyponatremia, and hemoconcentration (decreased intravascular fluid and increased red cell volume) are the principal laboratory findings in pure salt depletion.

HYPERNATREMIC DEHYDRATION

In a second experimental situation, subjects lose salt and water but have limited access to water while continuing to ingest salt. Clinically, this pattern of dehydration typically develops in confused or somnolent patients who have lost water disproportionately to salt or for whom water has been inadequately replaced. Similar findings may occur in patients with an osmotic diuresis (secondary to diabetes mellitus, diabetes insipidus, or high-protein feedings), with postobstructive diuresis, and with fluid loss from burns. Since two thirds of body water is in the intracellular fluid compartment, equilibration from losses of extracellular fluid will result in water loss from cells, a trigger for thirst and the release of ADH from the hypothalamus. Thus, *pure water loss* (or *pure water deprivation*, or *hypernatremic* or *hypertonic dehydration*) is characterized early in its development by intense thirst. Indeed, the perpetuation of this condition in situations where water is available suggests a blunting of normal mechanisms of thirst or of the response to thirst. Since extracellular fluid volume is fairly well maintained in states of pure water deprivation, skin turgor, blood pressure and pulse are relatively normal.[11,21]

The clinical presentation in this condition has been likened to the symptom complex in hyperglycemia and other hyperosmolar states that cause brain-cell dehydration. Once significant pure water loss develops, mental-status changes ensue, beginning with mild confusion and progressing to obtundation and coma. Profound neurologic damage has been reported in children. The neuropsychiatric symptoms may affect the sense of thirst and further hinder the ability to replace fluids. Symptoms seem to be more severe when hypernatremia develops rapidly. Fatigue, muscular weakness and low-grade fever have also been reported with hypernatremic dehydration.

The major laboratory finding of pure water loss is hypernatremia.

DEHYDRATION IN THE TERMINALLY ILL

Dehydrated terminally ill patients usually present with mixed disorders of salt and water depletion, resulting typically from abnormal GI or renal losses, normal water losses from the skin, lungs, or kidneys, and failure to replace these losses. Isotonic dehydration, a condition that is generally overlooked in discussions of the symptoms of fluid and electrolyte disorders, may occur.

Clinicians with a special interest in the care of the terminally ill[4,9,15] describe thirst and dry mouth in dehydrated patients, but do not report encountering the other worrisome symptoms—headache, nausea and vomiting, or cramps—that are cited in some reviews of water deprivation. In the author's experience, thirst and xerostomia are the only seriously troubling symptoms commonly encountered in dehydrated terminally ill patients. These symptoms may be satisfactorily relieved by amounts of fluid too small to significantly reverse metabolic abnormalities[7,25] or by maintaining moisture in the oral cavity with water, ice chips, or various forms of artificial saliva. Postural hypotension may be bothersome in ambulatory patients. Bed-bound patients report primarily lethargy, drowsiness, and fatigue, but these symptoms are rarely a source of much distress. Mental status changes that foster and perpetuate salt and water deficiencies may obliterate the awareness of suffering. Indeed, patients who become dehydrated may be too apathetic to be bothered by symptoms produced by this disorder. Personal observations of terminally ill patients suggest that nausea and vomiting are frequent causes but not regular sequelae of hyponatremic dehydration or other forms of dehydration.

The decision to administer fluids to a dehydrated patient is often determined by the symbolic or emotional meaning of such measures to the patient, family, and caretakers. However, insofar as the physical comfort of the patient guides management (or until more systematic studies are available), dehydration in dying patients should be viewed as a disorder with relatively benign symptoms. Successful treatment of the discomfort of thirst and a dry mouth, as described in Section E, probably does not require rehydration. Administration of salt and water by enteral (oral or, sometimes, rectal[15]), subcutaneous,[6] or intravenous routes should be considered for the purpose of restoring health and prolonging life, and may be easily justified in selected patients (e.g., those who still enjoy meaningful well-being but cannot ingest liquids). Correction of hypernatremia or hyponatremia may occasionally be indicated to provide symptomatic relief. However, when the goal of management is the relief of suffering, treatment generally can be confined to simple comfort measures in the form of mouth care.

REFERENCES

1. Arieff AI, Schmidt RW: Fluid and electrolyte disorders and the central nervous system. In Maxwell MH, Kleeman CR (eds): Clinical Disorders of Fluid and Electrolyte Metabolism, 3rd ed. New York, McGraw-Hill, 1980
2. Arieff AI, Guisado R: Effects on the central nervous system of hypernatremic and hyponatremic states. Kidney Int 10:104–116, 1976
3. Arieff AI, Llach F, Massry SG: Neurological manifestations and morbidity of hyponatremia: Correlation with brain water and electrolytes. Medicine (Baltimore) 55:121–129, 1976
4. Baines MJ: Control of other symptoms. In Saunders CM (ed): The Management of Terminal Disease. Chicago, Year Book Medical Publishers, 1978
5. Beecher HW: The Measurement of Subjective Responses. New York, Oxford University Press, 1959
6. Berger EY: Nutrition by hypodermoclysis. J Am Geriatr Soc 34:199–203, 1984
7. Black DAK, McCance RA, Young WF: A study of dehydration by means of balance experiments. J Physiol (Lond) 102:406–414, 1944
8. Brenner BM, Rector FC Jr: The Kidney, 2nd ed. Philadelphia, WB Saunders, 1981
9. Cassileth PA: Common medical complications. In Cassileth BR, Cassileth PA (eds): Clinical Care of the Terminal Cancer Patient. Philadelphia, Lea & Febiger, 1982
10. Edelman IS, Leibman J, O'Meara MP, Birkenfeld LW: Interrelations between serum sodium concentration, serum osmolarity and total exchangeable sodium, total exchangeable potassium and total body water. J Clin Invest 37:1236–1256, 1958
11. Elkinton JR, Danowski TS, Winkler AW: Hemodynamic charges in salt depletion and in dehydration. J Clin Invest 25:120–129, 1946
12. Epstein FH: Signs and symptoms of electrolyte disorders. In Maxwell MH, Kleeman CR (eds): Clinical Disorders of Fluid and Electrolyte Metabolism, 3rd ed. New York, McGraw-Hill, 1980
13. Fishman RA: Neurological manifestations of hyponatremia. In Vinken PJ, Bruyn GW (eds): Handbook of Clinical Neurology, 28. Amsterdam, Elsevier, 1976
14. Ladell WSS, Waterlow JC, Hudson MF: Desert climate: Physiological and clinical observations. Lancet 2:491–497, 527–531, 1944
15. Lamerton R: Care of the Dying, rev and expanded ed. New York: Penguin Books, 1980.
16. Leaf A: The clinical and physiologic significance of the serum sodium concentration. N Engl J Med 267:24–30, 77–83, 1962
17. Leaf, A, Cotran R: Renal Pathophysiology. New York, Oxford University Press, 1976
18. Marriott HL: Water and Salt Depletion. Springfield, IL, Charles C Thomas, 1950
19. McCance RA: Experimental sodium chloride deficiency in man. Proc R Soc Lond 119(series B):245–268, 1936
20. McCance RA: Medical problems in mineral metabolism. III. Experimental human salt deficiency. Lancet 1:823–830, 1936
21 Nadal JW, Pedersen S, Maddock WG: A comparison between dehydration from salt loss and from water deprivation. J Clin Invest 20:691–703, 1941
22. Rose DB: Clinical Physiology of Acid-Base and Electrolyte Disorders. New York, McGraw-Hill, 1977
23. Ross EJ, Christie SBM: Hypernatremia. Medicine (Baltimore) 48:441–473, 1969
24. Schroeder HA: Renal failure associated with low extracellular sodium chloride: The low salt syndrome. JAMA 141:117–124, 1949
25. Winkler AW, Danowski TS, Elkinton JR, Peters JP: Electrolyte and fluid studies during water deprivation and starvation in human subjects, and the effect of ingestion of fish, of carbohydrate, and of salt solutions. J Clin Invest 23:807–815, 1944

K.   Neuropsychiatric Symptoms and the Management of Brain Tumors

INTRODUCTION

Frank delirium and stupor are characteristic features of the terminal phase of many malignancies, particularly those that affect the brain directly or that cause failure of the liver, kidney, or respiratory system. A variety of subtle neuropsychiatric disorders are extremely common in patients with far-advanced cancer, although these symptoms, like mild weakness, are commonly either not severe enough to command attention or are ascribed to the general deterioration of health, the stress of being ill, and the effects of treatment. Sometimes notable are distinct nonfunctional behavioral and emotional disorders—apathy, lability, shallow affect, lack of inhibition, selective inattention, minimization of the consequences of illness, and apraxia—which are not included within gross diagnostic categories such as "acute brain syndrome" or "organic brain syndrome."[4]

Detection of the earliest signs of neuropsychiatric disorders allows the clinician to pursue a correct diagnosis, provide definitive treatment, offer palliative measures, and strengthen the support system so that the family can better tolerate the patient's disturbed mental state. Regular detailed attention to the mental status examination will sharpen the physician's awareness of the ubiquity of mood swings, mild behavioral changes, and slight intellectual impairment. Help may be provided by formal testing, using, for example, the Mini-Mental State Examination.[9] Subtle neuropsychiatric disturbances may first become apparent to the clinician as a vague sense of discomfort in the interview, as a feeling that the patient is eccentric, strange, unlikeable, or uncooperative. Suspect organic brain dysfunction when you, the family, or staff begin to avoid or dislike the patient; systematic mental status evaluation should follow.

Mood disorders—grief, depression, fear, and anxiety—are also commonly observed in dying patients. These emotional states, as discussed in Chapter 6, may be associated with disturbances in attention, memory, and other facets of the mental status and are occasionally mistaken for the "organic" conditions described in this section. Conversely, mood and behavioral changes associated with medical conditions may be incorrectly attributed to a psychiatric disorder. One psychiatric liaison service reported that 40% of referred cancer patients had organic brain disease; 26% had been given the diagnosis of depression but had an organic brain syndrome.[11]

PATHOPHYSIOLOGY[13]

While most gross disturbances of mentation are readily recognized and characterized, the entire array of neuropsychiatric disorders does not easily lend itself to a simple diagnostic system. Two classification schemes are useful in approaching neuropsychiatric disorders in the cancer patient. First, a number of neuropsychiatric syndromes can be considered, as described in Table 2K-1: stupor, coma, and related disturbances of depressed consciousness; delirium and other acute confusional states; dementia; anxiety disorders; the affective disorders; personality or other behavioral changes; and amnestic, delusional, and hallucinatory states.[12] Each of these syndromes implies a differential diagnosis and a characteristic treatment approach.

TABLE 2K-1
Neuropsychiatric Syndromes in Terminal Illness

Depressed consciousness, stupor, coma
Delirium and acute confusional states
Dementia
Anxiety disorders
Affective disorders
  Depression
  Mania (including steroid-related)
Personality changes—associated especially with metabolic disorders and tumor in the central
  nervous system (CNS)
Delusional syndromes—seen especially with stimulant drugs
Hallucinosis—seen especially with sensory deprivation, drug withdrawal, and seizure
  disorders
Amnestic states—especially Wernicke–Korsakoff psychosis
Dysphasia (mistaken for confusion)
Preexisting neuropsychiatric disorders

Second, the symptoms may be approached from a pathophysiologic or neuropathologic scheme.[7,8] Major diagnostic categories include the following:

Local or metastatic complications of the tumor. A first consideration is usually whether the neuropsychiatric symptom is a manifestation of cancer metastasizing to the brain or meninges; the management of brain tumors, cerebral edema, and seizures is discussed later in this section. Organ failure and infection are other common precipitants of confusional states.

Paraneoplastic syndromes, including both neurologic disease produced "at a distance" by the tumor (listed in Section L, Weakness) and neuropsychiatric manifestations of systemic paraneoplastic syndromes (especially the endocrinopathies noted in Section N).

Complications of treatment, including toxic effects of therapy[6] and nonspecific effects of pain, sleep deprivation, grief, and anxiety.

Symptoms unrelated to the cancer and its management, including those due to preexisting conditions.

Table 2K-2 presents an extensive list of diagnoses that may be considered in evaluating a neuropsychiatric disturbance. A knowledge of the patient's underlying illness and of the likelihood of various complications of the disease and its treatment can guide the physician in identifying which of the vast number of possible underlying conditions is producing neuropsychiatric symptoms. Drug-related conditions are especially worth considering as a cause for altered consciousness,[3] as illustrated below:

Case Example

A 65-year-old man with multiple chronic medical problems presented to the hospital with ataxia and two episodes of loss of consciousness. He was found to have a cerebellar tumor. The patient and family shunned any major med-

TABLE 2K-2
Common Causes of Confusional States in Terminal Illness

INTRACRANIAL PROCESS
    Meningeal
      Meningitis
      Carcinomatosis
      Subarachnoid hemorrhage
    CNS
      Tumor (primary and metastatic)
      Paraneoplastic syndromes—limbic encephalitis, multifocal leukoencephalopathy
      Radiation toxicity
      Seizure disorders, postconvulsive states
      Abscess, encephalitis
      Hemorrhage, thrombosis, embolism, thrombophlebitis, hypertensive encephalopathy,
        hyperviscosity syndrome, vasculitis (*e.g.*, disseminated intravascular coagulation,
        subacute bacterial endocarditis), superior vena cava syndrome
      Trauma
      Idiopathic dementia

DRUGS (toxic and idiosyncratic reactions)
    Sedative–hypnotics
      Barbiturates, glutethimide
      Benzodiazepines, meprobamate
      Chloral hydrate, paraldehyde
      Antihistamines
      Bromides
    Antipsychotics (often used for antiemetic properties)
    Antidepressants
    Stimulants
      Caffeine
      Amphetamines
      Methylxanthines (bronchodilators)
    Opiates
    Anticholinergics (including neuroleptic and tricyclic drugs)
    Alcohol
    Corticosteroids
    Salicylates, other nonsteroidal anti-inflammatory drugs
    Anticonvulsants
    Chemotherapy, especially:
      L-Asparaginase
      Procarbazine
      Intrathecal methotrexate
    Miscellaneous
      Cimetidine
      Topical and local anesthetics
      Antiarrhythmic
      Metoclopramide
      Digitalis
      Antihypertensive
      Sympathomimetics
      Hormones, oral contraceptives
      Disulfiram, metronidazole (alcohol reaction)
      Antiparkinsonian

TABLE 2K-2 *(continued)*

DRUG WITHDRAWAL
Barbiturates
Chloral hydrate
Alcohol
Stimulants
Corticosteroids

METABOLIC AND ENDOCRINE
Hepatic failure
Renal failure
Respiratory failure—hypoxia, hypercarbia
Acidosis, alkalosis
Hyper- and hypo-
  natremia
  kalemia
  calcemia
  magnesemia
  osmolality
  (including hyperparathyroidism, syndrome of inappropriate antidiuretic hormone, and
  disorders of steroid metabolism)
Cushing's syndrome, Addison's syndrome
Thyrotoxicosis, hypothyroidism
Hypopituitarism
Hypoglycemia (paraneoplastic, hepatic), hyperglycemia
Vitamin deficiency (B_6, B_{12}, thiamine)

HYPERTHERMIA, HYPOTHERMIA

SYSTEMIC INFECTIONS especially pneumonia, sepsis

CIRCULATORY FAILURE
Hypovolemia, anemia
Cardiogenic shock
Septic shock

NONSPECIFIC FACTORS (often aggravating confusion but not the primary cause)
Sleep deprivation
Stress, pain, discomfort
Anxiety, depression
Sensory deprivation, perceptual distortion, isolation
Debility, advanced age

ical intervention. He was sent home on phenytoin 200 mg daily. A good therapeutic level was noted on discharge. He continued a number of previous medications, including digitalis, quinidine, and cimetidine. Two weeks later, he became increasingly ataxic. Progression of the tumor was suspected. He was unable to attend follow-up appointments at the hospital. He eventually became unmanageable at home owing to falling, uncooperative behavior, and occasional belligerence. On readmission, his serum phenytoin level was $3\frac{1}{2}$ times the upper limits of a therapeutic level. Two weeks after the anticonvulsant was discontinued (and after the cimetidine dosage was reduced to once a day), his phenytoin level reached a low therapeutic range, and he returned to his baseline mental status.

PRINCIPLES OF MANAGEMENT

Many families are terribly disturbed by the patient's abnormal thoughts or behavior. Relatives may blame the patient for acting improperly, and they may feel shame, irritation, resentment, or frank anger. The husband who can no longer manage the monthly bills or discipline the children, the wife who loses interest in homemaking or leaves the gas stove on, or the elderly parent who cannot cooperate with feeding or bathing—all can come to seem hateful to the family.

Confusion, *per se,* does not require pharmacologic treatment. When neuropsychiatric symptoms trouble the family, yet do not bother the patient or lead to dangerous or noncompliant behavior, management requires discussion, explanation, and support, not necessarily drugs. Repeated discussions of how the patient's actions are being affected by the tumor may help the family attribute irritability, forgetfulness, self-neglect, and other improper conduct to the disease rather than to the willful misbehavior of the person with the disease. However, such a distinction—"It's not him, it's the illness"—is not readily made by many laypersons, especially those who are closely involved with the patient.

> *He's just behaving badly, taking advantage of us. If he really wanted to help out, he could.*

Similarly, when the semicomatose patient makes random or bizarre gestures, the family can be gently advised not to interpret these behaviors as conscious or meaningful, yet professional counsel may be ignored.

When confusion bothers the patient or is associated with worrisome behavior, further interventions should be considered. Confused patients—especially those exhibiting agitation, disorientation, misinterpretation of the environment, and an inability to repress primitive (often paranoid) feelings—can be overwhelmed by terror, suspiciousness, confusion, nightmares, and a distressing inability to focus attention; they deserve vigorous treatment. Troublesome behaviors (such as restlessness or agitation) also demand intervention when they interfere with household function, particularly sleep, or with important medical care, or otherwise seem dangerous to the patient and his or her support network.

Family resistance to pharmacologic treatment is common. Family members may object to the patient being "drugged" or labeled as "crazy." They may express concern about medications that "alter consciousness" or produce side-effects. The family can be helped to appreciate that confusion has a significant morbidity, including falls, self-destructive behavior, interference with therapy, and the patient's fright.

General Measures for Confusional States

Depressed Consciousness
In illnesses manifested primarily by drowsiness or apathetic disorientation, supportive measures include the following:

Handle tasks previously carried out by the patient (*e.g.,* feeding, bathing, skin care, mouth care, monitoring bladder and bowel function—see Section L, Weakness) and manage incontinence.

Prevent injury (*e.g.,* from automobile accidents, falls, medication errors and ingestions, burns and fires from smoking or use of matches) by limiting hazardous activities, and by using restraints and barriers (including locking doors and closets, changing locks, shutting off or removing knobs from stoves, removing matches).

Provide orientation (*e.g.*, explain to patients where they are, who you are, why they are drowsy, what is happening in the room).

Avoid medications that further depress consciousness.

Coma

In the patient with advanced stupor or coma, additional tasks may be considered:

Prevent eye damage—apply methylcellulose drops q4h prn, shut lids with an eye pad and tape.

Provide mouth care (see Section E).

Care for skin daily and turn frequently.

Maintain a clear airway and suction secretions.

Consider an indwelling urinary catheter or, in males, a condom catheter.

Discuss potentially disturbing symptoms with the family, including
Roving eye movements
Respiratory abnormalities (including hyperventilation or Kussmaul's breathing, Cheyne–Stokes, and other breathing patterns with periods of apnea)
Seizures, posturing, and other motor activity
The ability or inability of the patient to appreciate pain

Prescribe less attention to vital signs, nutrition, urinary output, nonessential medication, and other supportive measures that are unlikely to provide comfort. Explain to the family and other caretakers the appropriateness of such steps and discuss concerns about not feeding the patient, stopping intravenous fluids, etc.

Prepare the family for the death (see Chap. 11).

Delirium

In mental states characterized primarily by agitation or confusion, appropriate measures include the following:

Handle tasks previously managed by self-care, as described above.

Prevent self-injury, either by pharmacologic measures that lessen agitation or by the use of bedrails, poseys, and other physical restraints and barriers.

Counsel the family on avoiding injury (*e.g.*, being bitten by the patient, being struck if the patient is combative).

Provide a friendly, secure atmosphere, and orient the patient reassuringly to new events with the following:
Well-lit rooms
Clocks, calendars
Familiar faces and objects
Identifying who is in the room and what they are doing
Attempting to engage the patient in discussions about available memories, usually those of the distant past
Minimizing distractions and disturbances (*e.g.*, loud noises, unfamiliar faces, frightening procedures, strange rooms)

Avoid medications that impair orientation.

Avoid interruption of sleep.

Gently correct the patient's misinterpretations and misperceptions. Help the patient examine and clarify misidentified phenomena and, if possible, explain how the illness is causing confusion.

Your mind may be playing tricks on you. When you're sick like this, you can sometimes have trouble concentrating, or you tend to imagine things.

A sense of amusement about disorientation can be helpful for the family and caretakers, and some patients can laugh about their confusion, but beware that patients can be badly offended and become more suspicious when made the object of humor.

Pharmacologic Treatment of Confusional States[1,2,14]

Neuroleptic (antipsychotic) medications are the drugs of first choice for managing confusional states. They are useful in reducing bizarre, troubling thoughts and in controlling restlessness and agitation.

Many neuropsychiatric symptoms will appear or worsen in the night and will be less tolerable in the evening hours, when the family expects and desires quiet and rest. Unfortunately, outside support is also less available at this time. Therefore, maximal pharmacologic intervention is usually required at night.

Single nighttime doses are often effective, but additional prn orders for the treatment of insomnia and restlessness can be provided. Successful treatment does not necessarily abolish bizarre thoughts or behaviors, but should reduce their frequency, severity, and urgency and resolve major difficulties of patient management.

Haloperidol (Haldol) is usually the drug of choice. It is among the least sedating and least toxic agents in the neuroleptic class. Rapid control of acute confusional states is possible with little risk of life-threatening side-effects (*e.g.,* cardiovascular toxicity or respiratory depression). Extrapyramidal effects are relatively common with haloperidol and occasionally require the addition of antiparkinsonian drugs such as benztropine mesylate (Cogentin) or trihexyphenidyl (Artane). The infrequent development of acute dystonic reactions can be handled quickly with diphenhydramine (Benadryl) or benztropine mesylate.

Failure to control agitation with haloperidol usually represents a failure to administer adequate amounts of the drug. Low doses (0.5–1.0 mg po or IM) are reasonable when beginning treatment in an elderly, debilitated patient with mild agitation, but if no response is noted, the dose can be repeated hourly and can quickly be increased to 5.0 to 10.0 mg po or IM, the usual initial treatment for a younger, physically healthy but severely disturbed patient. The patient should be medicated hourly until the desired effect is achieved. Later, the dose is repeated prn recurrence of symptoms. Eventually, a total daily dosage requirement can be estimated (usually amounting to 50%–100% of the daily dose initially required to produce sedation), and it can be given over 24 hours in two divided doses. Additional prn doses should also be prescribed. Oral doses are roughly equal in potency to parenteral doses, but slower acting.

In the phenothiazine class of neuroleptics, thioridazine (Mellaril) is mildly sedating, has a low incidence of extrapyramidal reactions, and may be selected for patients who do not tolerate haloperidol. Because rapid (*e.g.,* hourly) administration holds greater risk of overdosage and toxicity, including cardiovascular effects, an interval of 2 to 4 hours between doses is preferable. Thioridazine has prominent anticholinergic activity, often causes postural hypotension, and has no antiemetic action.

When sedation or antiemetic effect is desirable, chlorpromazine (Thorazine) may be considered. Compared to thioridazine, chlorpromazine is an excellent antiemetic, may have less anticholinergic action but has similar significant cardiovascular toxicity, including postural hypotension.

Perphenazine (Trilafon) and prochlorperazine (Compazine) may be prescribed for antiemetic effects (see Section A) but are associated with a significant incidence of extrapyramidal reactions, which occur when high doses are employed to control psychosis and agitation. Perphenazine is occasionally useful for managing confusion because, like haloperidol, it causes relatively little sedation and hypotension.

NEUROLEPTIC MEDICATIONS

Haloperidol (Haldol)	0.5–10.0 mg po, or IM q1h (usual dose—1.0–5.0 mg po or IM q1h until symptoms abate, then 3–20 mg po qd in 2–3 divided doses)
Thioridazine (Mellaril)	25–50 mg po or IM q2–4h (usual dose—50–400 mg po qd)
Chlorpromazine (Thorazine)	25–50 mg po or IM q2–4h (usual dose—50–800 mg po qd)

Minor tranquilizers, particularly benzodiazepines, should generally be avoided in confusional states, since they may aggravate disorientation or produce "paradoxical" agitative reactions. However, the usefulness of these drugs in treating the alcohol and sedative–hypnotic withdrawal syndromes is well documented, and these sedatives may occasionally be effective in other agitated states, especially when anxiety is a major contributing factor (*e.g.*, some patients with hypoxia). In addition, a few patients with mild confusion or nocturnal restlessness do not tolerate neuroleptic agents well, usually because they suffer prolonged sedation, yet can be managed successfully with benzodiazepines. Short-acting agents—oxazepam (Serax) and lorazepam (Ativan)—are often preferable to longer-acting drugs—diazepam (Valium) or chlordiazepoxide (Librium). In contrast to the antipsychotic agents, benzodiazepines do not produce anticholinergic side-effects or cardiac toxicity. However, these agents may occasionally cause significant respiratory depression in patients with advanced pulmonary disease.

Physostigmine (Antilirium) 0.5–2.0 mg IM q30–120 min prn should be considered as an antidote to anticholinergic drug-induced delirium (*e.g.*, from scopolamine or tricyclic antidepressants).

Lithium may be effective in preventing steroid psychosis,[5] but has not been studied for use once such drug-induced mental status changes occur.

BRAIN TUMORS AND CEREBRAL EDEMA

Presentation[9]

Metastatic brain lesions frequently occur with lung and breast cancers and are relatively common with melanoma and renal cell carcinoma, but can also be seen with a variety of other tumors. Metastases typically develop in the cerebrum, but are occasionally found in the cerebellum and brainstem.

Intracranial metastases usually present with headache, seizures, and mental status changes. They may also be signalled by such nonspecific problems as nausea, vomiting, and lethargy, especially when cerebral edema and increased intracranial pressure develop. The headache of increased intracranial pressure is often generalized, may wake the patient in the early morning (after prolonged recumbency), and may be aggravated by coughing and Valsalva's maneuver. Brain tumors may also produce a variety of localized findings, such as inattention and other thought disorders, changes in affect, hallucinations, aphasia, visual disturbances, anosmia, numbness, weakness, reflex changes, ataxia, and incontinence. Subtle (and occasionally overlooked) neuropsychological disturbances include an erratic memory, childishness, agitation, irritability, easy frustration, and restlessness.

The diagnosis of a brain tumor in an advanced cancer patient is often made on clinical evidence and is confirmed by computed tomography (CT) scan.*

Management[15]

General Care

In addition to many of the general and pharmacologic measures cited earlier in the section, interventions may be targetted at the patient's specific neurologic deficits. For instance, patients with impaired intellect may benefit from establishment of a simplified, stable environment that requires less reliance on their diminished cognitive function. Caretakers can be instructed to provide and repeat careful, clear, simple instructions. Patients with hemianopsia should be approached from the side of normal vision, and may need to be reminded to attend to the other side. Diplopia may be more tolerable when one eye is patched. Physical therapy, braces, and various aids will assist the hemiparetic or ataxic patient.

Treatment of the Tumor

Cerebral metastases will frequently respond to radiation therapy, including, at times, implantation techniques and second courses.[10] Some cell types respond to chemotherapy, including intrathecal or intraventricular administration. Surgery is often required for the management of primary brain tumors and occasionally is employed for the initial diagnosis and management of metastatic tumors. Surgery is also used increasingly for patients with recurrence of disease after chemotherapy and radiation, and for the management of the presumed sole metastasis in otherwise disease-free patients, especially those with melanoma, osteosarcoma, or renal cell carcinoma.

Symptomatic Treatment

Shunting for hydrocephalus can be a beneficial palliative measure.

Glucocorticosteroids are given to patients who are candidates for the antitumor therapies noted above. In selected other patients, steroids may be administered with the goals of relieving symptoms from the cerebral tumor and edema and, perhaps, of prolonging survival. Such therapy will frequently diminish headache and vomiting. Variable, often excellent and prolonged, improvement can be anticipated for confusion, visual disturbances, and other neurologic symptoms.

A number of steroid regimens have been employed for managing cerebral tumors and edema, but rigorous studies are not available to compare various steroid mainte-

---

*Carcinomatous meningitis commonly presents with cranial nerve signs, but may also produce headache, aching or stiffness of the neck or back, nausea, weakness, confusion, and seizures. Lower extremity weakness and bladder dysfunction can occur without a sensory level. The diagnosis is facilitated by cytologic examination of cytocentrifuged cerebrospinal fluid (CSF). Radiation and chemotherapy (systemic and local) have been useful in selected tumors.

TABLE 2K-3
Use of Steroids for Cerebral Tumors and Edema

Steroid dosage should be guided by monitoring neurologic signs, papilledema, and mental status.

Begin with dexamethasone 4 mg po 4id with meal or snack.

If practical, prescribe either antacids or cimetidine 4id for patients who continue steroids for more than a week. Prescribe both drugs if the patient has a significant history of upper gastrointestinal (GI) ulcers or bleeding gastritis or is receiving other drugs likely to cause these complications.

Side-effects of steroids include hyperglycemia, hypokalemia, increased susceptibility to infection, and masking of fever and inflammation. Neuropsychiatric effects are common when steroids are prescribed at high doses. Steroid myopathy may cause weakness.

After about 6 weeks of steroid administration, adrenal insufficiency may develop when steroids are discontinued or tapered to low levels (*e.g.*, to dexamethasone 1–2 mg/day), especially if severe stress occurs.

If no significant response to steroids is noted after 1 week, discontinue treatment.

If a fair to excellent response occurs, continue steroids for 2 weeks more, then begin to taper the daily dose of dexamethasone each week by 2 mg until the dosage reaches 4 mg/day. The side-effects from steroids may be considerable even at this dose, and downward adjustment can be continued cautiously, but often leads to recurrence of significant neurologic deficits.

If symptoms worsen during tapering, the dexamethasone dose should be increased 4 mg/day.

Any worsening of the patient's neurologic condition can be treated with an 8–16-mg/day increase in dexamethasone. Doses of dexamethasone of around 100 mg/day are not infrequent after repeated periods of neurologic stabilization, tapering of medication, further deterioration, and escalation of the steroids. If the quality of life is such that continued treatment is pointless, the medication should be discontinued.

nance doses or tapering schedules nor to evaluate prophylactic treatment for steroid-induced ulcers. Table 2K-3 presents a method for administering steroids to patients with brain tumors and edema.

For patients in whom the life-prolonging potential of steroids is undesirable or for whom steroid therapy is contraindicated or unsuccessful, symptomatic management may include administration of analgesics and antiemetics. Mental obtundation supervenes in many of these patients, leading progressively, and with little suffering, to stupor, coma, and death.

Seizures

Prophylactic administration of an anticonvulsant is generally recommended when an intracranial tumor is present. The prevention of seizures is particularly important for ambulatory patients who might harm themselves if they lose consciousness (*e.g.*, those who are driving cars).

Seizures in the patient with advanced cancer are treated or prevented with the same anticonvulsant-drug regimens used for other epileptic patients. The presumed association of the seizure with a cerebral tumor and cerebral edema, however, generally means that steroid treatment should also be instituted. Treatment for generalized seizures should begin with phenytoin, starting with a loading dose (1.0 g over a day), followed by 300 mg qd in divided doses. If seizures continue to occur, the blood level should be checked: if the level is low, the dose of phenytoin should be increased; if the level is within therapeutic range, add a second drug—carbamazepine (Tegretol) 200 mg po bid or phenobarbital 90 mg po hs (after a loading dose)—and adjust subsequent doses as needed. Both carbamazepine and phenobarbital can be used alone for patients who are intolerant of or allergic to phenytoin. Carbamazepine is generally favored for partial seizures (e.g., temporal lobe epilepsy and focal motor seizures) and for patients who are refractory to treatment with phenytoin. Toxicity from anticonvulsant medications includes drowsiness and a variety of neurologic changes that can be incorrectly attributed to the progression of cerebral tumor or edema.

Status epilepticus, a rare occurrence, is treated acutely with intravenous diazepam 5 to 10 mg every 5 to 10 minutes until seizures stop; treatment with a first-line anticonvulsant agent should begin immediately.

Patients with progressive brain tumors commonly develop difficulties in taking oral medication. Since phenobarbital has a long plasma half-life (4 days), omission of the drug for a day is rarely a concern when therapeutic blood levels have been obtained. The plasma half-life of phenytoin averages about a day, but is markedly variable, and thus daily or more frequent doses may be required to prevent seizures. Carbamazepine must be given twice a day.

When anticonvulsants cannot be taken by mouth, three options are available: inserting a feeding tube, giving parenteral treatment, or stopping medication. Anticonvulsant suppositories are not available. For the patient who is irreversibly comatose or never had seizures, the medication can generally be discontinued. For patients with established seizure disorders, withdrawal of treatment is likely to lead to recurrent seizures or status epilepticus, and so the anticonvulsants should usually be continued, if at all practical, whenever survival for more than a few days is likely. Regardless of decisions made on behalf of the patient, prophylactic anticonvulsant administration should be considered for the comfort of family members who are likely to find seizures extremely upsetting. Because phenytoin is difficult to give parenterally and carbamazepine is available only in oral form, the drug of choice for chronic parenteral anticonvulsant treatment is phenobarbital.

A few words of advice to the family on the acute management of seizures can be enormously helpful in relieving anxiety:

> Ordinarily, you don't have to do anything for a seizure. In the hospital, we just stand back and let it happen, except to try to make sure the patient doesn't fall or hit any sharp objects. When the seizure stops, you can place him comfortably in the bed or wherever he is, and just let him wake up. Don't try to hold him down or put anything into his mouth until he's alert again, and don't be surprised if he is breathing hard or bites his tongue and has a little blood in his mouth. If you turn him on his side, he is less likely to let the secretions in his mouth slip into his lungs.

SELECTED REFERENCES

1. Anonymous: Drugs for psychiatric disorders. Med Lett Drugs Ther 25:45–52, 1983
2. Anonymous: Drugs for the elderly. Med Lett Drugs Ther 25:81–84, 1983
3. Anonymous: Drugs that cause psychiatric symptoms. Med Lett Drugs Ther 23:9–12, 1981
4. Bear D, Arana G: Neurological syndromes affecting emotions and behavior. In Guggenheim FG, Nadelson C (eds): Major Psychiatric Disorders: Overviews and Selected Readings, pp 365–372. New York, Elsevier Biomedical, 1982

5. Goggans FC, Weisberg LJ, Koran LM: Lithium prophylaxis of prednisone psychosis: A case report. J Clin Psychiatry 44:111–112, 1983
6. Goldberg ID, Bloomer WD, Dawson DM: Nervous system toxic effects of cancer therapy. JAMA 247:1437–1441, 1982
7. Henson RA, Urich H: Cancer and the Nervous System: the Neurological Manifestation of Systemic Malignant Disease. Oxford, Blackwell Scientific Publications, 1982
8. Hochberg F: Neurological aspects of systemic tumors. In Isselbacher KJ, Adams RD, Braunwauld E, Petersdorf RG, Wilson JD (eds): Harrison's Principles of Internal Medicine, 9th ed, Update I. New York, McGraw-Hill, 1981
9. Knights EB, Folstein MF: Unsuspected emotional and cognitive disturbance in medical patients. Ann Intern Med 87:723–724, 1977
10. Kurup P, Reddy S, Hendrickson FR: Results of reirradiation for cerebral metastases. Cancer 46:2587–2589, 1980
11. Levine PM, Silverfarb PM, Lipowski ZJ: Mental disorders in cancer patients: A study of 100 psychiatric referrals. Cancer 42:1385–1391, 1978
12. McEvoy JP: Organic brain syndromes. Ann Intern Med 95:212–220, 1981
13. Plum F, Posner JB: The Diagnosis of Stupor and Coma, 2nd ed. Philadelphia, FA Davis, 1972
14. Thompson TL, Moran MG, Nies AS: Drug therapy: Psychotropic drug use in the elderly. N Engl J Med 308:134–138, 194–199, 1983
15. Wilson CB, Fulton DS, Seager ML: Supportive management of the patient with malignant brain tumor. JAMA 244:1249–1251, 1980

L. Weakness and Fatigue

EVALUATION

Weakness and fatigue are nearly universal symptoms in late-stage cancer. Patients describe a variety of problems by using terms such as weakness, fatigue, tiredness, and lack of energy: generalized lassitude, weariness, and inability to sustain exertion; loss of motor power and easy muscular fatigability; spasticity or impaired mobility; ataxia; sleepiness or drowsiness; confusion (see Section K, Neuropsychiatric Symptoms); apathy, lack of interest, poor concentration, mental sluggishness, slowed motor activity, helplessness, and a sense of inadequacy (see Depression, Chapter 6); dizziness; and dyspnea. Careful questioning and examination are required to elucidate these forms of weakness and to distinguish episodic from constant symptoms. Two or more types of weakness frequently coexist. The following discussion focuses largely on loss of motor power and on neuromuscular fatigue.

Common causes of these symptoms are listed in Table 2L-1. *Localized* loss of strength may be associated with regional pain, swelling, spasticity, or similar problems that hinder neuromuscular exertion. Alternately, complaints reflect true motor weakness from localized neurologic or muscular disease. *Generalized* loss of strength and fatigue are frequent manifestations of many systemic processes, including drug toxicity. In advanced cancer, muscle wasting and the adverse consequences of disuse are common, as are paraneoplastic or remote effects of cancer, including cancer-associated asthenia.

While the neurologic literature suggests that flagrant carcinomatous neuromyopathies are rather rare, subtle presentation of these conditions can often be noted. Multiple paraneoplastic neurologic syndromes and classification schemes have been reported, including (1) degenerative conditions, which typically present with demen-

TABLE 2L-1
Conditions Presenting as Weakness and Fatigue

LOCALIZED WEAKNESS
Neurogenic
    Central nervous system (CNS) lesions (usually causing paresis and paresthesias and
        including carcinomatous meningitis and paraneoplastic syndromes)
    Peripheral nerve injury (especially entrapment or compression, but also paraneoplastic
        neuropathy and various metabolic, toxic, ischemic, and inflammatory etiologies [*e.g.*
        diabetic, alcoholic, B_{12} deficiency])
Muscular
    Myasthenia, localized
    Disuse atrophy
    Immobility due to swelling, stiffness, pain, tenderness, arthralgia, spasticity, etc.

GENERALIZED WEAKNESS
Neurogenic
    Polyneuropathy
    Carcinomatous neuromyopathies and cancer-associated asthenia
    Ataxia
    Spasticity, parkinsonism
    Neuropsychiatric—see Confusional States (Section K), Depression (Chap. 6)
Muscular
    Muscular wasting
        Malnutrition, weight loss
        Inactivity, disuse atrophy
        Myopathy—tumor related, treatment related (especially steroids)
    Myositis—polymyositis, dermatomyositis
    Myasthenia—myasthenia gravis and Eaton–Lambert syndrome
Systemic conditions
    Electrolyte abnormalities—K, Ca, Mg, PO_4
    Endocrine
        Addison's, panhypopituitarism
        Hypo-, hyperthyroidism
        Hyperglycemia
    Anemia
    Dehydration
    Renal failure
    Hepatic failure
    Cardiopulmonary failure
    Infection, inflammation, fever
    Malnutrition

tia or ataxia or with other neurologic deficits that might be attributed to intracranial
mass lesions, namely limbic encephalitis or bulbar encephalitis; encephalomyeloneu-
ropathy or progressive multifocal leukoencephalopathy; and subacute cerebellar
degeneration; and (2) conditions commonly presenting with peripheral weakness or
sensory changes, namely subacute necrotic myelopathy or subacute myelitis; subacute
motor neuropathy; pure sensory neuropathy; sensorimotor distal polyneuropathy; and
dorsal root ganglionitis. Unfortunately, their identification rarely assists in choosing
therapeutic measures.

MANAGEMENT

Specific treatments, especially for systemic conditions, pain and depression, can lead to dramatic resolution of weakness and fatigue. Section N reviews a number of reversible endocrinologic conditions that can present as profound weakness and that may be mistaken for advanced carcinomatosis and cancer-associated asthenia.

General measures to support the weak patient are outlined in Table 4-1, The Task of Physical Care. As patients become more debilitated, they can increasingly benefit from general measures to maintain comfort, to promote a sense of well-being, and to prevent the common sequelae of inactivity and inattention to self-care.

Mild Impairment

When weakness and fatigue first develop, the following suggestions for the patient may be offered:

1. Conserve energy for important events and chores.
2. Plan shorter excursions and tasks.
3. Plan for a rest period during the day.
4. Delegate responsibilities or get assistance, especially for less attractive chores.

The patient's or family's intuition and personal experience may tell them that bed rest is valuable or protective when one is sick. However, bed rest and immobility can promote muscle wasting and soreness, loss of conditioning, skin breakdown, disturbed sleep cycle, boredom, frustration, and a host of other problems. The physician should review the appropriateness of any limitations on physical activity and should encourage reasonable exercise. Patients who are inclined to "take to bed" or whose families encourage inactivity may benefit from suggestions to take walks, get out of the house, maintain participation in household tasks, continue independent self-care, and so on. Getting "tired out" from a pleasurable activity can be recommended:

> *This may leave you a little exhausted, but should help you keep up your strength.*

> *You're going to be somewhat limited by this weakness from the cancer, but you want to keep your muscles in shape by using them regularly.*

Trips for special occasions—movies, weddings, seeing home-bound friends or relatives—should be considered. The need for elaborate arrangements for the excursion—wheelchairs, portable oxygen, transportation, an attendant nurse, and so on—should be viewed as a challenge, not a deterrent.

Specific exercise prescriptions may be useful: the length and frequency of walks, range-of-motion exercises, and exercises for different muscle groups. Physical therapy consultation can be considered. The risk and likely consequences of falls (which are frequent inside and outside of institutions but much less commonly cause significant injury) or of other injuries should be weighed against the benefit, both physical and emotional, of mobility and independence.

Immobility may limit the patient's range of pleasures. A review of the patient's usual enjoyments may suggest which activities have been lost and which can be preserved. Many debilitated patients' lives consist largely of sleeping and watching the television, an unrewarding existence, which is occasionally relieved by the appearance of a visitor or a meal. Time for solitary reflection is rarely in short supply. Stimulation and diversion can distract the patient from the physical and psychosocial problems of advanced illness while improving the quality of remaining life. "Friendly visiting," especially to talk about oneself, is a favorite activity for many patients, while others prefer games, music, reading or being read to, drawing, and so on. Volunteers have been helpful when family members lack the time or ability to provide such diversion. Inexpensive cassette tape recorders are owned by many patients or can be purchased or borrowed, and tape libraries can offer musical or spoken programs to meet the wishes of most patients.

Moderate Impairment

When diminished strength and mobility impair the patient's activities of daily living, consider the following:

1. Aids for transfer and ambulation (*e.g.*, walkers or wheelchairs)
2. Aids for self-care (*e.g.*, bedside commode, rails in bathroom)
3. Outside help for the patient and for the support of family caretakers (*e.g.*, a home health aid for bathing)
4. Review of safety measures to prevent falling

"Compact care" is a term that describes efforts to maximize the patient's independence despite limitations in mobility. Objects that the patient can no longer reach by walking—a television, radio, or other entertainment, a commode or urinal, food and beverages, and various personal items—are brought to the room or bedside.

Severe Impairment

When patients become bed-bound or mostly bed-bound, consider the following measures:

1. Move important personal items to the bedside.
2. Check skin condition regularly; use heel guards, sheepskin, and massage.
3. Instruct on turning, positioning, and use of drawsheet and pillows.
4. Install rails, trapeze.
5. Provide aids for eating in bed—trays, flexible straws.
6. Institute bedpan, commode, urinal, incontinence care.
7. Begin exercises to maintain strength and mobility, including active and passive range-of-motion exercises.
8. Maintain oral hygiene.
9. Give massage for relaxation.
10. Review recreational activities.

Corticosteroids (*e.g.*, prednisone 5–10 mg po 2–3 times a day) are often useful as a "tonic" for tired or anorectic dying patients.

SPINAL CORD COMPRESSION

The early diagnosis of epidural cord compression proves to be quite difficult.[2,4,5] Many patients with this condition present with irreversible damage, whereas many others for whom this diagnosis is considered never develop significant neurologic problems.

Of those patients who develop compressive signs and proceed to significant cord injury, the vast majority will have back pain and evidence of metastatic disease on plain films of the spine, yet an uncertain, possibly small, proportion of patients with back pain, abnormal x-rays, and even myelographic evidence of epidural compression will suffer significant neurologic damage if not treated.

Pain localized over the spine is nearly a universal precursor of cord compression from epidural tumor and is usually a constant discomfort. The pain may be relatively acute or long-standing. Radicular pain, often worse in recumbency and aggravated by motion and straining, also occurs commonly. Weakness, progressing to paraplegia, may develop gradually or suddenly. Weakness without pain is rare. Urinary or fecal retention are signs of advanced disease and suggest that treatment is unlikely to successfully reverse neurologic damage.

On physical examination, significant cord compression is characterized by localized vertebral tenderness, pain on motion of the spine, weakness, sensory loss, and occasionally, sphincter dysfunction. Plain films of the spine show evidence of metastatic cancer in about 85% of patients with epidural metastases. A similar but less common syndrome of cord compression is produced by intramedullary metastases and is not associated with abnormal spine x-rays. While computerized tomography (CT) may be increasingly useful in assessing cord compression, myelography is currently the definitive diagnostic procedure.

Immediate treatment with steroids should be considered in all patients. Dexamethasone 10 mg IV, then 4 mg po q6h is the usual initial dosage, although higher doses (100 mg IV, then 24 mg po q6h) have been advocated.

When significant paresis has occurred, therapeutic results for epidural cord compression are often disappointing. Adequate prospective studies comparing radiation therapy and surgery are lacking. Radiation therapy provides definitive treatment with lymphomas and most solid tumors. Decompressive laminectomy may be chosen as the major modality of treatment when tumors are radioresistant or when symptoms develop after or during radiation therapy. When neurologic deficits progress rapidly (*i.e.*, over 1–3 days), surgery has been advocated as initial treatment, followed by radiation, but the outlook for good recovery is poor.

Cord compression in late-stage cancer can be approached as an emergency if the patient and physician are willing to proceed with myelography and either radiation or decompressive laminectomy in the hope of preserving function of the extremities and bowel and bladder innervation. Even when aggressive therapy holds promise of a few months or more of normal neurologic function, however, the prospect of hospitalization and either radiation or surgery may be more distasteful then living a bed-to-chair (or, often, bedridden) existence at home. Patients who are already severely debilitated or immobile will suffer further insult from paraparesis, but have much less to gain than do ambulatory patients from definitive treatment.

Patients commonly survive for at least a few months after epidural spinal cord compression occurs, regardless of whether treatment is initiated or successful. The patient who develops paraparesis will need an extensive program to prevent decubitus ulcers, maintain maximal mobility, establish a satisfactory bowel and bladder regimen, and adjust to a severely altered physical condition.[1] A wheelchair may allow for movement in and around the house and for travel outside the home. Physical therapy may be considered to learn transfer techniques, maintain range of motion, strengthen key muscles, prevent contractures, and select appropriate appliances.

SPASTICITY

A great number of drugs have been recommended for spasticity.[3,6] Dantrolene and baclofen are recommended when an upper motor neuron lesion is the underlying cause:

> Dantrolene (Dantrium) 25–100 mg po 2–4 times a day, beginning with 25 mg qd and increasing by 25-mg increments at 4–7-day intervals
> Baclofen (Lioresal) 5–20 mg po 3–4 times a day, beginning with 5 mg tid and gradually increasing by 5-mg dose increments

Common muscle spasms may respond to benzodiazepines (*e.g.*, diazepam 2–20 mg po 2–3 times a day) or agents such as the following:

> Cyclobenzaprine (Flexeril) 10–20 mg po 2–3 times a day
> Methocarbamol (Robaxin) 1.5 g po 4id for 2–3 days, then 1.0 g 4id

SELECTED REFERENCES

1. Dietz JH: Rehabilitation Oncology. New York, John Wiley & Sons, 1981
2. Gilbert RW, Kim J, Posner JP: Epidural spinal cord compression from metastatic tumor: Diagnosis and treatment. Ann Neurol 3:40–51, 1978
3. Merrit JL: Management of spasticity in spinal cord injury. Mayo Clin Proc 56:614–622, 1981
4. Rodichok LD, Harper GR, Ruckdeschel JC et al: Early diagnosis of spinal epidural metastases. Am J Med 70:1181–1188, 1981
5. Rodriguez M, Dinapoli RP: Spinal cord compression with special reference to metastatic epidural tumors. Mayo Clin Proc 55:442–448, 1980
6. Young RR, Delwaide PJ: Drug therapy: spasticity. N Engl J Med 304:28–33, 96–99, 1981

M. Infections, Fevers, and Sweats

INFECTIONS

The oncology and infectious disease literature deals extensively with the prophylaxis and management of infections in those cancer patients who can still benefit from aggressive measures to eradicate their malignancy. In many instances, the infectious agent is an unusual or hospital-acquired organism, the patient has an extensive history of exposure to antibiotics, and the host defense system is severely compromised by the malignancy or its treatment. In such situations, the patient's impaired inflammatory response may make the diagnosis difficult, while the course of an infection is likely to be rapidly fatal. Elaborate inpatient diagnostic and treatment regimens are appropriate for many of these patients.

For the outpatient with late-stage advanced cancer, compromised host defenses may also influence the presentation and course of infections, but profound granulocytopenia is uncommon (except in terminal patients with hematologic malignancies), while concerns about unusual organisms or sites are usually much less urgent than when the patient is undergoing more aggressive treatment. When a patient has been managed at home, the likelihood is greatly reduced that an infection is due to bacterial organisms that are resistant to multiple antibiotics.

In a large autopsy series from a cancer hospital, one half of deaths from nonhematologic malignancies were due to infections.[3] Septicemia, pneumonia, pyelonephritis, and peritonitis were the common diagnoses. Infections are also common terminal events in home care. For patients with far-advanced cancer, the physician may recognize infection as either a source of discomfort, which is appropriately evaluated and managed with only rather simple measures, or as a humane, even welcome, terminal event. In a recent report on "nontreatment" in an extended-care facility, 72% of febrile cancer patients were neither hospitalized nor treated with antibiotics, compared with 36% of febrile patients with other diagnoses.[1] However, as was well-known in the preantibiotic era, infectious diseases such as pneumonia or even sepsis are not uniformly fatal; 40% of patients who were not hospitalized or treated with antibiotics survived the immediate febrile illness.

The common sites of bacterial infection in the chronically ill—lungs and urinary tract—are also the site of the majority of infections for terminally ill patients in the home. The physician's familiarity with the problems of the compromised host is usually less helpful for managing the late-stage cancer outpatient than an awareness of the likely sites of infection for various advanced malignancies: cholangitis from tumor involving the liver or porta hepatis; aspiration pneumonia when swallowing or coughing are impaired; intra-abdominal abscess or bacteremia from obstructed bowel; cystitis or pyelonephritis from urinary tract obstruction or instrumentation; and so on. A careful history and physical examination, supplemented by examination of a sputum or urine sample, are usually sufficient for the diagnosis. Chest x-rays and blood tests rarely add essential information. A single oral agent will almost always provide adequate antibiotic coverage. In addition to the usual antibiotics, chloramphenicol 3 g a day in four doses is a good drug for combating gram-positive and most gram-negative organisms, and especially anaerobes.

FEVER AND SWEATS

Fever and sweats are two systemic symptoms that are commonly associated with infections and that may deserve vigorous management, even if their underlying cause is not treated. In the absence of infection, fever is occasionally seen with lymphomas and with some nonmetastatic solid tumors such as renal cell carcinoma. In advanced cancer, additional noninfectious causes of fever include metastatic tumor (especially to the liver), drug reactions, dehydration, and adrenal insufficiency. Sweats occur in similar circumstances and may or may not be associated with febrile episodes.

In adults, fevers below 103°F (39.4° C) often produce no discomfort. Even higher temperatures may be well-tolerated if they are not prolonged or complicated by dehydration. Much of the discomfort accompanying febrile illnesses results from the chills and sweats associated with fluctuations in the temperature, not from an elevated temperature *per se*. Because intermittent or prn medication for fevers can provoke such variations in temperature, antipyretic treatment should generally be given regularly. Four-hourly regimens of aspirin and acetaminophen will almost always suppress a fever and its major fluctuations; six-hourly regimens will often be satisfactory. Nonsteroidal anti-inflammatory agents may also be effective antipyretics. In a small series of cancer patients with fever of unknown origin, lysis of the fever in response to naproxen 250 mg po bid was highly suggestive that the elevated temperature was due to the neoplasm rather than to an infectious process.[2] See Medications for Fevers and Sweats.

Tepid baths or sponge baths with either water or a water–alcohol mixture can be used to treat an elevated temperature.

MEDICATIONS FOR FEVERS AND SWEATS

Aspirin 325–1000 mg po q3–6h—available as a liquid and as rectal suppositories
Acetaminophen 325–650 mg po q4–6h—also available as liquid or as rectal suppository
Indomethacin (Indocin) 25–50 mg po 3–4 times a day—other nonsteroidal anti-inflammatory agents are presumably similarly effective, and may have advantages in terms of patient tolerance and duration of action (see Chap. 1)
Additional agents:
    Steroids (*e.g.*, prednisone 5–10 mg po 2–3 times a day)
    Cimetidine (Tagamet) has suppressed sweats in patients with Hodgkin's disease

---

SELECTED REFERENCES

1. Brown NK, Thompson DJ: Nontreatment of fever in extended care facilities. N Engl J Med 300:1246–1250, 1979
2. Chang JC, Gross HM: Utility of naproxen in the differential diagnosis of fever of undetermined origin in patients with cancer. Am J Med 76:597–603, 1984
3. Inagaki J, Rodriguez V, Bodey GP: Causes of death in cancer patients. Cancer 33:568–573, 1974

N. Endocrine Aspects of Advanced Cancer

This section offers a brief reminder of a few endocrine conditions that produce symptoms similar to the systemic manifestations of a terminal illness and that might easily be overlooked in the late stages of cancer. Some endocrinopathies—adrenal insufficiency, hypothyroidism, Cushing's syndrome, and the syndrome of inappropriate secretion of antidiuretic hormone (SIADH)—can mimic far-advanced cancer by producing profound weakness or apathy; the detection of these conditions, like the recognition of severe depression, can lead to measures that literally snatch the patient from the jaws of death. Hypercalcemia, another fairly common phenomenon in late-stage cancer patients, produces mental status changes and constipation—symptoms often attributed to advanced illness or the effects of drugs. Convenient means for detecting and palliating many of these syndromes are available.

Adrenal insufficiency in advanced cancer may result from metastases to the adrenals, removal of or damage to the glands from cancer treatment (including the use of aminoglutethimide), or suppression of function due to exogenous or endogenous steroids. Adrenal metastases are relatively common and, increasingly, are being diagnosed with the use of computerized body tomography, but adrenal insufficiency from metastases is rarely recognized.[1]

Typical symptoms and signs of adrenal insufficiency include weakness and fatigue, pigmentation, weight loss, gastrointestinal (GI) complaints (anorexia, nausea, vomiting, and abdominal pain), hypotension, tachycardia, and mental status changes. Hyponatremia and hyperkalemia are common. A simple screening procedure for adrenal insufficiency is now widely available, the cosyntropin (Cortrosyn) stimulation test—250 μg is given IM or IV, followed in 60 minutes by a blood sample for plasma cortisol. Cortisol levels below 18 μg/100 ml suggest the need for further investigation.

Hypothyroidism occurs after neck surgery or radiation, when patients on chronic thyroid replacement discontinue their medication, and because of hypopituitarism.

Hypopituitarism may lead to adrenal insufficiency or hypothyroidism and has been reported as a complication of cerebral radiation.[6]

Cushing's syndrome (of pituitary, adrenal, or ectopic origin) produces hypokalemia, myopathy, and a variety of other familiar metabolic derangements and can be screened for with the overnight dexamethasone suppression test.[3] Metyrapone (Metopirone) 250 mg can be given orally in doses adjusted to suppress the plasma cortisol level and reverse hypokalemia.[5]

The *syndrome of inappropriate antidiuretic hormone* produces hyponatremia and may cause symptoms when the serum sodium is less than 130 mg/dl. The diagnosis is confirmed when a normovolemic patient (who is not receiving diuretics and has normal renal, adrenal, and thryoid function) is hyponatremic and has an inappropriate natiuresis (*i.e,* urine less than maximally dilute or urine osmolality inappropriately high compared with that of plasma). This condition responds to water restriction but may be conveniently managed with demeclocycline (Declomycin) 300–600 mg po bid.[2]

Hypoglycemia may be a presenting manifestation of insulin-producing tumors, but occasionally develops with non-islet cell malignancies, especially mesenchymal tumors and hepatomas. Hypoglycemia may occur late in the course of a cancer and is often associated with tumors with extensive hepatic metastases. Treatment consists of dietary measures, intravenous glucose, and a trial of glucocorticosteroids.

Hypercalcemia is a relatively common manifestation of malignancy, and may cause both the earliest symptoms of cancer and its terminal complications. A number of etiologies for this disorder have been described, but patients commonly have either multiple bony metastases (with normal or elevated serum phosphates and normal or low serum parathyroid hormone [PTH]), or they have humorally mediated bone resorption (similar to that of hyperparathyroidism, often associated with hypophosphatemia and sometimes with an elevated level of immunoreactive PTH). Primary hyperparathyroidism can also coexist with cancer. In addition, hypercalcemia occurs with endocrine therapy for breast cancer and when popular nutritional treatments of cancer lead to hypervitaminosis D or A. Immobilization, diuretic therapy, and dehydration are frequent precipitants of symptomatic hypercalcemia.

Common manifestations of this mineral disorder are anorexia, nausea, vomiting, constipation, lethargy, weakness, and mental status changes, which range from mild personality alterations to coma. Polyuria and pruritus may also occur. Neuropsychiatric manifestations may persist for 2 to 6 days after normocalcemia is established.[8]

Hypercalcemia in the late stages of cancer is often a preterminal event, even when vigorous therapy is instituted. Some patients will have a prolonged, comfortable life after developing this disorder; others will die quickly despite treatment; and a few will survive, only to succumb soon to complications which, in retrospect, may leave the physician wishing that the patient had been left untreated, slipping quietly into coma and death.

Immediate treatment of hypercalcemia consists primarily of hydration with salt and water.[4,7] Additional therapy may be unnecessary. Under hospital supervision, a vigorous diuresis can be provoked by saline loading and the administration of furosemide. Steroids are commonly added intravenously (hydrocortisone 100 mg IV q6h) or orally (prednisone 40–60 mg qd), especially when initial hydration fails to correct the hypercalcemia. Mithramycin 25 μg/kg IV is slow-acting but reliable; it can be used if hydration and steroids prove inadequate, and can be repeated every 2 to 3 days. Finally, calcitonin 4 MRC units/kg IM or SC q12h will produce a rapid lowering of serum calcium for some patients and may work best in conjunction with steroids; higher doses (8 MRC units/kg IM or SC q6–12h) can be tried if lower doses fail.

Chronic measures for managing hypercalcemia include ensurance of hydration (3 liters of fluid daily) and of mobility. Limitation of calcium intake is probably useless, although dietary supplements of calcium and vitamin D should be avoided. Patients who are not hyperphosphatemic should be given a trial of oral phosphates—Fleet PhosphaSoda 5 ml 1 to 3 times a day or Neutro-Phos (or Neutro-Phos-K) 250 mg 2 to 8 tabs qd. Diarrhea often makes phosphate treatment intolerable; this side-effect is said to be minimized by giving small doses at long intervals and by diluting the medication in a large glass of water. Chronic use of steroids is often appropriate if the above measures fail; lower doses (e.g., prednisone 20–30 mg qd) should be tried once hypercalcemia is controlled. Nonsteroidal anti-inflammatory agents (e.g., aspirin or indomethacin) are also occasionally effective. Since the above measures will often not control hypercalcemia, continued use of mithramycin is commonly required—25 μg/kg IV as needed whenever the serum calcium reaches symptomatic levels (usually at least once a week)—although toxicity may ensue. Salmon calcitonin can also be continued, but must be given frequently and parenterally and can be expected to lose its effectiveness after a few days or weeks. Diphosphonates may be the agents of choice in the future.

SELECTED REFERENCES

1. Black RM, Daniels GH, Coggins CH et al: Adrenal insufficiency from metastatic colonic carcinoma masquerading as isolated aldosterone deficiency. Acta Endocrinol 98:586–591, 1981
2. Forrest JN Jr, Cox M, Hong C, Morrison G, Bia M, Singer I: Superiority of demeclocycline over lithium in the treatment of chronic syndrome of inappropriate secretion of antidiuretic hormone. N Engl J Med 298:173–177, 1978
3. Gold EM: The Cushing syndromes: Changing views of diagnosis and treatment. Ann Intern Med 90:829–844, 1979
4. Mazzaferri EL, O'Doriso TM, LoBuglio AF: Treatment of hypercalcemia associated with malignancy. Semin Oncol 5:141–153, 1978
5. Orth DN: Metyrapone is useful only as adjunctive therapy in Cushing's disease (Editorials). Ann Intern Med 89:128–130, 1978
6. Samaan NA, Bakdash MM, Caderao JB et al: Hypopituitarism after external irradiation: Evidence for both hypothalamic and pituitary origin. Ann Intern Med 83:771–777, 1975
7. Stewart AF: Therapy of malignancy-associated hypercalcemia. Am J Med 74:475–480, 1983
8. Weizman A, Eldar M, Shoenfeld Y et al: Hypercalcemia-induced psychopathology in malignant diseases. Br J Psychiatry 135:363–366, 1979

O. Anemia and Transfusions

In advanced cancer, anemia usually results from bleeding or decreased red blood cell production. In a large series of patients with nonhematologic malignancies who were autopsied in a cancer hospital, bleeding accounted for 7% of deaths.[1] Foremost bleeding sites were the gastrointestinal (GI) tract, brain, a major vessel, and the lung. Thrombocytopenia was an etiologic factor in 18% of hemorrhages.

Routine diagnostic studies for anemia—a complete blood count and smear, reticulocyte count, and serum ferritin or serum iron and iron binding capacity—may occasionally lead to identification of a treatable etiology for diminished marrow function. Strategies for managing hemoptysis, hematuria, and bleeding wounds are reviewed in previous sections.

When bleeding cannot be controlled and red blood cell production cannot be made adequate, the only available relief is transfusion—a treatment that entails moderate risk and cost as well as expenditure of a precious resource. Asymptomatic or mildly symptomatic anemia can generally be left untreated; debilitated, bedridden patients may tolerate hemoglobin levels of 6 to 7 g/100 ml and find no improved well-being after transfusion. Indications for transfusion include otherwise unexplained fatigue, weakness, and dyspnea, usually associated with hemoglobin levels below 9 g/100 ml, in a patient who might find an improved quality of life from relief of such symptoms. Transfusion is occasionally useful to bolster a patient's stamina for attending a special occasion (*e.g.*, a wedding or graduation). Blood can be administered conveniently in an ambulatory-care transfusion service or emergency ward and occasionally can be given in the home.

Patients with significant cardiopulmonary disease may require hemoglobin levels of 10 g/100 ml in order to feel well. Transfusion to such levels or higher may also be required as supportive therapy for patients undergoing surgery, radiation, chemotherapy, or treatment for a major, reversible infection.

Two units of packed red cells will often ensure adequate blood levels for a few weeks, sometimes for over a month. If the patient's symptoms do not respond convincingly to transfusion, the treatment should not be repeated.

Decisions to transfuse a patient with acute bleeding are difficult, and guidelines are few. On the the one hand, death from exsanguination can be gruesome (especially when extensive hemoptysis, hematemesis, or hematochezia occur or frank bleeding develops from a neck tumor or other wound), while, on the other, it can be viewed as a simple and painless terminal event as the patient drifts into shock. Transfusion is sensible when an intervention to control the bleeding is planned or when spontaneous cessation of bleeding can be anticipated soon. Prior to beginning transfusions, decision-making may be facilitated by setting a clear upper limit to the amount of blood to be given, usually in the range of 2 to 4 units. Transfusions are senseless if they only prolong an acute exsanguination or momentarily delay a timely death.

SELECTED REFERENCE

1. Inagaki J, Rodriguez V, Bodey GP: Causes of death in cancer patients. Cancer 33:568–573, 1974

P.   Oncologic Emergencies

Many unforeseen conditions that arise in the patient with advanced cancer will require immediate action, either for maintaining the patient's comfort or for preventing serious sequelae. Most of these problems (e.g., severe pain or vomiting) are not included in traditional lists of oncologic emergencies.[5] Some conditions, such as hypercalcemia, would best be labeled as "potential emergencies"; they may require immediate action at times, but can be managed in a more leisurely fashion when detected early in their natural course or when severe manifestations have not developed. Moreover, many of the conditions regularly labeled as oncologic emergencies may be viewed as acceptable terminal events for the patient with far-advanced cancer and may be treated symptomatically or not at all. Even when a patient is considered terminal, however, the physician should recognize these potentially urgent conditions and formulate a treatment plan—standard emergency procedures or comfort measures—based on an understanding of the pathophysiology of the condition and the full range of possibilities for management.

Common oncologic emergencies are listed in Table 2P-1. The following sections review a few urgent conditions that are not regularly encountered in general medical practice and that have not been discussed earlier in the text.

SUPERIOR VENA CAVA SYNDROME

The superior vena cava syndrome may be the first sign of a cancer, and discussions of its management often focus on establishment of a diagnosis as well as on treatment.[2,3] Patients may present with an insidious or a rapid onset of dyspnea, facial swelling or swelling of the trunk and upper extremities, and, less often, dizziness, syncope, chest pain, cough, and dysphagia. Central nervous system (CNS) manifestations include headache, visual disturbances, and altered mental status. Physical examination typically reveals thoracic and neck vein distention with cyanosis or plethora, facial edema, and tachypnea. Horner's syndrome and vocal cord paralysis are noted rarely. Definitive diagnosis is often made on clinical grounds, supplemented by a chest x-ray that demonstrates an intrathoracic mass. Tomography and computerized tomography (CT) may provide further diagnostic information, and venography is occasionally indicated.

Radiation therapy is the treatment of choice for the superior vena cava syndrome due to malignancy. For the patient who is either not a candidate for radiation therapy or for whom such definitive treatment is rejected, management can include trials of elevation of the head, high-dose steroids, and diuretics. The natural course of this condition and the usefulness of medical treatment have not been well studied.[4]

PATHOLOGIC FRACTURES

Pathologic fractures are particularly troublesome when they occur in major weight-bearing sites (e.g., the femur and acetabulum). Some investigators have concluded that the presence of painful lytic lesions that are large or have destroyed a substantial

TABLE 2P-1
"Emergencies" in Advanced Cancer

Any severely distressing symptom, especially pain
Cardiovascular
  Cardiac tamponade
  Superior vena cava syndrome
Pulmonary
  Hemorrhage
  Obstruction
  Embolus
  Respiratory failure
Gastrointestinal
  Obstruction, perforation, hemorrhage
Urologic
  Obstruction, hemorrhage
Gynecologic
  Hemorrhage
Neurologic
  Cerebral edema and herniation
  New or frequent seizures
  Spinal cord compression
  Infections—meningitis, abscess
Orthopedic
  Pathologic fracture
  Metastases causing significant destruction at major weight-bearing sites
Infections, especially pneumonia, bacteremia, sepsis, and any infection in the severely
  compromised host
Metabolic/endocrine
  Hypercalcemia
  Hyponatremia, hypernatremia
  Hyperkalemia, hypokalemia
  Hypoglycemia
  Hyperuricemia
  Lactic acidosis
  Acute adrenal insufficiency
Hematologic
  Severe thrombocytopenia, leukopenia, anemia
  Thrombotic and hemorrhagic states; DIC
  Hyperviscosity

portion of the cortex of a critical, weight-bearing area should be promptly treated with prophylactic orthopedic stabilization, perhaps followed by irradiation. Other investigators have recommended radiation alone.[1]

In terminally ill patients, surgical prophylaxis will rarely be considered, but radiation treatment for painful bony lesions often provides prompt relief with relatively little inconvenience. Radiation can also be considered after a fracture has occurred. Alternate methods of managing fractures include the use of immobilization and analgesics. Stabilizing devices may lessen pain and increase mobility. Physical therapy consultation may be helpful for both established and threatened fractures.

SELECTED REFERENCES

1. Cheng DS, Seitz CB, Eyre HJ: Nonoperative management of femoral, humeral, and acetabular metastases in patients with breast carcinoma. Cancer 45:1533–1537, 1980
2. Parish JM, Marschke RF, Dines DE et al: Etiologic considerations in superior vena cava syndrome. Mayo Clin Proc 56:407–413, 1981
3. Perez CA, Presant CA, Van Amburg AL: Management of the superior vena cava syndrome. Semin Oncol 5:123–134, 1978
4. Schraufnagel DE, Hill R, Leech JA et al: Superior vena caval obstruction: Is it a medical emergency? Am J Med 70:1169–1174, 1981
5. Yarbro JW (ed): Oncologic emergencies. Semin Oncol 5:123–227, 1978

Appropriate Treatment Limits in Advanced Cancer **3**

Edwin H. Cassem

When cancer is advanced, both neglect and overzealous treatment of patients are hazards: neglect, because any treatment may seem likely to accomplish so little; overzealous treatment, because "doing everything" may seem easier than denying a patient some treatment or diagnostic procedure. Physician fallibility is emphasized by advanced cancer. Am I missing something correctible? Might we find it if we reexplored? Shouldn't I at least bring the patient in for an Xray? If the patient develops pneumonia, is this the time to forego antibiotics? Can such a simple treatment be denied a patient? When is a feeding tube inappropriate? A competent patient can simplify these questions by refusing further diagnostic workup or treatment. When he is not competent, what can be done when family members disagree about what is appropriate?

Cancer is called advanced when in someone's clinical judgment it is no longer reversible. Setting treatment limits in advanced cancer is not an option but an obligation. There is always more that can be done. Just as neglect of the patient is unthinkable, use of every available technological means to counter organ failure is not sanctioned, even medically. No patient, semicomatose from glioblastoma and in failure from cardiomyopathy, is a candidate for cardiac transplant. Nor would any physician be willing to prolong the resuscitation of the advanced cancer patient (if it were even possible) until brain death occurs. The foregoing hyperboles illustrate that the advanced cancer patient and the health-care team face inevitable choices. Some judgments are quite difficult to make. This chapter will discuss certain ethical principles that can guide these decisions, will outline a methodology for decision-making, and will discuss specific situations that commonly vex patients, families, and physicians.

MEDICAL ETHICS APPLIED TO ADVANCED CANCER

Ethics is a philosophical discipline of which medical ethics is one part. For the practical purpose of considering appropriate limits of treatment of patients with advanced cancer, three principles may be extracted.

First Principle

The first principle of all ethics can be stated in the tautologic form, "Good must be done and evil avoided." Each branch of ethics then specifies the good and the evil unique to it. In medical ethics, the first principle is traditionally stated so that the negative half is primary: *primum non nocere*, "first do no harm." The good to be done by the physician is stated in a twofold manner: the doctor must restore health and relieve suffering. As Slater has pointed out,[1] problems of treatment limitation arise when these two duties conflict: for some patients the more we do to restore their health, the more suffering we cause them. When a young woman with breast cancer metastatic to the liver and lungs and negative estrogen-binding receptor protein presents herself for treatment, almost anything done to attack her malignancy has a 90% chance of making her feel worse without any therapeutic impact on the cancer. By definition, the patients discussed in this book are beyond restoration of health, if that is construed as "cure." As the disease worsens, the treatment goal shifts toward avoidance of undue procedures, preoccupation with side-effects, and attention to comfort. Nevertheless, portrayal of this shift does insufficient justice to the spirit of optimism that should pervade an outpatient treatment program. A good motto, fully in keeping with this first principle of medical ethics, would be *palliate everything, exacerbate nothing.* Appropriately aggressive in tone, it addresses that necessary eagerness to maximize the patient's health, while including judicious caution for minimizing suffering.

Second Principle

The second principle stresses the primacy of the patient's will in the decision-making process and is sometimes stated, "Let the will of the patient, not the health of the patient, be the supreme law." Based on the patient's legal right to privacy, this principle affirms the patient's right to refuse any treatment. In other words, from the point of view of a contract, the first principle guarantees that the physician recommends a decision that is medically best for the patient, whereas the second principle guarantees that the patient is free to accept or reject it. The patient's right to receive treatment or to demand a specific treatment are separate, distinct issues.

However, four factors may impair the patient's ability to choose competently.

1. Pain and other physical symptoms may be so intense that the patient would rather die than consider any procedure. Prolonged, severe discomfort can distort a person's ability to make rational decisions, sometimes leading the patient to reject helpful measures or to grasp at useless ones. Immediate relief of such suffering should be sought. Afterward, a better determination can be made of whether the patient genuinely desires to refuse treatment.
2. Treatable depression may make it impossible to take a patient's treatment refusal at face value. For example, a rather healthy patient with recurrent colon cancer is found with acute fever, cough, increased sputum production, and clinical signs

of pneumonia. He has been severely depressed for 1 month and had expressly stated on several occasions that he wished he were dead and wanted to die. He refuses transfer to the emergency ward and when asked whether he understands that this could result in a fatal outcome, replies that he not only understands this but wants to die. The problem is that he wanted to die before he ever got the pneumonia, so that this refusal of treatment seems more related to his prior depression than to his pneumonia. Aggressive treatment of depression is part of appropriate palliation.

3. An emergency may arise in which the patient cannot express an opinion, when the physician must act in accord with the patient's best interests.

4. The patient may become incompetent by reason of delirium, dementia, coma, or some mixture of the three. In such a case the dialogue about treatment choices is then ordinarily conducted with the patient's next of kin, whose obligation is to judge what the patient (not they) would want done.

Dialogue with a competent patient can be viewed as a discussion of the risk–benefit ratio of a specific treatment course. The physician's responsibility is to spell out the nature of the treatment, the probable benefits to the patient, and the cost. The patient's responsibility is to state whether he will take these risks for that benefit. Moreover, the patient almost always expects the physician to express his best clinical judgment about the balance of good and bad and to offer a recommendation for or against the option. For a patient whose recurrent bladder cancer was becoming progressively symptomatic, the question of further surgery may arise. The physician might say:

> At this point, it is worth raising the question about another exenteration. The second procedure was an ordeal for you. It was quite painful, and we had a good deal of trouble controlling the infection and hemorrhage. After those 5 weeks in the hospital, in spite of a pulmonary embolus, you managed to get back on your feet and got around reasonably well for 3 months. A third procedure almost surely guarantees even more trouble with pain, infection, hemorrhage, and other complications. I am reluctant to recommend it.

After further dialogue about these realities, one patient would say, "On no account would I go through that again," whereas another might reply, "Even if there is a remote chance for a bit more decent quality time, I'd like to take it." Or the decision might be to reconsult the surgeon. There are no fortune tellers in medicine, only fallible clinicians, and so second opinions are welcome. However, patients appreciate being able to count on the physician's honest judgment to protect them from foolish and costly risks.

Third Principle

Stopping a treatment is ethically no different from never starting it. Granted, discontinuing a mechanical ventilator for a comatose patient is much more difficult psychologically than never starting it, but ethically and legally, the two acts are equivalent. Let us suppose that 2 months after achieving an excellent remission from a lymphoma, a 25-year-old man is brought to the emergency ward comatose and without spontaneous respiration. Initial examination does not reveal a cause for his deterioration, or, if the cause is known (e.g., hemorrhage), whether it can be reversed. Does one intubate him? If, at that point, God appeared and announced that the patient had

sive, infiltrating brainstem involvement that left him beyond treat-
ians would thank Him, dispense with intubation and resuscitation,
e patient dead when asystole came. Lacking this diagnostic inter-
ur, they intubate and sustain him in the intensive care unit. Two weeks
_y have come to the same diagnostic conclusion and the patient has remained
coma, his breathing sustained by the ventilator. Now, however, when someone
points out that the ventilator is no longer necessary, an accuser is likely to emerge,
announcing that discontinuation of the ventilator is tantamount to murder, since the
patient will die when it is disconnected. But what justified the initial use of the ventilator was the possibility of the patient's coma being reversible. It is this that continues to justify use of the ventilator. Once it is clear that the coma is not reversible, the
ventilator is no longer necessary. In this patient, moreover, it cannot be justified and
should be discontinued. Emotionality clouds and prevents effective use of this principle. Any medical treatment is justified by the benefit it is thought to have. When it
is begun and later found to provide no such benefit, it ceases to be necessary.

A PROCESS FOR MAKING TREATMENT CHOICES

No universal criterion or formula exists whereby a specific choice can be made. At
times, medical knowledge (expertise) clearly dictates the options. For instance, in
evaluating a gastrointestinal (GI) bleeder, it may be quite clear that definitive means
for treating the hemorrhage have been exhausted or have no possibility of working, as
in considering a third gastric or esophageal reconstruction for a patient whose second
procedure made such a conclusion unmistakeable. Many decisions seem much less
clear. Choice then becomes a process that requires a dialogue, and one should not
pretend that a problem has only one solution that can be given independently of the
choosers. The physician may find practical the following points for guiding a dialogue.

Opening the Dialogue: The Rationale and the Facts

How can one tell a patient he belongs in a "Do Not Resuscitate (DNR)" category, and
yet not rob him or her of hope? Honesty requires the admission that it may be impossible. The physician needs some way of introducing a discussion of carefully chosen
options. The earlier in the course of treatment this occurs, the more comfortably it is
likely to proceed. There is no need to start the discussion with direct focus on the
incurability of the disease. To the young woman mentioned above who was found to
have stage IV breast cancer, the physician might say

> Since we will have to be making decisions about the treatments that are best
> for you, let me describe a philosophy for choosing. First, no matter how com-
> plex the technology of the treatment, if it is sure to help, it will always be
> available to you. At the same time, many of our treatments for cancer are dan-
> gerous and harmful. I refuse to use treatments just because they are there. If
> a treatment were proposed for you, for example, which I thought would only
> hurt and not help you, I will tell you that I'm against using it and why.

The point of this opening is to reassure the patient that her doctor intends to protect
her from inappropriate treatments. It is not a small favor. Moreover, this introduction
is brief in order to invite some response. The opening words should be followed by
silence, allowing the patient to lead the discussion into further topics. If given the

chance to begin wherever he or she wants in responding, the patient often will do a good deal of the remaining work of specifying goals and preferred methods of evaluation and treatment. Some of them will even spell out their wishes about resuscitation and respirators. By contrast, the physician who tries to deliver an uninterrupted didactic lecture is likely not only to fail but also to get himself into unnecessary trouble, owing, for example, to the patient's misinterpretations of something in the lecture. The opening statement, then, states or restates the concern about doing no harm to the patient, and is made deliberately brief to give the patient the opportunity for self-disclosure. An additional element in the dialogue might be an invitation to the patient to share responsibility for the choice:

> *Whenever we start one of these potentially harmful treatments, I need to know that you have some idea of what you are getting into and that you agree to it.*

Clinical facts often seem incomplete for clarifying difficult choices, but when reviewed in detail with the patient and family, can be powerful and helpful. An elderly woman with small cell carcinoma metastatic to the brain, responsive only to pain, had suffered a series of episodes of aspiration pneumonia. Someone had suggested use of a gastrostomy tube, but it had not been placed. After another episode of pneumonia, more extensive than the last, the patient was hospitalized for intravenous antibiotic therapy at her family's insistence. After 10 days, she was still spiking fevers. When the physician expressed his plan for switching the patient to oral antibiotics and returning her home to die, the family was initially horrified and thought this "was practicing euthanasia," by which they meant neglectful homicide. The doctor then reviewed her course: diagnosis, lobectomy, radiation, 6 good months, discovery of brain metastasis with slow but relentless deterioration, inadequate gag reflexes, and increasingly frequent pneumonias not prevented by placement of a nasogastric tube. To prevent aspiration, she already required round-the-clock suctioning, a procedure manifestly uncomfortable to the patient. After explaining that the nasogastric tube failed to prevent aspiration because of the nearly constant aspiration of oropharyngeal secretions, the physician then spelled out what might be required to stop the aspiration definitively: surgical placement of a gastrostomy tube, tracheostomy, and perhaps closure of the vocal cords and upper trachea. The family began by thinking the therapeutic intervention relatively simple: How could anyone refuse the patient antibiotics? Itemizing the details and consequences of the treatment and, especially, putting it into the context of the entire illness erased their doubts about the appropriateness. "We'd never want to put her through that, Doctor."

It helps to think ahead. Suppose, in desperation, the patient decided to ask for a trial of a phase I drug and is placed on it. After 1 week, he feels neither better nor worse. What should be done if he has a sudden cardiac arrest? The physician who prescribed the drug, fearing it may have caused the arrest, may automatically assume the patient should be resuscitated. Such an assumption is erroneous and would be motivated primarily by guilt. The decision to resuscitate depends, as argued above, on the chances of the treatment being sufficiently successful to satisfy the patient. If the phase I drug caused ventricular tachycardia, which would be reversed by administration lidocaine or countershock, the doctor might reasonably try these without questioning their appropriateness. If an asystolic arrest, however, appears to be the result of the natural disease process, it would be much more difficult to justify initiation of cardiopulmonary resuscitation (CPR). The decision may not be easy, but guilt feelings about use of a potentially dangerous agent, to which the patient agreed, are extraneous. The situation is similar to that of choosing high-risk surgery over a lingering illness. Even if death occurs, it is a risk that the patient chose to take and, in fact, that he preferred over living as he was prior to surgery.

Discussing the future does not guarantee that the patient will not change his or her mind about CPR or about the general amount of suffering that is an acceptable price to pay for a little more time or for the hope of "getting back to baseline" briefly. If the woman with stage IV breast cancer chose to forego any treatment, discussion could proceed as follows:

> *Of course, our goal will be to keep you functioning as well as possible at all times and to avoid hospitalization unless necessary. You should call us and discuss any new symptoms or problems. If you develop something serious like a pneumonia, it might be more comfortable for you to be in the hospital; it certainly is always available to you. [Pause. She replies she'd like to avoid hospitalization at all costs.] I'll remember that and support it, although you can change your mind at any time. By the way, if something totally unexpected happened—say, if you fainted or something (more serious), your family is likely to zip you right in anyway.*

Whether the patient approves of her family doing this or not, this is an excellent opportunity to remind her that the family cannot be realistically excluded from these choices. Decisions will be much more harmonious, and usually more easily made, when family members are included from the start.

Consensus in the Midst of Differing "Values"

As respiratory distress worsens progressively, a choice must be made, for example, between giving more morphine for comfort and hospitalizing the patient for additional diagnostic tests or brief aggressive treatment. If the choice is made to give morphine and the patient slowly improves, was it the "wrong" choice? Decision-making in these patients is not based on the search for an absolutely "right" answer. It proceeds because some choice must be made. Agreement by all does not guarantee a pleasant outcome; death or suffering may be inevitable. At times, discussions of "values" are likely to be distractions from responsibility rather than means of achieving enlightenment or harmony. Not only are such discussions potentially divisive—people start them occasionally in order to provoke arguments which, though unpleasant, are usually easier than making tough choices—but they also tend to evade reality by dealing in absolutes or generalities. It would be well to recall here Ingelfinger's maxim: "Just as there are no atheists in foxholes, there are few absolutists at the bedside."[2] Cassem's corollary is that any absolutist at the bedside of an advanced cancer patient either cannot grasp the reality of the situation or has a psychological problem, usually both (see the sample dialogue below):

Family member:	*Remember, Doctor, everything must be done. Whatever life is present, no matter how little, must be preserved.*
Doctor:	*Everything?*
Family member:	*Yes, everything.*
Doctor:	*You mean, as his heart gives out while he's on the ventilator, we should take him to the operating room and hook him up to the heart–lung machine?*
Family member:	*The what? [Doctor explains]* *Oh, Doctor, you're being facetious.*

Doctor: *No, I'm telling you that we will have to make choices as we go along, and they won't be easy.*

This family member, like many laypeople, had little idea what the reality was going to be. The slogan "everything must be done," expresses an illusory hope that there are easy answers for difficult problems. It also expresses the fear that the doctor's philosophy (or religious values) conflict with hers. Gentle discussion about the reality of treatment options generally eases these fears. Resorting to such slogans, however, usually proves another old law stating that any philosophy that can be put in a nutshell belongs there.

Some patients and families fear that the physician has one of two desires: to clear by systematic starvation all nursing homes of the feeble elderly or to transform by torturing technology all dying cancer patients into frankensteinian monsters. Our job is to help them see that patients, families, and the health-care team must work together to choose treatments best for the patient. Even then, it will be difficult.

For practical reasons, physicians are generally advised to be cautious about defining "quality of life" for the patient, since an outcome repulsive to one may be acceptable to another. Mental anguish is subjective. Some religious persons "offer up" their sufferings as part of their commitment to a transcendent plan (e.g., God's will). The physician's philosophic or religious reasoning may not be of interest to the family— in fact, it may be viewed as hostile if it differs from theirs, especially at times of life-and-death crises. Keeping things basic, the physician is better off saying, "Look, my expertise is in the nature of body organs, how they go wrong, what has to be done to make them work better, and what dangers accompany drugs and other treatments we can use for that purpose." When the parents of a retarded child with terminal cancer already have a highly developed sense of their child's right to the best medical care, efforts to restrict treatment on the basis of retardation would be unkind and unjustifiable. Pointing out, however, that the child's inability to understand the purpose of a treatment can increase suffering is both necessary and helpful in a discussion of treatment limitation.

Common Obstacles to Reaching Consensus About Treatment Limits

Even when universal consensus about treatment limitations is reached, the choices, though guaranteeing the noble aim of minimizing suffering, remain tinged with tragedy. The patient is going to die. Loss, bereavement, and perhaps feelings of abandonment will follow. Strong feelings about the death of the patient probably account for most or all of the specific difficulties recounted below.

Hope may be carried by the patient in an exceedingly fragile vessel. Is there a danger that a discussion of limits, "DNR," and the like will shatter that vessel, cause the loss of hope, and produce despair? The strength of patients is commonly underestimated by their families and physicians alike. If the patient has equanimity in the face of terminal illness, it will emerge in early discussions about diagnosis or later ones about appropriate treatment. Sooner or later, the physician will encounter a patient who makes it quite explicit that not only is death frightening but that treatments are the "only hope." A woman in her mid-50s who, with the help of radiation therapy and combination chemotherapy, had survived with pancreatic carcinoma for 14 months, was hospitalized with bowel obstruction due to recurrence. She was receiving only 5FU at the time. Believing chemotherapy was not helping her, her oncologist informed her of his plan to stop it. "What will you give me in its place?"

she wanted to know. When he said that he did not intend to replace it with another drug because of the toxicities of other agents, she said "If you are not giving me something for my cancer, I will lose hope." Her oncologist, taken aback, said that her body "needed a rest from chemotherapy for a while," that chemotherapy can also do harm, that the good should not be outweighed by the harm, that 5FU had not helped over the last 3 months, and that he had pushed it to the point of lowering her white blood cell count—the body's way of signalling we had to back off. She countered that she had heard of streptozotocin; couldn't he use that? Familiar with the latest drug protocols, he replied that its record was poor, its toxicity significant, and he would not even consider it because he thought it would hurt her. Without treatment, she repeated, she would lose hope. Perplexed, he said that he would return to discuss it further the next day; since her white blood cell count was marginal, he would hold her 5FU (as he had in the past). The next day he asked her if she understood that new, untried drugs could cause her harm without making any impact on her cancer. She understood. Then why would she want such a drug? "If I don't have it I'll lose hope." Mystified, the physician gently asked a crucial question: "Hope *for what?*" The woman was momentarily speechless (this specific question had not occurred to her). "I don't know. It certainly is not for cure; I understood from the beginning that this can't be cured. . . . Maybe it is that I want to get home again and back onto the golf course." A new anticancer drug would make that *less* likely, the oncologist told her. "I know that whether or not you give me a drug you will still take care of me, so it isn't that." Although they talked longer, she could not figure out why she had felt so strongly. On the following day she told him that she felt much better and appreciated the prior day's discussion. "My sense of fear is gone; it's still not clear to me, but I've regained the feeling that I'll be all right." Curious, her oncologist asked what she would think if, without informing her, he had given her a placebo and told her it was streptozotocin. "Why, that would be a betrayal! I wouldn't approve of that," was her reply. The encouragement to spell out what she meant by hope seemed to have helped this patient considerably.

Is there a time when food should be forced on the patient? Should it ever be withheld? Almost as simple a given in nature as oxygen, food can likewise present vexing difficulties for those caring for advanced cancer patients. "Starvation? I can't approve that for anyone!" is an example of the spontaneous emotion generated by the question of withholding food. Reality, however, makes the question unavoidable for certain patients. Some patients' GI tracts become obstructed by extensive metastatic disease, and they cannot eat. In a few cases, a jejunostomy tube may bypass gastric obstruction. Total parenteral nutrition (TPN) is available, but it is an option that many cannot receive at home. Many patients (and physicians) perceive it as "extreme" and do not consider it, especially if they are already being cared for as outpatients. When a patient with intestinal obstruction has been admitted for further diagnosis, placed on TPN, and found to have untreatable extension of disease, then the question of stopping TPN can be a tense one, even when continuation of TPN makes no medical sense. A discussion with such a patient could begin gently with, "I wanted to discuss with you some reservations I have about TPN and what I see are its disadvantages." Mention each reservation, one at a time, giving the patient adequate opportunity to disclose his thoughts. Examples of topics that could serve sequentially to develop a dialogue include: having to remain hospitalized, lack of freedom of movement, possible aggravation of ascites, complications of the indwelling catheter, and possible (even disproportionate) contribution to tumor growth with consequent worsening of current symptoms. Some patients will quickly reject continuation (or beginning) of TPN. For others, the dialogue will produce the fear, "I will lose hope," as mentioned in the last paragraph.

Faced with a nutrition dilemma, the physician returns to the most radical of questions about all treatment: What *good* will it accomplish for the patient? For the advanced cancer patient, *no* procedure or agent can be given unreflective approval. Food is no exception. When illness cannot be reversed and the patient is dying, comfort usually takes precedence. With the conscious patient, the physician may have to argue softly against the benefits of calories. Calories do not necessarily increase comfort. If they do not, what justifies their use? (The principle here remains the "first" one: every treatment must be justified; only those treatments are justifiable whose benefits outweigh the risks.) The risk of ordering administration of calories is that of increased suffering. The benefits are maintenance of the energy requirements of body organs and single cells. In the patient for whom aggressive treatment is maintaining only marginal aeration or even pain control, will added calories alleviate or worsen the situation? The answer to this question justifies or disqualifies their use. Moreover, a hard-core medical judgment is required by this question. Both the patient and family need this judgment to anchor their own perspective, which seldom if ever allows them to foresee specific medical complications the way the physician does. Discussions of calories far more commonly arise between doctor and family after the patient has ceased to be competent or even conscious. Some estimate of confidence in the judgment is also owed the family by the physician. Thus, "I have begun to have some (moderate/strong/severe) reservations about the potential effects of feeding here. His pain/breathlessness/potential for further hemorrhage is relentlessly mounting." When the medical formulation is "I cannot in conscience recommend them," the family benefits from hearing it. By communicating this, the doctor fulfills the medical part of the care contract: to state as specifically as possible the medical judgment of risks and benefits likely to follow initiation or continuation of a medical treatment. Families may naturally say, "We want to save him as long as possible, Doctor; even a little life is something precious to cling to." A sympathetic reply would be, "I understand how dear he is to you and only wish I could make him better. Since that is no longer possible, as his physician I must examine every treatment suggested for him in hopes that it will benefit him. I want only the best for him. I am opposed to this treatment because it seems to guarantee him only more suffering."

Often we assume that hydration is essential for comfort, even when caloric intake is not. However, this should not be taken for granted. Dehydration often produces little discomfort, especially among terminally ill patients whose cause for inadequate fluid intake is advanced debility and/or altered mental status. Unless the patient is vomiting or the cancer and its treatment directly prevents the passage of liquids into the intestines, the development of dehydration often reflects "poor intake" brought about by general weakness, drowsiness, and so on. Such patients may still experience thirst, but the other sequelae of dehydration—postural hypotension, poor skin turgor, and anorexia (especially in the case of hyponatremic dehydration) or fatigue and mental-status changes—do not commonly produce discomfort. Thirst and a dry mouth can usually be alleviated by simple mouth care, especially lubrication. Thirst may also be relieved by amounts of water (taken by mouth) that are much smaller than those required to reverse dehydration significantly. Thus, intravenous rehydration may not be necessary as a comfort measure for many patients, especially those for whom the prolongation of life is not a goal. Its usefulness as a comfort measure is overrated. It will prolong the life of some patients, and may at times be desirable for improving alertness and energy. The patient who is generally well but cannot swallow or retain enough liquids to compensate for current fluid losses will generally benefit from enteral or parenteral fluid administration and, perhaps, nutrition.

Substituted Judgment

"Substituted" judgment is the judgment given by one person for an incompetent person. It is called "substituted" because it is meant to convey what the incompetent person would have wanted in this situation, not what his family or guardian would want. Family members may not understand this. The physician can explain the concept and ask whether the patient ever made any comments on what he would want were he comatose or in the present circumstances: "You or I may want something different for him, but it is his wish we'd really like to know."

No family member wants to think a treatment decision is made because everyone just "gives up" on the patient. Since this is never a legitimate reason, a thoughtful review can emphasize how the doctor and family did not give up. The family may start this dialogue with the question, "How do you really know that he won't get better?" The best answer spells out the flesh and blood specifics of treatments, responses, complications, and the turning points that marked the patient's deterioration. For example, an answer could be as follows:

> That's an excellent question, one I've asked myself repeatedly. Remember how $2\frac{1}{2}$ years ago when he was robustly healthy, he had a seizure and we found his astrocytoma? The neurosurgeon removed most of his right frontal lobe, and he then received 6000 rads of radiation therapy to his brain and a course of CCNU, the chemotherapy. Remember how a year later he still rated himself as "95% effective" and continued to do better than we ever predicted, until last summer, when he just seemed to lose all his pep? It was then the CT scan showed dilated ventricles, and those lumbar punctures were done to remove spinal fluid, but it didn't help. By September, the neurologists concluded that he had "radiation dementia," and much to all our dismay, he continued to decline. By October, he was incontinent and deaf and speechless. Even then they told us there was "little to offer" for treatment. That was 4 months ago, and you have been absolutely heroic about caring for him at home. He had been eating when fed until 3 months ago, when we noticed he had trouble swallowing and developed aspiration pneumonia. That cleared with antibiotics. We put in that feeding tube, but he got pneumonia again last month. Again he cleared with antibiotics. Now he has pneumonia again. That is why we must review the wisdom of what we do to him. But this also reviews for you my perspective and that of the consultants who have seen him; all of us agree he won't get better.

Reviews of illness are particularly important for all individuals involved in the discussion of treatment limitation.

Taking responsibility for decisions to limit treatment is burdensome for all involved, including the physician. Anxiety may cause him to present his opinion in such a way that the family feels that all or undue responsibility has been placed on them. Shortly after a 16-year-old boy was officially pronounced brain dead, the family physician said to the youth's parents: "Well, it's up to you. We can disconnect the respirator now or continue for a little longer." Although the only humane treatment of the dead is provision of dignified passage to burial or cremation, this family interpreted the doctor's words (who later said that they quoted him incorrectly) as a request that they "sign the death warrant" for their son. This rather extreme example illustrates how useful it is for the family to hear the physician's explicit opinion. "For my part, I can't in conscience recommend intubating her if she deteriorates further, but I'd want to know if she'd disagree with that," is the sort of statement that aids the dialogue with a family.

Generally, families are quite sensible about limiting treatment, especially when they are well-informed. Moreover, they tend to be grateful for care and concern shown them and are rewarding to deal with. Conflict is part of life, however, and can also appear as death approaches. When vehement protest about treatment limitation comes from a family member who has lived for the past several years emotionally (and often geographically) remote from the patient, and the protest is at variance with the wishes of the rest of the family, the behavior is usually pathologic, based on long-standing conflict with the patient. Such a relative may present with disruptive, hostile complaints—meant to convey to the world what a devoted son (or brother) he has been, demonstrated by the extremes he will go to to "save" the patient. Even for a psychiatrist, these patients are almost impossible to deal with on an individual basis. A meeting with the entire family will most efficiently clarify the discrepancy in family opinion and make it much more difficult for this remote member to misrepresent family wishes. One might open such a meeting with the following:

> I'm pleased that we could all meet so that we can discuss what course of treatment will ensure the very best for Mrs. Jones. It is very helpful that you are here, too, Mr. Jones. You would not have come all this distance if you, too, were not very concerned that your mother get the best possible treatment. Now let me review the course of her illness and where we stand.

The Request to Accelerate Death

For some patients and families, death's arrival seems painfully delayed. Even when relatively pain free, a patient may feel that life is so diminished as to be an imposition rather than a blessing. What can be done for the patient who says, "I want to die now"? A 42-year-old unmarried businessman with recurrent lymphosarcoma had specified to his physician that he preferred comfort measures to further aggressive attempts to slow the progression of his disease. Pleural effusions had been tapped on three occasions to relieve his shortness of breath. A fourth was accepted and performed during an office visit, after which the patient said, "I am quite comfortable at this point. I'd like you to help me die as soon as possible." His doctor asked whether he had anything specific in mind. Explaining that he tolerated disability and dependency poorly and that he had all affairs in meticulous order for death, he added that he had assumed physicians had ways to accelerate death in a comfortable and dignified manner. "How would your family view this?" asked his doctor. His parents were dead, and his only sibling, a younger sister, was fully sympathetic—as were his network of friends, a small but devoted group who had impressed the office nurse by their support and availability throughout the patient's illness. The patient was not satisfied that in the future a new pleural effusion or other mediastinal complications might be allowed to progress while he was kept adequately comfortable with morphine, even though the morphine itself might somewhat hasten the moment of death. "Can't you just inject enough morphine to guarantee a rapid death before I ever get to that point?"

His physician expressed sympathy for the patient's fears of an uncomfortable or undignified death, then stated her own limits in treatment: that she liberally gave medicine for comfort but would not administer any agent to induce death. Expressing irritation, the patient left but returned to the dialogue in subsequent visits. The physician noted that the patient refused to bring in his sister or any close friends for discussion of the point, that he denied being suicidal or depressed (nor was he clinically depressed), and that he never took an overdose of his hydromorphone, of which by her calculation he had about 100 tablets. Nor would he consult any other physician, including, in particular, the psychiatrist she recommended. This she suggested after he asked her about potassium chloride injection, pointing out to him, "I know this is very difficult for you. You have coped superbly—in fact, I have no idea whether I myself could cope half as well were I in your situation. Because it is a matter of continuing to cope, I'd like you to see one of my colleagues, a psychiatrist, who has helped others to get the most out of their coping skills." When he refused, she explored another option. "You probably feel that my treatment limitations are only another burden to bear. Would you like to see another doctor?" "Do you know any doctors who inject potassium chloride for dying patients?" he asked. "No," she replied, "but there are many good oncologists who could review your treatments to see if there is anything I could do better." "I don't want another doctor," he said, confirming his positive attachment to her, which she had felt all along. "The way I look at this as your physician," she said, "is that the illness, like so many things in this world, is bigger than both of us. I am only a physician. Society, wisely, I think, does not license me to kill, even out of motives of mercy. But I have become quite good at minimizing discomforts associated with these illnesses, and I would very much like to remain available to you as each new difficulty presents itself."

The physician in the foregoing example modeled a response when confronted by the request to accelerate death. She stated her own treatment limitations humbly and honestly; explored the meaning of the request in terms of the patient's family, depression, and suicide; suggested psychiatric consultation to decrease emotional distress and increase coping efficiency; was open to another opinion; expressed admiration for the patient's coping ability; and reaffirmed her desire to help, her ability to minimize suffering, and her intention to remain available to the patient (and family) for each difficulty as it would arise. Her soft answers averted his anger at not being able to control her. Her openness helped to explore all the implications of his request. Perhaps most important, her restatement of her commitment to caring for him diminished his fears of abandonment, loss of respect, and ultimate failure to cope with his illness.

Documentation

Whenever decisions are made about treatment limitation, the medical record should include an explicit statement of the reasons that led to them, the patient's comprehension of and agreement with them, and the understanding and reactions of other persons significant to the patient, usually the family. The more explicitly this is done, the better the record. Despite contemporary fears of litigation for neglect, malpractice, and homocide, complete honesty is recommended. In the life-and-death struggles with advanced cancer, no therapeutic stone is left unturned to minimize harm and maximize comfort for the patient. Nothing about this goal need be hidden or apologized for. Failure to make orders explicit on the order sheet only jeopardizes care of the patient.

As Death Approaches

Treatment-team members often hear the question, "What will death be like? How will it come?" Sometimes it is quite possible to forecast the mode of death, as by infection, hemorrhage or slow lapse into coma. Often behind these questions is the fear that the death will be violent, painful, or humiliating. Since this is usually not the case, it helps to reassure patient and family of this. Cicely Saunder's gentle image of cancer death has been helpful to many: "It is like a candle going out."[3] Management of this phase of illness is described in detail elsewhere in this volume. Once a decision to limit treatment is made, however, it is important to help the family realize that preparing for a comfortable death is the major task at hand. No further trips to the emergency ward means that we now must cope with the life-threatening process at home. If one stops at the limitation decision itself (*e.g.,* no more antibiotics), the family and patient may not have progressed to this next concern: What will they do to cope with the infection? What can they expect? How are they to handle it? Reassurance that the team is as available to them now as it was during the more aggressive treatment phases is essential.

Decisions can change. Death is a natural process, and the course toward it can be punctuated by transient improvement. If a patient recovers spontaneously from aspiration pneumonia without antibiotics, it does not mean the decision to withhold them was "wrong." It was the best possible at the time. Patients and families can be warned ahead of time of these realities. The mature and noble vigil to which health-care professionals commit themselves in the care of their dying patients can adjust to these changes with no less equanimity and thoughtfulness than has been shown throughout the illness.

REFERENCES

1. Slater E: New horizons in medical ethics. Wanted—a new approach. Br Med J 1:285–286, 1973
2. Ingelfinger FJ: Bedside ethics for the hopeless case (Editorial). N Engl J Med 289:914, 1973
3. Saunders C: Care of the dying: The problem of euthanasia, 1–6. Nurs Times 55:960–961, 994–995, 1031–1032, 1067–1069, 1091–1092, 1129–1130, 1959

SUGGESTED READING

Cassem NH: Treating the person confronting death. In Nicholi, AM Jr (ed): The Harvard Guide to Modern Psychiatry, Cambridge, Harvard University Press, 1978
Cassem NH: Procedural protocol when illness is judged irreversible. In Cassem NH: Psychiatry. In Rubenstein E, Federman DD (eds): Scientific American Medicine, New York, Scientific American, 1980
Veatch RM: A Theory of Medical Ethics. New York, Basic Books, 1981

Psychosocial Support

Part Two

The Task of Physical Care   4

HOSPITAL-IN-THE-HOME

The Family as Caretakers[21]

When a person with advanced cancer is discharged from the hospital, all the regular chores of the nurses, nutritionists, and housekeeping staff are transferred to the patient and family. A myriad of important tasks, readily delegated in the hospital to specially trained therapists, technicians, pharmacists, clerks, administrators, messengers, maintenance and supply personnel, and volunteers is now transferred to the household. The family, unlike hospital employees who work in shifts and have regular vacations and days off, distributes these chores among a few people who are now "on-call" 24 hours a day, 7 days a week.

Many patients maintain some responsibility for their own care, insofar as they are capable. When the patient is debilitated and dependent on others, however, a "primary caretaker,"[11] "chief carer,"[22] or "responsor"[8] usually emerges—a person who does most of the physical chores or at least assumes major responsibility for managing the patient's care. A spouse or daughter typically becomes the primary caretaker for older patients; younger patients are usually cared for by their mothers. Daughters-in-law, sons, siblings (usually sisters), fathers, roommates, or friends may also take on this responsibility. The primary caretaker's job is occasionally shared by a few persons.

If patients' social networks are limited, neighbors, volunteers, or health-care professionals may assume the primary caretaker function. The emotional involvement and commitment of such persons may be quite different from that of family

155

members or close friends, yet their interest in serving or their sympathy for the ill person's plight may make them devoted caretakers.

Isolated individuals who lack social supports and dedicated help may seem ill-suited for home care. However, many such persons are quite intolerant of institutional care. They may insist on continuing to look after themselves, seeking to die on their own homeground, whether this be the YMCA, a boardinghouse, or a solitary home or apartment. The professional caretaking team can support this wish for independence.

> Mr. A had been living in a boarding house for many years when he developed inoperable cancer. He was a quiet, pleasant man who had little to say to anyone and spent most of his days alone or on the benches at a nearby city square. He had never been married. He maintained occasional contact with a brother, his only living relative.
>
> Mr. A's room, located on the third floor of an old walk-up, was not much bigger than a large closet. A pay telephone was located down the hall. He had been placed on a strict low-sodium diet to relieve the swelling in his legs, but he continued to live on salty canned foods, which he usually ate cold or sometimes cooked on a hot plate.
>
> Mr. A's major physical problems were weakness and the swelling of his legs—problems that did not cause much discomfort but that left him unable to get up and down stairs. He wanted to stay in his own room, saying he liked it because "it's my place." As long as he was helped to be reasonably comfortable, he had little concern about dying.
>
> As Mr. A's condition worsened, his brother repeatedly asked him to move in with family. His brother also offered to provide better accommodations elsewhere. Mr. A refused the proposals, saying that he was happier in his room and retained a sense of independence there. He was grateful when his brother agreed to do the grocery shopping and to bring an occasional meal.
>
> The patient was seen periodically by a physician and visiting nurse. His connection with the outside world was mostly by way of telephone conversations with a "patient advocate" in the neighborhood health center. She arranged for "meals-on-wheels," transportation to see the oncologist, and delivery of medications. She personally performed a few errands and helped straighten out his insurance forms and bills. Most importantly, she was available by phone, maintaining regular contact and assuring Mr. A that someone was ready to assist with any problems that might arise. Even though he seemed terribly isolated in his room, Mr. A had a sense of being helped, of not being utterly alone.
>
> Mr. A eventually became bedridden, barely able to sit up on the side of his bed. He refused hospitalization. He was provided with a urinal and bedpan. Arrangements for further assistance from a home health aide were initiated, but Mr. A was found dead the following day.

The presence of family in the home does not ensure the availability of a primary caretaker. The family may be negligent, incompetent, or physically and emotionally unable to provide assistance. Also, the responsibility for home care of the elderly falls, in great part, on the elderly themselves, many of whom are disabled.[2,18] The physical well-being and morale of an aged spouse or parent often is a crucial factor in the ability of an ill person to remain at home.

The continued successful management of a terminal illness at home usually depends more on the motivation of the primary caretaker than on his or her physical or intellectual capabilities or on the medical condition of the patient. In ideal circumstances, the primary caretaker role is assumed willingly and eagerly. Many factors, however, can enter into the choice of a caretaker. In some cases, the patient or family simply designates a particular person who seems best suited to the task. Similarly, the patient and family may exclude another candidate for this role because of his or her ill health, strained financial resources, job responsibilities, need to care for small children or other relatives, inconvenient home size or location, and so forth.

Even though the tasks described in this chapter may seem burdensome, many family members do not find their responsibilities oppressive. Obligations are often assumed without question, as if to say, "In our family (or community), this is what one does for one's parents (or child, spouse, neighbor, etc.)." Even when exhaustion develops, the nature and limits of the obligation are often unquestioned.

Other family members balance an awareness of their encumberment with a sense of duty and a desire to help. With death imminent, caretakers may be strongly motivated by feelings of obligation toward the ill person or by a desire to repair a relationship before its ostensible conclusion. When the provision of physical care is an avenue for expressing gratitude and affection, and especially when the dying person conveys appreciation, the job feels "therapeutic" and can be the source of great personal fulfillment. The act of caring may momentarily divert attention from grief, allowing for satisfying action in the face of ultimate helplessness. Nevertheless, many families set limits on their obligations; when home care is difficult, they may readily accept outside help to relieve the burden of caretaking, or they may consider institutional care.

Feelings of guilt and ambivalence about the tasks of care are particularly evident in some families. Caretaking may seem to expiate old sins, to atone for past neglect and disharmony. Extreme dedication to the dying person may reflect a preoccupation with old emotional injuries. The adult who becomes the excessively devoted primary caretaker for a mother or father has often not been a "favorite child," but rather one who never sensed that he or she got enough from the dying parent (and now tries to gain it) or never felt adequately valued by the parent (and now tries to establish his or her worth). Any limiting of responsibilities (*e.g.*, taking time off, getting help) may seem heretical, bringing the family member's devotion into question. Deep involvement in caretaking may also be an attempt to divert oneself from recognizing the impending loss, bespeaking a profound sense of inability to go on alone after the death. Mental-health consultation can be helpful in such instances.

The Transformation of the Home

Ward reports that 39% of patients who died at home spent a week or less unable to get out of bed without assistance, while 41% spent greater than 2 weeks in bed, 17% greater than 4 weeks, and 6% greater than 3 months. Only 13% were never bed-fast.[22] When a patient's mobility is significantly impaired, the home may be reorganized to create a "sick room" where the patient spends most of his or her time. Convenience for the entire family often dictates that this room—usually the living room or dining room—be on the ground floor. Furniture is rearranged to create storage space for medications, dressings, equipment, and supplies. The telephone, television, radio, tape deck, or record player may be appropriated for the sick room.

A recreation or rest area may be created for the patient near the bedside, and furnished with a special chair or couch. The nearest bathroom is reorganized for the patient's needs, while portions of other rooms (*e.g.*, a sink, bureau, refrigerator shelf) may be used for patient care. The phone numbers of the doctors, nurses, and hospital are often displayed prominently by the bedside or phone, while additional sites may be set aside for medication lists, charts, and instruction sheets.

Often, the kitchen or another room not frequented by the patient becomes a "backstage" area.[7] Its use is similar to that of a hospital staff room. Family and friends retreat there to get away from the work, for moments of rest and quiet, for eating, drinking, and smoking, for pursuing personal tasks unrelated to the caretaking job, and for talking about the patient away from the bedside, beyond the dying person's sight and hearing.

New Chores and Responsibilities[1,2,12,16,17]

The patient and family are unlikely to be familiar with many of the caretaking chores—complicated pharmacologic regimens, injections, management of tubing and dressings, monitoring of the patient's condition (e.g., pulse, urinary output, oral intake), positioning in bed and transferring from bed to chair, and helping with evacuation of bowels and bladder. Remarkably, families commonly show a willingness and interest in learning such chores and a devotion to doing the job well. A lack of technical competence is rarely a barrier to good physical care at home. With patient and sympathetic teaching, most families can learn to handle these chores properly. The job done at home is often as good as or superior to institutional care, although perhaps provided at great personal cost to the family. The physician can often encourage and support the family's painstaking efforts with honestly enthusiastic comparisons of the home to an intensive care unit.

Queasiness or revulsion about managing wounds, handling urine and stools, or confronting disfigurement are surprisingly rare or are readily overcome among families who choose to keep the dying at home.

> *A patient summoned her grandson in the middle of the night to help her with the bedpan. Bashfully, she asked, "Oh Jimmy, do you mind?"*
>
> *"Oh, Grandma," he replied, "it's three in the morning. Pee is pee. Let me have that bedpan."*

The experience of caring for young children prepares some family members for the physical management of a helpless adult. Taboos about adult nakedness and touching, which ordinarily shape family behavior decisively, are often discarded. The sight of the dying person's body may be—especially for a relative or intimate friend—an overpowering experience and an uncomfortable reminder of approaching death:

> Maman had an open hospital nightdress on and she did not mind that her wrinkled belly, criss-crossed with tiny lines, and her bald pubis showed. 'I no longer have any sort of shame,' she observed in a surprised voice.
>
> 'You are perfectly right not to have any,' I said. But I turned away and gazed fixedly into the garden. The sight of my mother's nakedness had jarred me. No body existed less for me: none existed more. As a child I had loved it dearly; as an adolescent it had filled me with an uneasy repulsion: all this was perfectly in the ordinary course of things and it seemed reasonable to me that her body should retain its dual nature, that it should be both repugnant and holy—a taboo. But for all that, I was astonished at the violence of my distress. My mother's indifferent acquiescence made it worse: she was abandoning the exigencies and prohibitions that had oppressed her all her life long and I approved of her doing so. Only this body, suddenly reduced by her capitulation to being a body and nothing more, hardly differed at all from a corpse—a poor defenceless

carcass turned and manipulated by professional hands, one in which life seemed to carry on only because of its own stupid momentum. For me, my mother had always been there, and I had never seriously thought that some day, that soon I should see her go. Her death, like her birth, had its place in some legendary time. When I said to myself 'She is of an age to die' the words were devoid of meaning, as so many words are. For the first time I saw her as a dead body under suspended sentence.[3]

Calm, confident behavior on the part of professional caretakers serves as a model for the family in carrying out its chores. The physician's patience, tolerance, and encouragement help laypersons develop expertise and self-assurance. When the professional staff, as a result, perhaps, of unfamiliarity with home-based self-care, is skeptical about the family's ability to do the tasks properly or, owing to arrogance, feels that nonprofessionals should not attempt such work, the family's confidence is, of course, less likely to be promoted.

Some burdens of care are commonly intolerable to even the best motivated family members.[20,23,24] Restlessness and crying out during the night are particularly troublesome, although these problems can often be managed with nocturnal sedation. If disturbances occur on successive evenings and if the primary caretaker does not share the night duty with others or must work during the day, the sleep deprivation may become intolerable. Equally trying is the wandering about the house of a confused or unsteady patient, especially when this or other disturbing behavior threatens the quiet of night, interrupts sleep, endangers the patient or others, and occurs when needed assistance is not available. The patient can usually be restrained or sedated, but the prospect of dangerous meddling (*e.g.*, with gas, fire, or breakable objects), or of struggle, escape, or a fall may be unbearable for some families.

When the primary caretaker and family are overwhelmed by the burden of physical care, they may become intolerant of chores that previously would have seemed acceptable. Alternately, they can become intolerant of physical tasks when the emotional climate in the home has become unmanageable. Failure to palliate the patient's physical suffering or to address the family's emotional distress may lead the family to feel overwhelmed by the work of caretaking. A new task or a worsening problem becomes the "last straw."

While families may tolerate brief disruptions in their lives in order to care for a dying patient, the prospect of providing home care for a prolonged illness may be frightening or unacceptable. The family may incorrectly conclude that progressive disability means an increasingly intense burden on the caretakers. In fact, physical caretaking may become easier as death nears. Clarification of the likely course of the illness, of future caretaking needs and the availability of help, and of the anticipated survival time may be useful (as discussed in Chapter 5), along with a reminder that institutional care can always be reconsidered.

Role Shifts

When a person is sick, his or her household responsibilities will shift to other family members. A husband might for the first time have to take on the tasks of cooking, shopping, cleaning, clothes-washing, and baby-sitting. A wife might for the first time have to manage household repairs, finances, legal matters, or a family business. Adults may acquire additional dependents; older parents, enjoying the relative freedom of an "empty nest," may find grown children or grandchildren returning to the household. Children may suddenly assume adult responsibilities. Family members usually exhibit an impressive willingness and capacity to take on these new roles and responsibilities.

Family caretakers are likely to have less time for work, hobbies, recreation, rest, socializing, and personal pursuits—activities that may normally contribute to a sense of well-being and happiness for themselves and others. When the patient requires a good deal of attention, the primary caretaker may not even find time to shop, pick up prescriptions, or run errands. The demands of a complicated medical routine may interfere with the family's ability to relax, share pleasant moments, engage in intimate conversation, or otherwise provide the mutual support that can be so important during a terminal illness.

A "ripple effect" may occur as family members find increasing difficulty in fulfilling their usual obligations or personal needs and as they either neglect their responsibilities or shift some of the burden to persons outside the immediate caretaking circle. Friends and relatives may take on new tasks or suffer from lack of attention. If a major change in the patient's needs occurs, the reverberations in the family's social circle may strike suddenly; if the patient gradually requires more attention, the ripple of repercussions may widen insidiously:

> Mrs. B, a 70-year-old Italian-speaking woman, came to the office for the first time in the early summer, complaining of being too hot. She had spent a few years living in the United States with her daughter's family and had been living in the same room during those years. The weather had not been unusually warm during the current season.
>
> Mrs. B felt that she would be fine if she had a fan. Her daughter, who ordinarily took her shopping and would have helped her with such a purchase, had been very busy. On further questioning, the patient indicated that she had gotten out of the house much less than usual, and that she had been reluctant to ask for help from her overworked daughter. Both the patient and her daughter were upset about the younger of three children in the household, a 5-year-old boy who was dying of a slowly progressive illness. The child's mother was carrying out an heroic, nearly full-time nursing program at home. The dying child's father was undergoing testing for physical symptoms (which later proved to be psychophysiologic in origin), while the two healthy children were having adjustment problems at school.
>
> Mrs. B's immediate problem was readily resolved by a fan (and by additional ventilation). The underlying problems were slowly and partially alleviated by helping the mother attend to her other dependent family members and to herself while still caring for the sick boy.

Difficult and uninterrupted responsibilities, confinement, and a lack of normal pleasures or time for reconstitution, especially when complicated by physical exhaustion and sleep deprivation, will be tolerated only for a limited period. Breakdown in coping by the caretakers may be evident as poor care for the patient, intolerance of minor physical or emotional problems, impaired physical health, a growing sense of helplessness and desperation, and inappropriate calls for professional assistance. The emotional consequences of new or shifted responsibilities in the family circle are commonly first manifested as anxiety, fatigue, irritability, and depression among those persons most heavily burdened, as adjustment problems in children, and as marital distress. When the family is overburdened, a feeling of guilt about not doing more for the patient is frequently expressed as anger at the community health team for neglecting or not caring for the patient or as accusations that the hospital staff has sent the patient home inappropriately or without proper help.

In conclusion, while institutional care (as discussed in Chapter 10) places significant burdens on the family—the time and effort of traveling back and forth to the hospital; of waiting, often helplessly, for long periods of time; of being a visitor in an unfamiliar, often frightening, environment; of being separated from each other—home care, too, may be physically, emotionally, or financially devastating. Although home care may be seen as a simple, less costly alternative to institutional care, the commitment of human resources can be extensive and, in some cases, exhausting. The long-term consequences of these stresses are difficult to appreciate and have not been systematically studied. As discussed in the following section, far-reaching, many-faceted problems in home-based management can often be detected and acted upon by the clinician before they become intolerable or lead to breakdown in family life or patient care.

MANAGING THE BURDEN

> Sometimes I wonder if health professionals
> realize how little we laymen know, and what a
> very small amount of practical information it
> takes to transform us into very capable
> managers and helpers.[9]

In approaching the physical symptoms of terminal illness, specific problems often respond to specific solutions: one person's cough yields to codeine; metoclopramide proves to be the "magic bullet" for another person's vomiting. In approaching the burden of physical care in the home, the family doctor is more likely to face a host of large and small interrelated social problems that are eased not by a single action but by an array of timely interventions. Occasionally, one crucial finger in the dike is needed, but the physician is more often surveying a leaky dam, attending to the bigger or more readily fixed leaks with whatever patching material is on hand, while watching for and trying to avert a major burst in the wall.

Human "support" systems have been compared with the structural supports of a bridge.[4] Like an engineer examining a weakened bridge, the physician first seeks an understanding of the nature of the damage to the family system. Which problems reflect an acute insult to a previously well-functioning structure? What problems are long-standing features of the family? How is the stress directly affecting the various family elements? How is the stress transmitted? With such an analysis, a variety of remedies can be applied at those points where strain can be relieved, where supporters can be strengthened.

Evaluation of Resources and Anticipation of Problems

As soon as home-based management is considered for a debilitated, dependent patient, a detailed appraisal should be undertaken of the job of providing care and of the family's resources. Medical social workers are often the central professionals in this process of evaluation and planning. For hospitalized patients, discharge planning

TABLE 4-1
A Checklist of Considerations for Home Care: The Physical Setting and Tasks

Housing	Satisfactory physical setting for care?
	   Comfort, cleanliness, spaciousness
	   Safety and comfort of the neighborhood
	   Access for patient, family, friends
	Consider housing assistance programs (mortgage
	   maintenance and rental supports)
	Consider special housing for independent or assisted living
	   Handicapped housing
	   Senior citizens' housing
	   Foster homes

Room	Where will patient be? Rearranging rooms. Where will others sleep and carry on their lives?

Bed	Rent, buy, or borrow
	Elevated, adjustable
	   Mechanical or electrical adjustments
	Side rails, trapeze
	Mattress—foam, air, water, or regular
	Bedding—sheepskin, plastic sheets, underpads
	Care in bed
	   Changing bedding
	   Moving, turning, washing
	   Special skin care (preventing and treating decubiti)
	   Cradles, bedding frames
	   Positioning

Mobility	Transfer techniques—lifting, mechanical devices
	Special chairs, couches
	Assistance in ambulation—canes, crutches, walkers,
	   wheelchairs, rails, ramps
	Safety hazards (*e.g.,* loose rugs, obstructions)
	   Aids (*e.g.,* railings, bars)
	Exercise (active and passive); physical therapy

Dressing	Bedclothes and normal clothes Laundry
Grooming	Hair and nails Makeup
Bathing	Techniques for bed baths Aids—flexible shower heads, long-handled brushes Safety equipment—grab bars, shower and bathtub seats, adhesive strips to prevent slipping
Skin care	See Chap. 2, Section H
Oral hygiene	See Chap. 2, Section E
Bowel and bladder function	*Continent*—use of bedpan, urinal, bedside commode, elevated toilet seat Access to bathroom Bowel regimens, suppositories

Table 4-1 *(Continued)*

	Incontinent—incontinence pants, underpads, plastic sheets, hampers, diaper service External or indwelling urinary catheter; drainage systems and their management

Feeding	Shopping or ordering food; "meals-on-wheels"
	Preparation
	    Soft and liquid diets
	    Tube-feedings
	Assistance in eating
	    Bedside fluids, snacks
	    Special utensils, straws
	Alcohol
	Food Stamps and other nutritional support programs

Medication	Purchase and delivery; storage and safety; refilling
	    monitoring, recording, adjusting
	    Self-administer vs. given by family
	Aid in swallowing—mashing pills, mixing with food,
	    liquid preparations
	Suppositories
	Topical treatments
	Injections

Medical supplies and equipment	Purchasing, borrowing, or renting; delivery; storage; use;
	    safety
	    Gloves, syringes, needles, sterile dressings, solutions
	    Catheter equipment
	    Oxygen nebulizers, suction equipment
	    Intravenous therapy, hyperalimentation

Attending	Professional or "skilled" help vs. "unskilled" help
	    Visiting nurses
	    Physical therapy, speech therapy, occupational therapy
	    Home health aides
	    Homemakers, chore services
	    Companions and volunteer services
	Training nonprofessional helpers (*e.g.*, to change dressing,
	    give injections, monitor vital signs)
	Availability of help—constant vs. intermittent
	Regular, anticipated chores (*e.g.*, dressing changes, meals,
	    skin care, medications) vs. intermittent needs (*e.g.*,
	    snacks, "as needed" medications, some transfers)
	Calling for help—telephones, buzzers, bells
	Night call
	What to do when questions arise? Caretakers absent?
	Handling emergencies

Diversions, entertainment, recreation	Hobbies, books, TV, radio, tapes, records Personally important objects—photographs, paintings, gifts, souvenirs, and mementos Family access and visitors Excursions

(Continued)

Table 4-1 *(Continued)*

Pastoral care

Legal aid

Financial aid	Who is familiar with the availability of and eligibility for services and the process of obtaining help?
	Hospital-based and community-based social-service agencies
	Sources
	Third-party health insurance (*e.g.*, Blue Cross–Blue Shield, Medicare, Medicaid, and other private insurers)
	Social Security, General Relief
	Area Agency on Aging
	United Fund and other community charities
	Special funds—American Cancer Society, local and national philanthropies, hospital funds
Out-of-home help	Sites
	Senior Citizens' center (for meals, recreation)
	Day-care
	Respite care
	Rehabilitation services
	Transportation

should not be a rushed, last-minute process. In order to train and support the family caretakers and to enlist additional help, time for preparation is required. A checklist of common considerations in planning is provided in Table 4-1.

Professionals familiar with home care can often foresee difficulties long before the family recognizes a serious problem or begins to feel overwhelmed. The physician who anticipates and repeatedly explores the stresses of caretaking with the patient and family will be in a position to recognize problems before they become excessive, shielding the family from an overwhelming burden. Services should be provided to prevent or rapidly treat a breakdown in coping with the burden.

Meticulous planning includes an awareness of and preparation for potential losses of support and for the fatigue and turnover in personnel that commonly occur during a long, taxing illness. Sensible and dependable arrangements to delegate duties should be established, so that no person is left with excessive chores and responsibilities. Undependable help may be more troublesome than no help at all.

Almost every family can benefit from some teaching, support, special equipment, or outside assistance.[16,19] Clear, detailed instructions about nursing care and about the use of equipment and supplies are necessary, and should be reviewed periodically. Medication regimens often need to be reviewed weekly, sometimes more frequently. Regular communication between professional caretakers ensures that consistent instructions are presented to the family.

Standard home-health equipment (*e.g.*, a hospital bed or wheelchair) is usually readily available and can be rented cheaply. Third-party insurance may pay for equipment; special funds (*e.g.*, from the American Cancer Society) may sometimes be obtained. Occasionally, a community service organization will maintain a store of equipment for lending.

Outside Help

Help from outside the family is regularly required. While such services are usually welcomed and appreciated, occasional problems arise. Assistance from the welfare department, a volunteer agency, or a charity may carry a stigma (although some beneficiaries, particularly those with private health insurance and pension plans, may have a strong sense of entitlement to aid). The family may tend to be critical of outsiders' competence. Distrust or dislike may develop. Some families perceive outside help as evidence of their own failure to be devoted or competent. Moreover, nurses and aides often develop close relationships with the patient, and jealousies may arise. A devoted wife may feel resentful when a home health aide is praised by the patient or physician. The outside helper who is eager to compensate for whatever the patient lacks from his or her relatives may need a gentle reminder not to rob the family of their sense of central importance.

The physician must be familiar with community resources and the capabilities of various service providers. The following services may be sought:

The *visiting nurse* (home-care nurse) performs nursing chores, shows the family how to handle nursing tasks, and provides suggestions about managing care in the home, including how to use equipment and obtain further help. The visiting nurse is usually the health-care professional who has most contact with the family and is most intimately involved with day-to-day care. Regular nursing visits can be tremendously reassuring to the patient and family. The nurse, providing the bulk of professional help in a home-health or hospice program, is in a position to set the style of care and can often make community care successful when optimal physician involvement is lacking. Much of this book relays information that will be familiar to an experienced home-care nurse.

Visiting nurses generally supervise ongoing care and make brief, task-oriented visits. In Boston in 1983, a visit cost $38; a "sliding" fee scale is available, and many health insurances cover such "skilled" nursing services.

For patients who require continuous professional nursing, "private duty" nurses are available from some community and private agencies. In Boston in 1983, home nursing costs about $16 per hour. Health insurance in the United States usually does not cover such services. Professional nursing (and less skilled nursing-aide services) are often difficult to obtain at night in the United States. In Great Britain, "night attendants" are sometimes available through the National Health Plan.

Home health aides bathe the patient, change the bed, manage dressings, assist in transfer, and relieve the family by assuming the care of the patient for part of the day. They may not be licensed to give medications, change dressings, or perform certain nursing chores. The current home health aide rate in Boston is $8 to $13 per hour, and 100 hours per month is covered by most federal health insurances but not by private insurance. In the near future, Medicare patients in accredited hospice programs will probably be eligible for more extensive home-health services.

Homemakers clean, cook, shop, and perform many other household chores. Direct "hands-on" care is usually forbidden. The current charge for homemakers in Boston is about $8 per hour.

Friends and *volunteers* (particularly volunteers trained by hospice groups) can help with chores such as shopping, transportation, and errands. They may also sit with the patient and provide companionship, perhaps allowing the family to get away.

Other *community resources* may help meet family needs. Neighbors, members of local churches, the police and fire departments, local business people and professionals (particularly lawyers and funeral directors) can be enlisted (*e.g.*, for help with an excursion, obtaining a haircut or special merchandise, or planning an estate or funeral).

Consultation with a *medical social worker* or the regular participation of a social worker in team deliberations is routinely advisable for identifying family needs, enlisting community resources, and providing personal counseling. Assessment of financial resources, insurance coverage, and eligibility for services is often managed by the social worker.

Each home-care team should include a person familiar with insurance coverage, welfare regulations, local services to the elderly and disabled, community charities (including the American Cancer Society), and private sources for funds. In a crisis that promises to be brief, rules about eligibility for services may be stretched, or exceptional resources may be mobilized: the visiting nurses may make extra visits, a nighttime home health aide will be covered by third-party insurance, or a community fund will pay for essential equipment. Terminal illness, however, often generates prolonged demands for such special services.

The MGH–Chelsea Memorial Health Care Center employs a patient-care representative who maintains frequent contact with homebound patients and families. This *ombudsman* provides a friendly, accessible entrée to the health-care system and can provide help with transportation, bills, insurance, appointments, medication refills, day-care, elderly services, baby-sitting, housing, and a host of other community resources. The patient-care representative sometimes finds city employees, service personnel, and local businessmen who can help with unusual problems.

A person who has been through a similar experience can sometimes provide *peer counseling.* Thoughtful, practical advice and support from such a layperson may be better heeded than professional counseling. Mutual-help support groups or an introduction to a carefully chosen individual can be helpful.

Geriatric services have developed a variety of programs to help families care for an ill relative in the community (*e.g.,* "Supporter Endurance Training"[14] or Alzheimer's family groups). Similar services can be developed for advanced cancer patients.

Although many patients and families are not interested in reading about the topic of terminal illness and home care, written materials appeal to some. For example, Mary K. House's lovely article, "Home Style Nursing," reviews the physical management of a patient in the home and goes on to offer the following practical advice: keep up your spirits; don't be a martyr, indulge yourself, take help; take good care of yourself; get out; use caretaking responsibilities as an alibi or an excuse when needed; celebrate when an occasion arises; and exploit moments of well-being.[10] Gerda Lerner's *A Death of One's Own* is also appreciated by some families.[13] A few popular guides—how to care for a dying person at home—have been published, but they tend to be idiosyncratic in viewpoint or bothersomely inaccurate. Mace and Robins's book on Alzheimer's disease, *The 36-Hour Day,* has been well-received by families and professionals and touches on many topics relevant to patients with advanced cancer.[15]

A Note on Visitors

Friendship is highly valued at a time of distress. Visitors for a homebound patient are often greeted eagerly. However, even the best-mannered and most well-intentioned visitors can pose a problem in the ill patient's home, as in the hospital, because of a conflict between the family's wish to observe the social conventions of being welcoming hosts and their need to attend to caretaking and personal wants. A visitor can disrupt complicated care schemes and may seem to put new demands on the family for attention or service. The hosts, even when they feel exhausted, do not comfortably put aside the habit of making conversation, inquiring about the guest's health and fortune, or offering food. Occasionally, visitors may seem insensitive, acting inappropriately cheerful or troublingly gloomy. Beleaguered family members may also resent the well-meaning visitor who has the luxury of sitting with the patient, coming and going as he or she pleases, while they scurry about with dressing changes or worry over an intricate medication schedule. Thus, even a guest who is trying to help may seem to add to the burden.

The physician can assist the family in looking out for themselves, encouraging them to decide who they want to have as visitors, when the visits should take place, and what the visitors should do. The family may need the doctor's prompting or even explicit sanction to exclude certain visitors, to excuse themselves from social amenities, and to request help from or place demands on their friends. The physician might say:

> *Let your friends bring the food and fix the coffee in your kitchen while you stay with the patient.*

> *You need to establish visiting hours. Tell them the doctor said so.*

> *Help the visitors out by telling them what you need. They seem to be trying to show their concern, but somehow they're causing more problems for you.*

Lessening the Overall Burden

Outside help is often not obtainable to meet the family's specific needs. A full range of home-health services may not be available in the community, or such services may not be affordable. Health-insurance coverage often seems to have been designed with little appreciation of the needs of dying patients in the community. Consequently, a lack of relatively inexpensive home assistance, such as that provided by late-night nursing aides, may force the physician and family to resort to costly institutional care.

When specific, appropriate services cannot be obtained, the physician may attempt to reduce the family's burden by aiding them in those chores, perhaps minor, for which help is available. By lessening the overall caretaking responsibilities and giving the family some sense that they do not bear the burden alone, the remaining tasks may become more manageable. For instance, a wife who can comfortably bathe her sick husband and change his bed may still benefit from a home-health aide who takes over these tasks and watches the patient for a few hours a day. The wife can use the free time for personal needs and may find that other, more troublesome, tasks— for example, responding to calls and giving medication in the middle of the night— seem more tolerable.

Encouragement and Setting Limits on Responsibility

The professional caretaker faces two potentially conflicting tasks: to encourage the family to provide care in the home and to help them recognize and set realistic limits on their responsibilities.

Regular praise from the physician makes the burden of caretaking more tolerable. The family's frustrations and sacrifice are more bearable when recognized and appreciated. The physician can foster a sense of meaning and mission in tasks that otherwise might seem mindless, thankless, and unending, and he or she should share delight in the caretaker's achievements:

> *You must have earned a nursing degree by now!*

> *Have you ever been through something like this before? Did you ever dream you would become so good at it?*

> *I know you'll be able to look back at this ordeal with pride that you did so much for your husband.*

> *You certainly have done a marvelous job here. Even though your mother seems grumpy and ungrateful at times, I know she must appreciate your kindness and good care.*

> *I don't know how you put up with it. I admire your patience.*

> *I know your husband [who is semicomatose or demented] can't thank you for the wonderful things you have been doing, but I want you to know how touched I am by your devotion and by how well you take care of him. I hope he somehow appreciates it.*

Family members can also be helped to acknowledge each other's skill and devotion.

In offering such encouragement, the physician runs the risk of stifling disgruntlement and of fostering unrealistic commitments. Families also need the opportunity to vent frustrations and to set reasonable limits on their responsibilities. Much of the care of the terminally ill revolves around deeply sensed commitments. In the context of terminal illness, particularly a brief one, "appropriate" limits may be difficult to set, and might not, of course, be judicious in other settings. In general, however, families should be urged to take time off from their caretaking burdens and to accept outside help, especially when there are signs of fatigue or "burn-out." A sense of unlimited duty can be tempered:

> *Nurses work 8-hour shifts and have regular days off. Do you really think you can be at this job constantly and still do it well and remain sane?*

> *Don't let yourself get exhausted over this. You'll need your energy for other matters.*

> *We've seen lots of families who can manage these sorts of duties for a few weeks or a month, but then it begins to wear them down. You'll need outside help if you want to keep this up without it driving you crazy or making a mess of your whole family.*

The family's unique role as concerned, close, and loving persons in the dying patient's life needs to be distinguished from their role in performing the tasks of care. Some people immerse themselves totally in the mechanics of caretaking, avoiding awareness of sadness and impending loss. Time should be set aside for moments of peacefulness and sharing, of communion:

> *He needs you there as his friend, for all the things you do for him and mean to him without even trying. You can't do that if you're exhausted or always running around changing bedpans.*

The home should not become merely an efficient institution, staffed by family members. Ideally, the family should have time and energy to devote to special meals, parties, or excursions with the patient. Also, the family's continued attention to other parts of its life—work, friends, recreation—helps maintain the social supports that will be important after the death.

The patient's wishes and needs for caretaking may conflict with those of the family. Some patients, for instance, will expect constant attention when they apparently require only intermittent care. The physician can help as a mediator:

> *I think your husband is getting exhausted. Can you help him decide to get away in the afternoons for the next few days? I know you can be well cared for without him, even though his company is very precious to you.*

> *Your wife wants to do everything she can, but it seems important for her to keep working, both for her own well-being and to keep the family going. We can get you the help you need when she's away, but she still needs your OK to leave.*

The Patient's Acceptance of Help

The patient may have strong feelings about accepting physical care from the family or from outsiders. The physician should listen for expressions of such feelings and inquire directly about these concerns:

> *How do you feel about the help you're getting at home?*

> *Have you ever gotten help like this before?*

> *How is your family managing with the nursing job? Do you think they're doing it well? Do they seem tired? Irritable?*

Patients may be acutely aware of the stresses reviewed in this chapter and may request hospitalization or nursing-home placement to protect their family from exhaustion. Sick persons may make heroic efforts to appear comfortable or cheerful so as to make life easier for relatives and friends or to avoid being dependent or demanding. Pain, despair, and frustration may be concealed. A patient who believes he or she has been treated with great generosity—for instance, by accepting an offer to live with a relative—may feel that no further requests for help are permissible. Some patients exaggerate their distress in order to justify continued attention.

A patient may not easily tolerate the passivity, physical intimacy, or dependence imposed by illness or by the outside helpers' style of care. A sick person can often be assisted to feel more independent at home, to be more his or her normal self rather than an object of care (see Chap. 10). Opportunities should be sought for the patient to give as well as to receive. Some patients may not want even small sacrifices made on their behalf and may require some assurance that help is offered willingly. The usual unspoken allegiances within the family—"I'll care for you if you need help"—may need to be addressed more explicitly—"I want to help you now"—lest the patient develop an intolerable sense of being burdensome:

> *Does it sometimes seem like too much to ask of them?*

> *Your family seems eager to help you and happy to have you here, but I gather you feel that you're imposing on them?*

> *How would you feel if you were well and another member of your family were sick?*

Sometimes, paid professional services are preferred by the patient because they do not entail emotional reciprocity. Alternately, patients may prefer the attention of relatives:

> *Would you rather the nurse took care of this?*
>
> *Who do you want to supervise the medication? Change the dressings?*
>
> *You may find it a little strange to have an outsider helping you here, but I think your family needs the assistance right now. Would you try it out? I think you'll soon be more comfortable with the new aide.*

Another set of problems arise when nonprofessionals—the family or outsiders—are not trusted with certain tasks. Such distrust may not be readily expressed. Patients may simply refuse help in order to avoid what to them appears to be poor care:

> *Does it seem that they are doing things right?*
>
> *Are they doing better than the doctor yet?*

Organizing the Team

Formalized arrangements should be considered for organizing the tasks of care. Ideally, a primary caretaker is designated to oversee management of the hospital-in-the-home and to serve as the central contact person between professionals and the family. Similarly, at least one professional will periodically need to review the care process and identify key responsibilities. Major topics for consideration are the quality of care and the supervision of skilled tasks, the coordination of services, an assessment of the family and patient's coping with the physical and emotional burdens, communication among the entire team, and the need for additional services. Multidisciplinary team conferences are extremely useful for achieving such a review. Family members may be asked to join in these sessions.

Family meetings may be used to organize schedules and assign responsibilities. Such gatherings can provide the opportunity to acknowledge service and to help the family set realistic expectations and limits regarding caretaking. In families that function well under the stress of caring for the dying, the meeting may foster an exchange of gratitude. Family members who have withdrawn from the process of care, perhaps as a result of intolerable anger or guilt or a sense of the burden being overwhelming, may be drawn in to support the main caretakers with a limited commitment. Family squabbles are inevitable, but conflicts can sometimes find better resolution or even be put aside in the face of a terminal illness. Resentments can be aired productively. Also, as discussed in Chapter 6, some authors on the care of the terminally ill see the crisis of dying as an opportunity for major transformations in relationships within the family, for reconciliation and growth. A sense of guilt and of having limited time will push many families to new alliances and understandings, to changes that promise at least temporary improvement for the patient or the family.

In families that seem to be having a hard time coping, participation in a meeting is often difficult to enlist. Key members may not attend, and the discussion of problems may only increase tensions and harden resentment. Mental-health consultation, not solely focused on improving the performance of tasks, may be indicated and may eventually lead to improved physical care.

Respite Care

Should the family become fatigued, a brief admission to a hospital or chronic-care facility may provide temporary relief. Such relief may be essential if home care is to continue over long periods of time. At the outset of discharge planning and whenever the burden of care at home intensifies, family members should be informed about the possibility of respite admissions. Simply knowing that such an escape from the daily routine is possible can ease the mind of the caretakers and patient alike, making the burden seem bearable. The opportunity for admission is often not used.

The criteria for admission should be explained, so that the family neither expects hospitalization according to whim nor suffers the reprehensible notion that the patient can never return to the hospital, that terminal cases are not allowed back. Advanced cancer patients are often sick enough to justify hospital admission in accordance with usual institutional standards and third-party–payment regulations. The occasion of hospitalization allows the physician to perform tests or give treatments not readily managed in the home.

Patients who severely dislike the hospital will usually accept respite admissions if they are given to understand that the family needs relief and that the arrangement is only a temporary one. Patients need to know that institutionalization is not the first step to abandonment and "social death."[5,6] The availability of hospice inpatient units (or other settings designed to provide appropriate care for the terminally ill) would presumably ease the family and patient's concerns about brief institutionalization.

Respite hospitalization itself may create new burdens: traveling to the hospital, long hours visiting, and long periods of the day spent outside the home. As part of respite care, the family should be encouraged to enjoy a true vacation. Patients who are given proper information and support can often tolerate a few days alone while the family gets a rest.

SELECTED REFERENCES

1. Calkins K: Shouldering a burden. Omega 3:23–36, 1972
2. Cartwright A, Hockey L, Anderson JL: Life Before Death. London, Routledge & Kegan Paul, 1973
3. de Beauvoir S: A Very Easy Death, p 23. O'Brian P, translator. New York, Warner Paperback, 1973
4. Gaites C: Personal communication, 1979
5. Glazer B, Strauss A: Awareness of Dying. Chicago, Aldine Publishing, 1965
6. Glazer B, Strauss A: Time for Dying. Chicago, Aldine Publishing, 1968
7. Goffman E: Asylums. Garden City, New York, Anchor Books, 1961
8. Golodetz A, Evans R, Heinritz G et al: The care of chronic illness: The "responsor" role. Med Care 5:385–394, 1969
9. Hine VH: Dying at home: Can families cope? Omega 10(2):175–187, 1979–80
10. House MK: Home-style nursing. JAMA 240:2472–2474, 1978
11. Lack S, Buckingham RW: First American Hospice. New Haven, CT, Hospice, Inc., 1978 (available at Hospice, Inc, 765 Prospect St, New Haven, CT 06511)
12. Lamerton R: Care of the Dying (rev and expanded ed). New York: Penguin, 1980
13. Lerner G: A Death of One's Own. New York, Simon & Schuster, 1978
14. Levine NB, Dastoor DP, Gendron CE: Coping with dementia: A pilot study. J Am Geriatr Soc 31:12–18, 1983

15. Mace NL, Robins PV: The 36-Hour Day: A Family Guide to Caring For Persons with Alzheimer's Disease, Related Dementing Illness, and Memory Loss. Baltimore, Johns Hopkins University Press, 1981

16. Martinson IM: Home Care for the Dying Child—Professional and Family Perspectives. New York, Appleton-Century-Crofts, 1976

17. Parkes CM: Evaluation of family care in terminal illness. In Pritchard ER, Collard J, Orcutt BA et al (eds): Social Work and the Dying Patient and Family, pp 49–79. New York, Columbia University Press, 1977

18. Parkes CM: Home or hospital? Terminal care as seen by surviving spouses. J R Coll Gen Pract 28:19–30, 1978

19. Rosenbaum EH, Rosenbaum IR: Principles of home care for the patient with advanced cancer. JAMA 244:1484–1487, 1980

20. Sanford JRA: Tolerance of debility in elderly dependents by supporters at home. Br Med J 3:471–473, 1975

21. Strauss A: Chronic Illness and the Quality of Life, St Louis, CV Mosby, 1975

22. Ward AWM. Terminal care in malignant disease. Soc Sci Med 8:413–420, 1974

23. Ward AWM: The impact of a special unit for terminal care. Soc Sci Med 10:373–376, 1976

24. Zarit SH, Reever KE, Bach-Peterson J: Relatives of the impaired elderly: Correlates of feelings of burden. Gerontologist 20:649–655, 1980

Feeling Secure 5

INTRODUCTION

Even when the physical symptoms of illness are well-tolerated and the burden of providing physical care in the home is manageable, the patient and family are constantly confronted with unfamiliar medical problems and with an uncertain, potentially frightening future. Unless the feeling of insecurity is diligently managed, care at home will be disrupted by crises that are both terrifying and avoidable, while minor medical events may lead to anxious calls, emergency-ward visits, and demands for hospitalization.

This chapter begins with a review of the common sources of normal anxiety in caring for a serious illness in the community. Fundamental questions about clinical practice are raised: What makes illness frightening and how do professionals allay these fears? A heightened awareness of these familiar, yet rarely explicated, issues can help the physician more successfully attend to the needs of the terminally ill and many other patients. Methods are explored whereby the physician can help the patient and family truly "feel at home." The promotion of a sense of security is analyzed as a function of how services are structured and how the clinical encounter is conducted. The elicitation of "attributions" and the thoughtful provision of explanation and reassurance are described as techniques for enhancing a sense of security amid uncertainty.

THE PROBLEM OF INSECURITY

Interpreting the Patient's Condition

Commonplaces about the home being a secure setting for the dying tend to disregard the patient and family's anxiety about managing new problems there. While laypersons can be taught to perform sophisticated medical and nursing tasks and to feel self-assured in carrying out these chores, they lack the professional training and expertise that, ideally, allows one to remain relatively calm in the face of serious illness. Physicians and nurses develop a sense of confidence from long training in the treatment of medical problems and from having dealt successfully with many crises in the past. Laypersons, however, when confronted with a new problem, may be unable to assess its significance or to distinguish the serious from the trivial. Not only are they subject to anxiety about the crises, large and small, that health professionals recognize as worrisome, but they also may interpret other phenomena—a change in the color of urine or slight irregularity of the pulse—as ominous. They may be haunted by the prospect of ignoring a serious problem or of overreacting to a minor one. As eager novice caretakers, they can become highly attentive to signs and symptoms that experienced health professionals have learned to dismiss. Their heightened awareness leads them to worry about matters that they ordinarily would have ignored. Such vigilance can be exhausting.

Expecting Problems

The course of any illness is unpredictable to health professionals and laypersons alike: "prognosis is perilous." Late-stage cancer, with its protean manifestations, is fraught with unwelcome surprises. While the health professional develops a somewhat comfortable sense of which problems are likely to arise, the lay caretaker lacks the experience to limit the range of possibilities.

Even when current problems are being comfortably managed, the patient and family may be plagued by the fear of future unmanageable crises, occurring far away from help:

> I once heard about a man whose bowels just spilled out of his belly, and I kept wondering if it might happen to my father. I'd check the bulging around his colostomy and worry about it.

> I've always been afraid of choking or drowning, and I worry whether I will fill up with fluid from the inside and be unable to breathe.

Anything imagineable is possible. The uncertain trajectory of the illness can be as wearing as the certainty of the final outcome.

The Sense of Responsibility

Anxiety arises not only from difficulty in making sense of current events, but also from a lonely and sometimes disproportionate sense of one's personal responsibility. The patient and family who say, in effect, "This is the doctors' and nurses' problem," are unlikely to become deeply apprehensive about the changes in the course of an illness. Most patients and family members, however, feel that, "If something happens, it's up to me to take care of it." Physicians ordinarily foster some degree of personal responsibility among laypersons for managing an illness, yet such duties are not easily borne alone. At home, the family may feel isolated. Help is far away. Responsibilities may seem overly burdensome, especially when the family members who are most confident about patient care are absent, or on nights and weekends when the physician is not in the office.

Vulnerability and Helplessness

> The syllogism he had learnt from Kiesewetter's Logic: "Caius is a man, men are mortal, therefore Caius is mortal," had always seemed to him correct as applied to Caius, but certainly not as applied to himself. That Caius—man in the abstract—was mortal, was perfectly correct, but he was not Caius, not an abstract man, but, a creature quite, quite separate from all others . . . "Caius really was mortal, and it was right for him to die; but for me, little Vanya, Ivan Ilych, with all my thoughts and emotions, it's altogether a different matter. It cannot be that I ought to die. That would be too terrible."
>
> Leo Tolstoy, "The Death of Ivan Ilych"[28]

Everyone contemplates, at moments, the possibility of personal tragedy, yet most people live from day to day with a dominant confidence in the future. Tomorrow is largely viewed as a predictable scenario, evolving out of a familiar past and somewhat shielded from great harm or loss. In contrast, people who have recently encountered a serious illness often display a heightened sense of vulnerability and helplessness. The sudden death of a friend or public figure, the development of an ailment in a relative, new knowledge about a devastating disease, the actual experience of having an illness—all these tend to challenge the common faith that one will remain well and that success in coping with the present shall prevail in the future. Disease introduces a new sense of the trajectory of life.

> The bridge underneath is ever so slightly
> Tearing a suture of itself in secret;
> And what is most feared is about to happen:
> The stage-set of a world taken for granted
> Will drop from the sky, robots of ashes
> In clouds grow solidly real, and murders
>
> That always before occurred at a distance
> Strangle the neck at home.
>
> Howard Moss, "Elegy for My Sister"[18]

For the cancer patient and family, the unwelcomed intrusion of illness and its inexorable progression, perhaps accompanied by a growing awareness of the inevitability of death, damages the everyday veneer of living—the myths that we control our destiny, the assumptions that we will escape catastrophe and live on.

Cancer patients are often fearful patients. Frightening processes have taken hold of them, threatening to destroy the body and the self. Patients undergo disagreeable or painful treatments in strange settings and suffer unexpected side-effects. Ill health unremittingly tears them away from their usual lives, from the routines that give each day its texture and meaning. Life with cancer can feel like being on a roller coaster, accelerating out of control as new problems arise, then slowing down momentarily as problems stabilize or as adjustment occurs, then rushing forward again with another crisis.

As the everyday sense of order is undermined, the patient and family may cling to people, places, and objects that give comfort, solace, and a sense of permanency or stability, yet they sense the tenuousness of these ties. Far-off disasters, perhaps encountered in the newspaper, can take on a new immediacy or poignancy. Possibilities for accidents crowd into awareness. Aches or blemishes that previously would have gone unnoticed or would have been dismissed become worrisome signs. The cancer patient's envisioned future can become a nightmare, full of dreadful surprises. Anxiety, insecurity, and vulnerability amplify each other and can flood the patient and family with intolerable feelings.

According to a physician, Kenneth Cohn, who is also a cancer patient:

> Any event that occurs unpredictably regardless of the cause, should be expected to produce feelings of helplessness and outrage.[3]

Some people in this predicament will react with anger—"It's not fair." Others become bewildered, wondering, "Why me?" Still others respond with guilt: "What did I do to deserve this?" "What did I do wrong?" When helplessness, dependency, and vulnerability are preoccupations, concerns about abandonment or of being too great a burden to others are common: "Will the doctors get fed up? Am I asking too much of my family? Am I being a pest?" In such a state of vulnerability and helplessness, a feeling of security is difficult to achieve.

A CLINICAL APPROACH TO PROMOTING SECURITY

The promotion of a sense of security for the patient and family, as they try to live well with an illness, is a daily task of the clinician.

Support and the Structure of Services

The regular presence of a familiar, concerned, competent physician and of a well-coordinated team of caretakers is the foremost antidote to insecurity. Cliches about needing a doctor to whom you can turn in a crisis have everyday relevance in the care of the dying. A sense of security in the home is established as trust develops in the consistent attention, availability, and skill of the health-care team. Successful management of symptoms, the provision of emotional support, and careful heed to the burden of caretaking are the groundwork for creating this feeling of safety. Specific suggestions for structuring services are described below.

Regular Contact

In the hospital, constant supervision is available to the patient and family. At home, the same protection is needed. Regular visits by the physician or nurse must suffice to ensure that everything is being attended to properly and that concern from the health-care workers is ongoing. Confidence is inspired not only by the completion of technical medical tasks, but also through empathic listening and counseling, information-sharing, and the reassuring effect of the professional's presence.

The frequency of visits should not be dictated solely by the usual medical indications, especially early on in the relationship. Regular housecalls or office visits, often one or two a week, should be offered initially in order to ease the patient's and family's anxiety. A visit to the home within a day or two after discharge is generally recommended.

The frequency of visits can later be tapered as trust develops, communication improves, and a sense of family competence and confidence becomes more evident. However, visiting should not be solely occasioned by requests from the family or by the development of a crisis. Most patients and families are reluctant to call the physician unless they are significantly disturbed. Waiting to be called often means waiting until matters are getting out of hand. Regular or "prophylactic" visits allow the physician to prevent problems from erupting. When a housecall can be scheduled in advance, the patient and family should be notified, since the anticipation of a visit will often help them bear mounting anxieties.

Regular visiting reduces the number of inconvenient emergency calls. Furthermore, when the frequency of visiting is determined, in part, by concerns for promoting security, the conduct of the visit will not be dictated solely by pressing medical concerns. The physician will be able to say that everything is fine, and there will be more time for dealing with psychosocial problems.

Regular telephone calls also help maintain security and require a smaller commitment of time from the physician than visits. Telephone calls can be used to gauge the need for housecalls. The conversations promote a sense of continuing involvement of the physician between visits. Suggested times for a telephone call are soon after any significant change in the patient's condition or medical regimen and before any weekend or holiday. Again, prophylactic calls prevent problems from becoming severe and avert emergency calls or visits.

Consistency and Dependability

The perseverance, dependability, and dedication of the physician set an important model for the family and other caretakers. Small breeches in the reliability of the physician may threaten the patient and family with a severe disruption of their sense of security. Missed or cancelled appointments, tardiness, and broken promises may be devastating.

Trust between doctor and patient may be slow to develop. Termination of the previous doctor–patient relationship, if not managed carefully, may have left the patient wary of the next physician.[6] Poorly coordinated arrangements of care, which require that patients have a different doctor in the home, office, and hospital, or that they switch physicians as their disease evolves, will mitigate against the development of trust and may undermine the patient's confidence, especially when collaboration between caretakers is faulty.

Team care can be hazardous if the patient and family receive inconsistent or contradictory information from various health-care providers. Discordant messages can be avoided by regular team conferences, the development of familiarity among team members of each caretaker's style of practice, and the inclusion in case records of notes about information-sharing. Each patient should have a clearly identified personal doctor. When one physician "signs out" to another, the on-call doctor's name should be provided to the patient and family, and the covering physician should be made familiar with the major medical and psychosocial issues of care.

Availability

> The value of a general practitioner in a village is largely that he is alive, that he is there and available. People know the number of his car, and the back view of his hat . . . The doctor's physical presence meets an emotional need.
>
> D. W. Winnicott[29]

In most households caring for a dying person, the doctor's and nurse's telephone numbers are prominently displayed. The ready availability of assistance and the opportunity to share responsibility with the professionals will help the patient and family remain confident in carrying on in the home.

The physician must be easily reached by telephone. The process for reaching the doctor by telephone should be reviewed carefully with the patient and family. If delays or difficulties with paging systems are common, the family is best warned, and told either to wait patiently or to use an alternate method. Coverage arrangements for nights, weekends, and holidays should be explained.

Optimal care requires 24-hours-a-day, 7-days-a-week physician and nurse coverage by phone and, when necessary, by visiting. When visits are indicated, they should be scheduled with little delay. Ideally, the doctor will come to the house promptly whenever needed or requested. Martinson's model program for dying children included a promise in writing to the family that the nurse would visit whenever the family desired.[14]

As relationships are being established, the patient and family may test the doctor's availability by making calls or requesting visits for relatively unimportant matters. "The word of action is stronger than the word of speech"[21]; the physician's response in such trials is more convincing than any promises. Later in the course of an illness, frequent or seemingly unnecessary telephone calls and the presentation of multiple concerns are often signs of escalating apprehension and of intolerance of home care.

Occasionally a family will fail to seek the physician's services when these are needed. A routinely scheduled visit will reveal serious, neglected problems. Sometimes these families are merely diffident, and require encouragement to call. Often, such neglect reflects a state of helplessness, poor capability of monitoring the patient's condition, or subversion of home care.

Discharge Planning

The transfer from an institution to the home commonly provokes a crisis of confidence. Discharge should not suggest neglect or a loss of interest or attention from trusted health-care providers.

If planning is initiated well before discharge, home services can be carefully arranged and coordinated. Before leaving the hospital, the patient and family can be instructed thoroughly in any new tasks. Worries about the availability and dependability of services in the home can be addressed. A thorough search for fears and concerns is useful as soon as home care is considered and often deserves to be repeated periodically throughout the discharge-planning process:

> How do you feel about going home? (or about taking the patient home?)
>
> What do you think it will be like?
>
> Do you foresee any problems?
>
> What would you do if a problem arose?

Physicians who cannot follow their patients after discharge from the hospital can ease the transition and the sense of loss by helping arrange continuing care and by "giving blessing"—conveying a sense of confidence in the new medical team. Any expression of continued interest—a request for a follow-up phone call, a willingness to see the patient again, a single housecall (even if regular visits are not offered)—eases this transition.

A Note on the Use of Hospitalization

Institutional care should be considered when insecurity is an overwhelming problem. While care at home may be initially favored for the patient's and family's comfort and security, their feelings may change. Temporary hospitalization may be useful for riding out a crisis or for reconsidering long-term institutional care. Patients and families should be offered the option of institutional care and be encouraged to reflect on where they feel happiest and most secure.

When a dying patient's condition changes dramatically, physicians sometimes resort routinely to hospitalization. Admission to the hospital is often an easy method for physicians to handle crises, but it may not best serve the patient or family, nor is it necessarily cost-effective. Home care is often still feasible when fresh fears are promptly addressed, new burdens are alleviated, and acute symptoms are quickly palliated. Suggestions that the patient be admitted may merely reinforce the laypersons' concerns that the crisis is severe and unmanageable.

Tasks in the Clinical Encounter

The following clinical approaches will help the patient and family feel secure.

Transfer of Information

Knowledge about illness and its management, when tactfully and thoughtfully provided by the health professionals, endows the patient and family with the expertise to cope with new problems and to face an uncertain future with greater confidence. Information-sharing is important not simply because it allows for appropriate technical care but also because it imparts a sense of control for the lay caretakers, making the future more predictable and manageable. The act of explanation conveys the physician's appreciation of lay concerns and, if used properly, is reassuring.

With adequate supervision, family members can become expert and confident in managing many caretaking tasks, including highly technical procedures, and can come to appreciate the appropriate occasions for seeking outside help. When properly supported, the family members will often make declarations such as, "I'm going to get a nursing degree," reflecting a pleasant awareness of their new competence.

The usefulness of information-sharing has been demonstrated in a number of medical settings.[4,24] For instance, Egbert performed a randomized, controlled study in which surgical patients who received standard treatment were compared with a group who were told prior to surgery what to expect in the postoperative period and were encouraged during the postoperative period and advised on how to remain comfortable. The patients who received this extra attention required less narcotics, experienced less pain, appeared in better physical and emotional condition, and were discharged an average of 2.7 days earlier than the control group.[4]

Effective information-sharing requires that the physician commit adequate time for explaining and for listening to questions and concerns. Learning is often slow, and facts need to be repeated. Intended messages may be misinterpreted. Careful listening allows for detection and correction of misunderstanding.

But what is to be explained? Explanations are never complete. The physician has an enormous store of knowledge, but time for communication is precious, and the layperson's ability to absorb new information is limited. Moreover, some well-intended explanations may have little therapeutic value. The use of jargon and technical terms may confuse or mystify, rather than empower the layperson. A common professional error is "overexplanation"—an overly detailed elucidation of the basis of decision-making and probabilities of various outcomes. Overexplanation often results from a physician's self-absorption in describing his or her clinical reasoning or reflects a notion that, in order to defend against malpractice suits, informed consent should convey every imaginable contingency. Attention to unlikely events—the 1% chance of a complication, the rare development of a side-effect—is often not desired by the patient and family and may only serve to make them uneasy.

Explanations should be brief and focused, followed by ample opportunity for discussion. The laypersons' responses to an explanation, especially their questions, can guide the physician to topics that require clarification and to concerns that deserve more attention. Questioning and listening, not lecturing, are the basis for good explanations. Discussion after the news is delivered is as important as the initial message.

General guidelines for the goals and content of explanations can arise from asking two questions:

1. What do the patient and family *need to know* to provide good care?
2. What do they *want to know?*

The answer to the first question arises largely from clinical experience with the course of illness and with the lay caretaker's needs for instruction in carrying out the treatment plan. The answer to the second question arises largely from appreciation of the layperson's view of illness and from meticulous attention to the attributions and concerns of the patient and family. In the following sections, suggestions are offered for gauging explanations to the layperson's needs and concerns.

Anticipation of Problems and Rehearsing Responses

The physician can often anticipate future problems: changes in pain; progression of confusion, stupor, and coma; the development of pneumonia or a urinary tract infection; the course of advancing organ failure; or the side-effects of medications. A few words of warning will help the patient or family feel that matters are under control and will prepare them to react calmly. A review and rehearsal of how to manage the problem will help them act appropriately when the difficulty arises, innoculating them against panic:

The urine will turn orange with this medication.

If the pill for constipation does not work by tomorrow night, keep giving it to him, but add 2 tablespoons of milk of magnesia. If I've given him a little too much and he gets diarrhea, stop the pills for a day. I'll write this down.

He is likely to get more of these black and blue marks, even if he doesn't hit himself. We don't have any more treatment for them beyond what he has already been given. They look terrible but they don't hurt. You don't need to worry about them. Is that OK?

Let's go over again what pneumonia is like. If his drowsiness remains this severe, he may very well get pneumonia, an infection in his lungs. You'll know it when it happens because there will be a big change—he'll start coughing, bringing up phlegm, and breathing fast, and he may get a fever.

> *There's nothing you'll need to do about it immediately, but I think we should talk over the phone if you think he has pneumonia.*

When information-sharing helps the layperson make sense of the experience of being ill and empowers him or her to act rationally, it provides a sense of control and security. New events, rather than seeming like threats, become occasions for effective action. In general, preparation for crises is reassuring to the patient and family, and the vast majority of anticipated problems will be manageable at home. The family later says,

> *It happened just the way you said it would, and we knew just what to do.*

The future, of course, cannot be predicted, and, too often, physicians offer useless and incorrect prognoses:

> *You've only got a few months to live.*

> *The disease is going to get worse quickly, and I'll be surprised if he's still around by Christmas.*

Since such declarations are often conveyed with a sense of certainty and gloom, the layperson feels hopelessly condemned. Even vague predictions may be taken literally and can be interpreted as definitive pronouncements: "a few weeks to live" becomes "I'll die in 2 weeks." The patient and family, however, may want to know what to expect and are entitled to our informed guesses. They can often profit from sketches of what may occur in the future.

> *I don't have a crystal ball, but as time goes on people with brain tumors like this often have problems with drowsiness or confusion. Pain is uncommon and is easily manageable. The confusion can be frustrating.*

> *It seems that weakness is your major problem now and will probably continue to be troublesome. You're not eating well, and it seems that you're mostly going to be suffering from this tiredness and an inability to do things for yourself.*

As reviewed in Chapter 7, Sharing Bad News, hopefulness—an emphasis on how problems are manageable or bearable—is usually consistent with honesty. When death is imminent, more exact predictions are often feasible, as discussed in Chapter 11.

What about especially dreaded and gruesome complications, such as exsanguination from erosion of a neck tumor into the carotid artery? The physician's explanation will not necessarily bolster a sense of security but the laypersons are entitled to this information in deciding how to proceed with care:

> Doctor: *Occasionally, severe bleeding can develop when these tumors damage blood vessels in the neck.*
>
> Patient: *What could we do?*
>
> Doctor: *Not much. The bleeding can be frightening but there's no pain involved, and you're likely to just pass out quickly.*
>
> Spouse 1: *Well, I don't think I could stand being in this house again if he bled to death here.*
>
> Spouse 2: *I don't like to think about it, but I guess we'll just have to do our best at home and see what happens.*

Reassurance[22]

Reassurance is an almost universal, though unstated, request of the patient who seeks the physician's service. Even a patient who knows he is dying and who expects blunt truth-telling from his doctor will appreciate the allied qualities of feeling reassured and encouraged:

> It's not a sign of the cancer worsening.

> Congratulations, your condition seems stable again this week.

> We've had a set-back, but we have some treatment to make the best of it.

Physicians often provide reassurance without conscious effort. For instance, the physicians' demeanor can have a profound effect on the patient and family's sense of security. Ideally, a sense of *aequanimitas* is conveyed—the physician appears dependable, purposeful, confident, able to bear uncertainty, tolerant, unruffled, yet sympathetic and responsible.[20] The physician's manner can communicate a feeling of order and control in a world that constantly threatens to become chaotic and unmanageable. A thorough, competent evaluation of the patient's condition and a thoughtful explanation may constitute adequate reassurance to many patients. The successful handling of repeated crises also contributes to confidence in the future.

The physician who relies on the routine of the clinical visit, the power of the professional demeanor, and a few words of global reassurance, however, may fail to address the patient's specific attributions and concerns, and thus runs the risk of neglecting to provide adequate reassurance. Indeed, global statements of reassurance can be frustrating and demeaning when they seem to gloss over the specific issues that worry the layperson:

> Everything seems fine.

> You have nothing to worry about.

Similarly, advice is not reassurance:

> Don't get upset by this. Be calm.

> You shouldn't let these matters worry you. Leave everything to me.

Such statements may incite doubts rather than settle them. Successful reassurance begins with an appreciation of attributions.

Eliciting and Addressing Attributions

OVERVIEW. Laypersons inevitably form attributions—notions about the cause, meaning, and consequence of their condition and its management. Symptoms, signs, diagnostic actions, therapies, and the behavior of the health workers are always interpreted by the patient and family, and a personal meaning is assigned. This personal meaning may be congruent or discrepant with the professional viewpoint.[5,10–12]:

> He gave me an appointment to come back in 4 weeks, so I must be doing fine.

> He didn't seem worried about the pain, but I'm sure it's a sign of the cancer getting much worse.

Lay notions may be realistic or unrealistic. Realistic concerns are best handled by making specific plans to deal with anticipated problems. Insecurity is thus treated by the sharing of worries and by rehearsing how to respond to problems. Unrealistic concerns can often be treated with a gentle dismissal:

I can appreciate your concern, but I don't think you have to worry about that. His pain will probably get better rather than worse now.

I'm not worrying about him choking. He's breathing well and his airway is clear. Nothing is happening with the cancer that should cause him to suffocate.

I don't think we need to be concerned about that problem now. If his kidneys shut down, we'll have lots of warning and I can tell you what to do.

The process of eliciting and addressing attributions is tremendously useful in the daily work of the clinician. Although most physicians are vaguely aware of the process, training for this clinical task is generally lacking. Few descriptions of the technique of eliciting and responding to patient attributions and of its usefulness are available. Medical students are usually trained to focus on the essential "facts," the "dimensions" of the symptoms, while lay attributions may be viewed as distractions. Indeed, the patient's viewpoint can mislead the physician into accepting an incorrect lay construction of the illness as, for instance, when a man who is having a heart attack requests and gets help over the phone for his "indigestion." The following sections offer a detailed discussion of attributions.

ATTRIBUTION THEORY AND THE LAY PERSPECTIVE ON ILLNESS. "Attribution theory" is a concept used in social psychology to understand how persons assign meaning to events. "To attribute" is to engage in the cognitive process of ascribing meaning (*e.g.,* "he attributed the blackout to a blown fuse,") while an "attribution" denotes the meaning assigned (*e.g.,* "his attribution for the blackout was a blown fuse, although he also considered a power failure").

The term, "attribution," has been usefully adapted in clinical medicine to describe the layperson's process of interpreting the events surrounding an illness ("He attributed the dizziness to his high blood pressure") or to describe a lay diagnosis ("His attribution is that the weakness is a side-effect of his medication"). Patient attributions convey elements of what are commonly called "the personal meaning of illness," "illness beliefs," "illness representation,"[13] or the "patient's perspective,"[10] and are a feature of what Mishler calls "the view of the patient life-world."[16] A broad use of the term, "attribution," may be offensive to social psychologists, who restrict the concept to the construction of causal explanations.

Persons normally and automatically ascribe meaning to the events in their conscious world. Symptoms and signs are such events. For the layperson, the process of assigning meaning to bodily sensations is analogous to the physicians's process of making a diagnosis or prognosis. For instance, a patient who begins to sneeze might assign a *predisposing cause* ("I let myself get rundown," "I've always been susceptible to bad colds"), an etiology ("I must be getting a cold," "I'm allergic to the cat"), *pathophysiology* ("Something is irritating my nose"), a likely *course* ("This is going to knock me out for a few days," "It will go away when I get away from this dusty room"), and *seriousness* or *significance* ("I better take good care of myself or I'll get pneumonia," "No big deal"). An attribution may lead to a *response* to the symptom ("This cold is like when my aunt got pneumonia last week, so I better see the doctor," "If it doesn't go away in a few days, I'll buy some cold pills"). In coming to a doctor, the patient's notions about the diagnosis, prognosis, and treatment may lead him or her to have *requests* about diagnostic and therapeutic efforts[5,10–12]:

I should be checked for an infection.

I need an x-ray.

This condition might be from a glandular problem, so I should see a specialist.

I want to be sure this won't go on to a serious problem.

I need a doctor who I can talk to about feeling so badly.

Strictly speaking, attributions are ideas or explanations, not affects, but they reflect mood and personality, and they often imply an area of concern or fear. The elicitation of attributions, although focused on cognitive data, is intimately allied with the elicitation of affective data and with the clarification of patients' wishes about how their problems should be approached.

EXAMPLES OF ATTRIBUTIONS. A brief consideration of the common lay theories of the cause of cancer reminds us that attributions are everpresent in the clinical encounter and that they reflect patients' views of their world, their illness, and their treatment.[2]

Cancer is commonly seen as a physical invasion. Lay (and professional) theories of the etiology of the disease may focus on *external* physical events (e.g., trauma, irritation, mechanical factors, infections, exposures, substances in the diet, medical treatments, losses, and excessive personal, social, occupational, or economic stresses). Chance, bad luck, and other magical influences may also be invoked. Such attributions often seem to project blame on malevolent external forces.

He was worried to death by his job and the responsibility for his senile parents.

I was kicked by a horse right in that area about 20 years ago.

It was the evil eye.

Cancer is also commonly viewed as evidence of a personal vulnerability or a psychological predisposition. *Internal* physical factors include fatigue, degeneration, heredity, and other forms of constitutional weakness that may cause or predispose to invasion by cancer. Psychological attributions invoke such factors as nervousness, being too guilty, or failing to express anger. A variety of moral, intellectual, or behavioral indiscretions are regularly cited, including improper eating, tobacco abuse, excess alcohol intake, not seeing the doctor, lack of proper rest, acting with incomplete medical information, and a host of other forms of negligence, sinfulness, poor judgment, or stupidity. Such etiologies often imply self-blame:

If I only had come to the doctor earlier, I wouldn't be in this mess.

We all told him to stop smoking.

Many attributions imply a combination of internal and external, as well as physical, psychological, spiritual, and existential factors:

What did I do to deserve this? Why is God punishing me?

The job was more important to him than his health, and that's why he let himself be poisoned by all those chemicals.

If he had eaten right, he would have been able to fight it off.

One person may hold multiple attributions about a single condition, some of which are highly realistic, others which are quite abstract and idiosyncratic.

I should have checked myself and seen the doctor before the lump got this bad, though I know the car accident really did this to me.

Surprising and seemingly bizarre attributions are frequently elicited, even among patients who are medically sophisticated, highly intelligent, or from upper social classes.

Symptoms often are associated with important personal meanings:

Weakness:	*I am no longer any use.*
Anorexia:	*If he doesn't eat, the cancer will get the better of him, and he'll die quickly.*
	He is rejecting our help by not eating the food.
Disfigurement:	*I am no longer myself. No one could stand me this way.*

For the dying patient, concerns about abandonment and of being overwhelmed rank second in importance only to fears of discomfort. The moment of death is not as frightening as the process of arriving there. Patients commonly fear being wrenched away from the people who help give life meaning and often are terrified of being alone and helpless and of losing control of bodily functions, thinking, or behavior. Attributions will reflect these concerns:

> *If I keep having these troubles, my family will get fed up, and the nurses will think I'm a bother.*

> *Is this a sign that I'm losing my mind?*

The appearance of any new problem implies a new set of attributions. Thus, the development of a significant symptom usually requires attention not only to the control of physical discomfort and the adequacy of the support system, but also to the insecurity of the patient and family, particularly to their attributions and fears. Bailey has stressed that home visits are usually initiated by an "intermediary"—someone other than the patient—and that a successful consultation should address the concerns and requests of the person requesting the help.[1] Worries about accelerated pain and suffering are often evident and need to be addressed. Fears of abandonment or of being too great a burden often reappear. New problems are reminders of the process of dissolution and impending death, and so a variety of concerns about dying may resurface. Fears of choking, exsanguinating, and of similar catastrophic events often come to mind but are not stated explicitly.

Attributions about diagnostic efforts and treatment also need to be addressed:

> *I think he is checking my urine for signs of the cancer spreading there.*

> *That must be a bad sign—they've stopped the hormone treatment.*

A respite admission is often misinterpreted by the patient. The physician can say,

> *I want to make it clear to you that we are not bringing you in to the hospital because of any secret plans to put you in a nursing home or because we think you have gotten worse or are going to die this week. This admission is for your family, not so much for you—to give them a break so they can continue to care for you well.*

Specific fears about the period immediately before and after death are discussed in Chapter 11.

ATTRIBUTION FORMATION. Myriad factors impinge on the attribution process of patient and family. Cognitive influences include the information received from the professional caretakers, previous experiences with illness, and ideas offered by fellow patients, friends, books, newspapers, and television and radio programs. The attribution process is also influenced by mood and personality. For instance, anxious or depressed patients may tend to assign grave meanings to events. "Defensive styles" for coping with anxiety can be described as habitual patterns of attribution: denial is a process of minimizing seriousness, projection assigns causality to outside forces, and so on.[8,23]

Mechanic's presentation on "medical student disease" provides a model of the attribution process, which can be applied profitably in daily medical practice.[15] This common psychosomatic illness occurs when a medical student interprets normal bodily sensatons or minor illness as a sign of a serious condition, often of a disease that has been recently encountered in school. Two factors seem important in producing this attribution. First, the student lacks the medical knowledge necessary to evaluate the symptom correctly. A second factor, however, is required to explain why a worrisome attribution was selected rather than a trivial one and why the symptom was taken seriously and brought to a physician's attention. Mechanic noted that medical student disease typically occurs at times of great anxiety, such as before exams. The heightened worry over one matter (the exam) seems to cause heightened worry in other areas (the significance of the body's sensations). Mechanic concludes that the illness is a reflection of incomplete knowledge and of stress. These two factors can be borne in mind when evaluating the misattributions of dying patients and their families.

ELICITING ATTRIBUTIONS.   The complaint that physicians do not talk enough to their cancer patients is variously said to result from doctors being uncaring or hurried, from their use of unintelligibile language, or their desire to conceal the truth. The complaint, however, also reflects the difficulty that patients experience in expressing their concerns and the lack of skill among physicians in eliciting those attributions that can guide explanations quickly to appropriate topics. The foremost impediment in properly addressing patients' concerns comes not so much in knowing how to explain well, but in first noticing or uncovering attributions.

Some patients and family members will present their ideas and concerns about illness directly, or their attributions will be obvious.

> *I figured the cancer was spreading.*

> *I guess that means he doesn't have long left.*

More often, laypersons are reluctant to share openly their notions about illness and to express directly their fears about what is happening or might happen in the future. They risk humiliation if the physician suggests that such ideas are naive, foolish, or presumptuous. Furthermore, when a layperson is thinking about serious and frightening matters, the acknowledgment of such concerns may be difficult; fears and troublesome thoughts may seem to be kept out of full awareness when they are not verbalized. Consequently, attributions are often expressed indirectly or are concealed. Sometimes, they are slipped in with other statements:

> *I couldn't get him to roll over in bed or eat a thing, so I just did the best I could, figuring the cancer had paralyzed him.*

> *He's lost all interest in food now. He doesn't eat a thing. He can't have long to go.*

Such serious concerns, mentioned offhandedly, could easily be ignored by an inattentive clinician.

Wife: *I don't want him to die of starvation.*

Doctor: *What concerns you?*

Wife: *Won't he suffer?*

Doctor: *People on starvation diets may feel bad, but I don't think they suffer.*

Wife: *Aren't we neglecting him?*

Doctor: *We're doing what's important, giving him lots of fluids and whatever really makes him comfortable.*

Careful listening to the patient and family will regularly suggest the nature of their concerns. Brief questioning can clarify these matters:

Wife of patient: *Is it OK to let him give himself the medication?*

Doctor: *Do you see any problems there?*

Wife: *Well, don't you think he might take too much?*

Doctor: *What do you mean?*

Wife: *Well, if he all of a sudden got fed up.*

At other times, attributions are presented indirectly or implicitly:

Spouse: *It seems to be making him sleepy.*

Doctor: *What do you make of it?*

Spouse: *I figure it's spread to his brain.*

Daughter: *I guess he won't have to worry about that anymore.*

Doctor: *How's that?*

Daughter: *I don't think he'll last much longer. The cancer's got him.*

Patient: *It's not much, but you begin to wonder.*

Doctor: *About what?*

Patient: *Aren't seizures like this?*

Attributions may be also expressed as denied thoughts or may be projected onto others:

I didn't think about it spreading or anything, but . . .

My aunt got real worried. She must think he doesn't have long to go.

Careful listening will help the physician appreciate many attributions. When attributions are not evident or concerns have not been stated, they routinely should be elicited. A brief exploration of the layperson's perspective on the illness will usually bring important concerns to the surface. Patient, tactful but persistent prodding may be required:

What do you make of your condition now?

What do you make of the situation?

How do you think the patient is getting along?

Have you had any thoughts about what this problem signifies? About what is causing it? What it is from?

Why do you think you have it now?

What ideas have you had about it?

How should it be diagnosed? Treated?

What does it seem to mean for the future? Does it seem serious?

What problems do you anticipate or worry about in the immediate future?

The patient's perspective may be sought on the following topics:

ETIOLOGY

What led up to the illness?

What predisposes to cancer?

Is it hereditary?

What does it mean for relatives?

What touched it off?

What initiated the abnormal growth?

What allows it to continue to grow or spread?

How can it be prevented?

What should the family do to protect themselves?

DIAGNOSIS

How is the illness diagnosed?

How is its extent determined?

What can be done to understand it better?

What is the significance of the tests?

How is the condition affecting the patient? Physically? Emotionally?

MANAGEMENT

How should it be treated?

What is the treatment for? How does it work?

What are its advantages and disadvantages?

What are its risks and benefits?

How does it affect the patient?

PROGNOSIS

How long has the problem been going on?

What is likely to happen next?

What kind of problems are likely to occur?

What do you foresee in the next few weeks? Months? Years?

Previous encounters with cancer, severe illness, death in the home, or any conditions similar to the patient's will often strongly influence attributions. Such experiences should be elicited when the diagnosis of cancer is made and often are worthwhile discussing earlier, when the diagnosis is first seriously considered. Such attributions can be reviewed as the disease progresses.

What have you heard about cancer?

Have you known anyone with this sort of problem?

Has anyone in your family ever been sick like this?

What was it like for them?

> *What kind of problems did they encounter? Pain?*

> *How was it managed?*

> *How were the doctors?*

> *How did the family respond?*

> *How were his last days? His death?*

Friends and the media are also important sources of information:

Have you ever seen or heard about people with cancer?

> *What have you read?*

> *What have you seen on TV?*

> *What have others told you?*

When asked, patients often initially deny having attributions, yet they will usually express their concerns if the physician waits silently and attentively for an answer:

> *No, I really had not thought much about it . . . though I did kinda wonder if it didn't mean there was spread to the liver.*

> *I really don't have any ideas here . . . that's what I came to you about . . . but I have heard about cases where the cancer didn't show up until a CAT scan was done.*

Sometimes, additional prodding is useful:

Physician: *What thoughts have you had?*
Patient: *Well, you're the doctor.*
Physician: *Yes, but everyone has some ideas about these things.*
Patient: *Well, it did occur to me that . . .*

When concerns are evident, yet not fully expressed, the physician can confront them more directly:

> *Are you worrying about . . .*

> *I expect you might be thinking about . . .*

This technique is most appropriate when fears are obvious, either because of the nature of the medical situation (*e.g.*, "You must be wondering what this weakness in your leg signifies") or because of previous knowledge of the patient's or family's concern (*e.g.*, "We talked a long time ago about your father becoming terribly restless before he died, and I wonder if that hasn't been on your mind again" or "You might be thinking that this chest infection is like the pneumonia which your roommate, Mr. _____, died of in the hospital last month. We discussed it then.")

One can imagine an approach to eliciting attributions that is overly confrontational, which heightens anxiety by focusing on deep fears and uncovering intolerable anxieties. Tact and sensitivity are impossible to prescribe. In general, however, patients and families are able to avoid overwhelming feelings and will react to inappropriate confrontations with denial or anger. They will almost always be grateful for straightforward help from a concerned physician who tries to address the many fears of which they are partially or fully aware. As the patient and family become accustomed to sharing their attributions during the clinical encounter, they typically save up a list of concerns for each visit, knowing that their fears will be acknowledged, addressed, and alleviated.

STUDIES ON ATTRIBUTIONS. A number of studies have attested to the powerful effect of information-sharing, reassurance, and encouragement on the clinical process, and some reports have attempted to correlate the patient's representation of illness with clinical outcomes.[13] Skipper, by providing information and support to mothers of children undergoing tonsillectomy, was able to show beneficial effects on the physiologic, psychological, and social responses to hospitalization and surgery.[24] Further studies are needed to define what kind of information is useful to patients and how personality and situational factors determine the value of such interventions.[9]

Attributions are important and manipulable factors in the experience of pain, anxiety, and other physical and psychological symptoms. For example, in a classic study on insomniacs, the explanation given with placebo sleeping pills was shown to make nocturnal arousal and sleep disorders better or worse.[27] Whenever arousal (or anxiety or fear) contribute significantly to the perception of symptoms, attributions about the meaning of the symptoms play a role in the severity of distress.

Many reports indicate that the provision of accurate expectations about *experimental* pain reduced the stress associated with the painful stimuli.[7,25] Moreover, in Johnson's study, experimental conditions that encouraged the subjects to attend to physical sensations did not affect the degree of distress.[7] This latter finding negates a common assumption that warnings about anticipated effects will increase a patient's discomfort. Similar conclusions have been described in clinical studies. Hypertensive patients receiving package inserts on the possible side-effects of their medications did not report significantly more side-effffects than uninformed patients, although they were more likely to attribute reactions to the drug.[17] Depressed patients who were warned about side-effects from tricyclic drugs neither complained more of side-effects nor discontinued therapy more frequently than did unwarned patients.[19]

THE CLINICAL IMPORTANCE OF ATTRIBUTIONS. Five major reasons can be cited for addressing attributions in the clinical encounter. First, many attributions are incorrect and can be gently dismissed or clarified. The family members who worry that the patient will choke or exsanguinate can often be reassured directly, once such fears are shared and their basis is understood. Events that may seem ominous to the layperson—a change in the color of a wound, a temporary increase in pain associated with an adjustment of medication—can be redefined as minor or insignificant matters.

Second, attributions that correspond with clinical reality, once shared, can often be addressed by further instruction and by rehearsal of remedial measures. If pneumonia is, in fact, a likely outcome of the illness, the family can be armed with the information and technology required to manage the complication: how the patient will feel, what physical signs will develop, and what needs to be done.

Third, the physician's task of explaining to patients and family members becomes much easier and more effective when attributions are shared. Rather than explaining everything imaginable or just explaining what seems important from the professional viewpoint, the elicitation of attributions guides the physician to the patient's and family's foremost concerns, pointing the discussion toward topics that are anxiety-laden and about which more information-sharing is needed. Reassurance can then be targeted appropriately. Moreover, when concerns are verbalized, they usually seem more manageable. A sigh of relief often accompanies the sharing of unacknowledged fears:

That's just what I was worrying about.

Fourth, attention to attributions helps reveal how the patient and family are tolerating the emotional strain of illness. Anxiety, particularly, is often not a forthright complaint, but is expressed in the quality of concerns. The physician's elicitation of attributions invites and acknowledges the laypersons' worries, providing a "cognitive" approach to emotionally laden matters.

Finally, shared attributions are a hallmark of a relationship of openness, trust, and confidence. Many fears are dismissed as irrational or are managed by anticipation, but even realistic terrors become more tolerable when these private, unspeakable concerns are shared rather than harbored. The physicians's interest in the patient's attributions reflects an appreciation of the personal meaning of illness, and constitutes a basic element of personal support.

Attributions are a feature of clinical work, regardless of whether they are recognized by the physician. The doctor who goes about his business without directly attending to the perspectives of the patient and family will be inadvertently modifying the layperson's attributions. Every clinical act—attention to symptoms and signs, tone of voice, facial expression, gestures, and new prescriptions and instructions—can be interpreted by the layperson in such a way as to confirm or deny an attribution, to suggest seriousness or triviality, to create new concerns, as well as to modify old ones. Insofar as this complicated attributional process is skillfully attended to, the patient and family's insecurity can be dealt with more effectively, and the physician gains increasing insight into the lay experience of illness.

Encouragement and Hopefulness

Family members often say,

> We just weren't sure we were doing things right. We just didn't know what to do until the nurse came.

They seek reassurance that they are doing their tasks correctly, but also want encouragement.

Patients or family members rarely complain that a doctor is too hopeful or too encouraging, except perhaps when they feel that the physician has been deceptive or has lacked good judgment. On the other hand, complaints are common that the physician is too hopeless or discouraging. Health-care professionals have the authority to confirm that a job has been carried out well and are in the unique position of being able to give praise and encouragement. They are often critical and demanding of themselves and others, and they forget to compliment the patient or family or to convey approval. Recognition and appreciation by the professional caretakers help the family build the self-esteem and sense of competency that are important ingredients for a feeling of security. Every visit can be an occasion for acknowledging the dedication and quality of care provided by the lay caretakers:

> *You're doing a great job.*

> *You're healing up fine there.*

> *You've been very sensible.*

> *You've been very tolerant.*

> *You've put up with a lot.*

> *Your mother should be grateful for all you have done.*

> *You've made a big sacrifice, and you should feel good about what you've been able to do here.*

A few words can often make a great deal of difference:

> In completing a first, brief visit to the home of a divorced, middle-aged man who was nearing death from cancer, the physician made a point of telling the primary caretakers—two teenaged children—that they were doing an excellent job: "I'm greatly impressed by your dedication and competence." On the next visit, a few days later, the patient was pronounced dead. In finishing up and saying goodbye, the physician was surprised to learn how important his praise had been. Relatives had been flooding the children with advice and criticism, while the stern professional manner of the visiting nurse seemed to imply also that the teenagers were ignorant and incompetent. The children had been trying hard to help their father, but were besieged by guilt, believing they were failing.

> Two years later, a student-researcher discussed the problems of caring for the dying at home with these two young adults. They again stressed how important the encouragement had been. "We really needed to hear that we were doing the right thing from the doctor."

Glib encouragement, based on an insincere or unrealistic evaluation, like bland nonspecific reassurance, is often not very effective. Clinicians, however, who have developed a sense that terminal illness is not intolerable and who view it, in part, as a challenging opportunity to find a satisfying life for the patient and family, can convey this attitude without bending the truth or consciously slanting facts:

> *Let's try this.*

> *We'll just have to see.*

> *It's a problem, but it's tolerable.*

Hopefulness is another quality that is important to cultivate. The many techniques available to the physician for relieving suffering, as described in this book, should give him or her confidence that medicine always has more to offer for the suffering patient. The physician learns to see the cup as half-full rather than half-empty—to be grateful for whatever relief is achieved, whatever function is maintained, whatever time can be enjoyed. No cure is guaranteed. The prognosis is grim, but it could be worse. Helplessness can be borne, perhaps with a sense of sadness or outrage, but also with a sense of strength and forbearance. Disfigurement, disability, profound fears, and wrenching emotions are acceptable. Being strong is not confused with an inability to acknowledge feelings or to take them seriously or to empathize with suffering. Any outcome is manageable and will offer opportunity for further help. The discomfort that remains after good treatment will be tolerable.

The British hospices embody an attitude that is simultaneously hopeful, yet also realistic and accepting of approaching death. The atmosphere on their wards seems an ideal antidote to insecurity. St. Christopher's Hospice radiates tranquility and quiet confidence. The staff seem eager to work with the dying, and they have the time and competence to make the patient comfortable. Familiar with dying, they seem unafraid of whatever comes next. The sick person on his deathbed is not hidden away, but rather looked upon as an example for fellow patients. While religious faith may play a role in developing such a mood of serenity, American secular systems of care—so often characterized by terror over terminal cancer and by fright and shame over dying—must measure themselves against this British example.

SELECTED REFERENCES

1. Bailey AJM: Home visiting: The part played by the intermediary. J R Coll Gen Pract 29:137–142, 1979
2. Bard M, Dyk RB: The psychodynamic significance of beliefs regarding the cause of serious illness. Psychoanalytic Rev 43:146–162, 1956
3. Cohn KH: Chemotherapy from an insider's perspective. Lancet I:1006–1009, 1982
4. Egbert L, Battit GE, Welch C, Bartlett M: Reduction of postoperative pain by encouragement and instruction of patients. N Engl J Med 270:825–827, 1964
5. Eisenthal S, Lazare A, Wasserman L: The customer approach to patienthood. Arch Gen Psychiatry 32:553–558, 1975
6. Friedin RB, Lazerson AM: Terminating the physician–patient relationship in primary care. JAMA 241:819–822, 1979
7. Johnson JE: Effects of accurate expectations about sensations on the sensory and distress components of pain. J Person Soc Psychol 27:261–275, 1973
8. Kahana RJ, Bibring GL: Personality types in medical management. In Zinberg NE (ed): Psychiatry and Medical Practice in a General Hospital, pp 108–123. New York, International Universities Press, 1965
9. Langer EJ, Janis IL, Wolfer JA: Reduction of psychological stress in surgical patients. J Exp Soc Psychol 11:155–165, 1975
10. Lazare A, Eisenthal S: A negotiated approach to the clinical encounter. I. Attending to the patient's perspective. In Lazare A (ed): Outpatient Psychiatry: Diagnosis and Treatment, pp 141–156. Baltimore, Williams & Wilkins, 1979
11. Lazare A, Eisenthal S, Frank A: A negotiated approach to the clinical encounter. II. Conflict and negotiation. In Lazare A, (ed): Outpatient Psychiatry: Diagnosis and Treatment, pp 157–171. Baltimore, Williams & Wilkins, 1979b
12. Lazare A, Eisenthal S, Frank A, Stoeckle JD: Studies on a negotiated approach to patienthood. In Gallagher EB (ed): The Doctor–Patient Relationship in the Changing Health Scene. Washington, DC, John E Fogarty International Center for Advanced Study in the Health Sciences, 1978; DHEW publication no. (NIH) 78–183
13. Leventhal H, Meyer D, Nerenz D: The commonsense representation of illness danger. In Rachman S (ed): Contributions to Medical Psychology, vol 2. London, Pergamon Press, 1982
14. Martinson IM: Home Care for the Dying Child. New York, Appleton-Century-Crofts, 1976

15. Mechanic D: Social psychological factors affecting the presentation of bodily complaints. N Engl J Med 21:1132–1139, 1972
16. Mishler E: The Discourse of Medicine: Dialectics of Medical Interviews. Norwood, NJ, Abler Publishing, 1984
17. Morris LA, Kanouse DE: Informing patients about drug side effects. J Behav Med 5:363–373, 1982
18. Moss H: Notes from the Castle. New York, Atheneum, 1979
19. Myers ED, Calvert EJ: The effect of forewarning on the occurrence of side-effects and discontinuance of medication in patients on amitryptiline. Br J Psychiatry 122:461–464, 1973
20. Osler W: Aequanimitas. In Osler W: Aequanimitas, 3rd ed, pp 2–11. Philadelphia, Blakiston Co, 1932
21. Osler W: Chauvinism in medicine. In Osler W: Aequanimitas, 3rd ed, pp 264–289. Philadelphia, Blakiston Co, 1932
22. Sapira JD: Reassurance therapy: What to say to symptomatic patients with benign diseases. Ann Intern Med 77:603–604, 1972
23. Shapiro D: Neurotic Styles. New York, Basic Books, 1965
24. Skipper JK, Leonard RC: Children, stress, and hospitalization: A field experiment. J Health Soc Behav 9:275–287, 1968
25. Staub E, Kellett DS: Increasing pain tolerance by information about aversive stimuli. J Person Soc Psychol 21:198–203, 1972
26. Stoeckle JD, Barsky AJ: Attributions: Use of social science knowledge in the "doctoring" of primary care. In Eisenberg L, Kleinman A: The Relevance of Social Science for Medicine, pp 223–240. Dordrecht, Holland, D Reidel, 1980
27. Storms MD, Nisbett RE: Insomnia and the attribution process. J Person Soc Psychol 16:317–328, 1970
28. Tolstoy L: Death of Ivan Ilych. In Great Short Works of Leo Tolstoy. New York, Harper & Row, 1967
29. Winnicott DW: The Child, The Family, and the Outside World. New York, Penguin Books, 1978

Coping with Loss 6

Susan D. Block

While psychological distress is a regular and, perhaps, inevitable feature of terminal illness and bereavement, the physician has an opportunity to facilitate adaptation and to prevent or palliate many of the emotional difficulties that afflict patients and families. This chapter describes "normal" and dysfunctional coping patterns of patients and families during the dying process and of survivors after the death. Its goals are (1) to help the clinician appreciate the themes and conflicts that characterize the process of adapting to loss, (2) to heighten awareness of signs of poor coping and treatable psychosocial distress, and (3) to provide an overview of treatment strategies and to guide the practitioner toward successful interventions.

Several basic assumptions underly the approach that will be elaborated in this chapter:

A secure, consistent, and trusting relationship between the patient and physician is often essential for eliciting the appropriate psychological data and is a prerequisite for management of all psychological issues.

Because the patient and his or her relatives are usually major sources of support or discouragement for each other, effective care must focus on the entire family. Family-oriented care is likely to optimize the care of the patient as well as to reduce the frequency of dysfunctional grief reactions among family members.

The responses of patients and families to terminal illness, death, and bereavement are mediated not only by individual differences, but also by ethnic and cultural styles of understanding and coping with these events. Attention must be focused on appreciating the unique experience of each individual, but the responses of patients and families also should be viewed within their cultural context.

The physician, patient and family will most effectively work together when they can develop a shared understanding of the patient's condition, prognosis, and treatment options. The development of a common ground of understanding facilitates the process of negotiating treatment goals and methods, and helps create an atmosphere of support and mutuality. Moreover, the patient's sense of responsibility and control over the negotiation process can be an antidote to the fear and helplessness that may accompany terminal illness.

All terminally ill patients can benefit from a supportive relationship and from some exploration of habitual coping styles, current fears and concerns, personal aspirations for the last phase of life, and the reciprocal relationship between physical well-being and emotional concerns. Such psychotherapeutic interventions are usually best provided by medical practitioners who are trained and supported by mental-health clinicians.

Some terminally ill patients seek psychotherapy to examine their feelings about their lives and for support in coping with the crisis of approaching death. Very few terminally ill patients are interested in a "personality overhaul" designed to change basic and long-standing character patterns and coping styles. Similarly, for family members, the crisis of illness may catalyze a desire for self-exploration, which can be facilitated by mental-health referral. Only a small fraction of terminally ill patients and their families develop sustained problems in coping that require intensive and focused interventions directly from mental-health practitioners.

THE PATIENT'S ADAPTATION

The dying person encounters paradoxical struggles: to maintain self and life in continuity with the past and yet to adapt to new realities; to hold on to life while letting go; and to maintain hope in the face of inevitable despair. Rather than being resolved once and for all, such tensions wax and wane and are continually redefined over the course of the illness. The patient's adaptation to the changing context of illness can be portrayed in terms of a number of overlapping themes or motifs. A clinician who is attuned to these issues can facilitate the patient's adaptation through techniques such as exploration, clarification, support, and confrontation.

Themes in the Emotional Lives of Terminally Ill Patients

Uncertainty and Control

The uncertainty and unpredictability of the course of terminal illness can create enormous stresses. Most people are accustomed to a certain amount of predictability in their daily lives and in the way their bodies function. Cancer creates havoc. How does one know which days will be good ones for a visit? How will treatment turn out? When will new symptoms develop? How and when will death come? Uncertainty places extraordinary constraints and demands on the patient.

The feeling that one's internal milieu is out of control often generates a frightening sensation of helplessness and vulnerability. Deep shame may arise from concerns about loss of physiologic control. Some patients fear that they will not be able to control their emotions under the stress of terminal illness.

As the illness progresses, the patient's sphere of control diminishes. Work, finances, and family issues are often being increasingly negotiated without the patient's involvement. Medical decisions are often made by others. Some patients are relieved to be unburdened of these weighty problems; others are panicked by a sense of fragility and dependency.

Serious illness forces the patient to relinquish usual roles and responsibilities and to accept the care of others. For those patients whose sense of self-esteem and personal worth derives from attending to others, the need to be taken care of may cause great conflict. Many patients find ingenious ways of continuing to care for others despite the limitations imposed by illness—helping family members grieve and plan for the future, investing energy into arranging financial affairs, or worrying about the physician's long hours. These "solutions" to the problem of helplessness and loss of control should generally be supported by the physician.

In contrast, patients who are eager to be taken care of and to assume a passive role may readily embrace the dependent stance of the sick role. The advice of worried family members and the medical system's encouragement of passivity may further reinforce a sense of inadequacy, helplessness, and fearfulness. Overly dependent patients may place extraordinary demands on the family—"who can say 'no' to a dying person?"—and their social and emotional functioning may seem worse than their medical condition warrants. Firm encouragement and support of the family in making realistic demands will help prevent further regression and may motivate the patient to function at a higher level.

An awareness of the patient's attitudes toward issues of control is helpful in negotiating decisions about the provision of care. For example, the patient with a strong need for control may be put at ease when the physician convinces family members that the patient can and should manage his or her own medications. Another patient might comfortably surrender this prerogative to family members and feel all the better for it.

Anger

Cancer often conjures up aggressive imagery—"fighting," "struggling," "invasion," and "killing the tumor." The illness can represent a betrayal of the body, an assault on personal integrity, a theft of health and life. Anger is a common and appropriate response to these insults. Anger can have enormous adaptive value, allowing patients to say "no" to death, to mobilize inner resources to live, and to fight for life itself. Adaptive anger may be expressed in such unrealistic but wishful statements as: "I'll die when I'm God-damn ready!" and "I've had it with being pushed around by this cancer. From now on, I'm calling the shots." Adaptive anger is allied with hope, determination, and defiance and may lead to improved survival.[11]

> Do not go gentle into that good night,
> Old age should burn and rave at close of day;
> Rage, rage against the dying of the light.
>
> Though wise men at their end know dark is right,
> Because their words had forked no lightning they
> Do not go gentle into that good night.
>
> Good men, the last wave by, crying how bright
> Their frail deeds might have danced in a green bay,
> Rage, rage against the dying of the light.

Wild men who caught and sang the sun in flight,
And learn, too late, they grieved it on its way,
Do not go gentle into that good night.

Grave men, near death, who see with blinding sight
Blind eyes could blaze like meteors and be gay,
Rage, rage against the dying of the light.

And you, my father, there on the sad height,
Curse, bless me now with your fierce tears, I pray.
Do not go gentle into that good night.
Rage, rage against the dying of the light.

Dylan Thomas*

Adaptive anger is generally not directed at anyone in particular or is appropriately aimed at a brusque radiation therapy technician or a late visitor. Dysfunctional anger is often directed at the wrong people, a process called displacement; it tends to be inexplicably diffuse and intense, and may feel out of control to the patient. Dysfunctional expressions of anger may include self-destructive behavior, refusal of treatment, heavy alcohol use, and displacement onto family members, health-care providers, and others. Such exaggerated anger can isolate the patient from important sources of personal support.

Rather than trying to soothe the patient's anger, the clinician should encourage the patient to talk about it, understand it, and accept it. The clinician must accept and tolerate the anger and work with the patient to clarify and validate its sources. Defensive responses to anger directed at the medical establishment (e.g., "There's no reason to be angry at me—I didn't cause your cancer") should be avoided. Pointing out the brighter side is also likely to be ineffective and alienating. At times, the professional staff may take the "heat," tolerating somewhat misdirected anger at themselves in order to allow the patient to maintain more reasonable relationships with friends and family members. When anger is out of control and threatens the patient's relationships with important caretakers or becomes dangerous to the patient, the clinician should attempt to set limits.

Young adults who are confronting death seem to become particularly angry. Unresolved conflicts about developmental issues such as body image and personal identity may make adolescents and young adults especially vulnerable to anger and depression when they encounter chronic illness. Adolescent omnipotence is drastically challenged by the approach of death. Struggles to achieve separation and independence from parents are sabotaged by illness-induced dependency. Work, relationships, and personal goals have usually not achieved a coherent form that can be mourned. The young adult is "stuck" in the early stages of grief—disbelief and anger—and cannot move forward. Jealousy, dependency, anger about being sick, and an unstable sense of self may lead to poor self-esteem, rage at healthy people (including physicians, nurses, and family members), and guilt over resentful feelings toward others. The patient's feelings are often further complicated by the reactions of health-care providers, who may identify intensely with their young patients. Aversion, despair, and profound helplessness in the family and in the professional caretaking staff may develop in response to the patient's distress. Awareness of these dynamics can help the clinician understand the patient's responses, remain involved, and provide necessary psychological support.

Guilt and Bargaining

In their efforts to understand why they became sick, patients often blame themselves (*e.g.*, "If I had only gone to see my doctor sooner, maybe I wouldn't be this sick," or "If I had listened to my wife and stopped smoking, I never would have gotten this lung cancer"). A patient's guilt may be a potent force in inducing compliance with medical treatments as a way of atoning for past lapses or as a means of bargaining for a good outcome (*e.g.*, "If I do everything the doctors tell me to do, then I'll be okay"). A sense of guilt may also allow the patient to tolerate the suffering that comes with the illness and its treatment (*e.g.*, "It was my fault I got this cancer, and this is what I deserve for not taking care of myself all these years").

The physician should make efforts to assuage unrealistic guilt (*e.g.*, "I got this cancer because of the abortion I had 30 years ago"), but should not offer false reassurance about realistic guilt, such as that over smoking in a patient with lung cancer. Rather, the patient should be encouraged to discuss his or her understanding of the connection between earlier behavior and the current illness. The clinician can offer realistic hope about the future and can emphasize the new opportunity the patient has to take care of himself or herself. Since patients often feel guilty if they do not respond to medical treatments, the clinician must strike a balance between emphasizing the control the patient does have over treatment outcome and cautioning that cancer is often difficult to control even with the best of treatment and the fullest possible cooperation from the patient.

Boredom

Being sick with cancer is boring. Lying in bed, being unable to enjoy food, undergoing tests and treatment, waiting in doctors' offices, and feeling too tired to take pleasure in seeing friends, all leave the patient feeling "weary, stale, flat, and unprofitable" (Shakespeare, *Hamlet*). Patients often have little energy. Sustained activity or concentration may be difficult. Mundane details that belong in the background of a life—moving one's bowels, turning over in bed—become major concerns and often require great effort. Time passes slowly and is hard to use well. Patients often are acutely aware of having too little time, yet lack the energy to accomplish their goals.

Secrets

Gaps in communication between patient, family, and physician make the process of dying more stressful and difficult for all. When patient and family are operating with different models of diagnosis, management, and prognosis, or if they are operating with the same models but do not acknowledge it, considerable tension and anxiety are inevitable. Each person tries to gauge without asking what the other is thinking and to modulate and monitor what is communicated. Families that have dealt with problems openly in the past tend to continue this pattern in dealing with terminal illness and appear to cope better than families with more "closed" communication[16]; open communication rarely develops for the first time in families facing terminal illness. There is some evidence that more open communication in families of patients with cancer may positively influence the patient's longevity.[54] An approach to encouraging the sharing of information is presented in Chapter 7.

To minimize gaps in communicaton, the clinician may want to discuss important information when the patient and family are all present. Such a practice conveys the message that distressing facts can be acknowledged, that they are not too terrible to hear, and that confronting issues directly offers most hope of productive solutions.

Loneliness

Dying is inherently a lonely process, even for those surrounded by great love and understanding. No one outside the experience can know what it is like—the private, unspoken griefs and disappointments, the fears, the weariness, the memories. While accepting the inevitable solitude of the patient, the clinician can try to understand the particular details of each individual's experience. This willingness to listen and an eagerness to understand is a powerful antidote to the patient's loneliness.

Alienation

As if the physical distress and losses of cancer were not burden enough, the terminally ill patient also confronts social isolation. A dying patient is often avoided because others believe that one can "catch cancer" as one catches the common cold. Avoidance of painful feelings, "not knowing what to say," and fears of helplessness may keep friends and relatives at a distance, adding to the isolation that arises with being unable to work and socialize freely.

Romanticization of cancer distances those living in the "Kingdom of the Sick" from those in the "Kingdom of the Well."[46] Where outsiders may see the terminally ill patient as extraordinary and ennobled by the illness, the patient is often mired in commonplace concerns and may feel pressure to live up to others' idealized expectations:

> Everyone is amazed at how well I cope. But really, what other choice is there?

> People want to talk to me about what it's like to be sick, but they somehow seem disappointed when I say it's mostly boring. It seems like they're expecting more. Like I'm supposed to all of a sudden get profound or something.

The physician's matter-of-fact acceptance of the patient's sick body may be potent salve for alienation. The laying on of hands and concerned questioning practiced by the physician communicates that the patient will not be abandoned, that he or she is still a worthwhile person, and that others can tolerate being physically and emotionally close. Comfortable touching of the patient by the medical staff can provide a model of behavior for family members who may be afraid of such contact.

Sexuality and Intimacy

Many terminally ill patients experience problems related to sexuality and intimacy. Between 50% and 100% of patients with surgically treated lesions of the gastrointestinal (GI), genitourinary, and pelvic area experience sexual dysfunction, and a high incidence of sexual dysfunction is reported in patients with breast cancer.[12] Cancer treatments themselves may cause organic sexual dysfunctions in a significant proportion of patients.[41] Illness otherwise impairs physical intimacy by causing fatigue, pain, and other physical symptoms, and by inducing negative effects on the patient's body image, self-esteem, and other facets of emotional well-being. Moreover, hospitalization or the need for help in the home may leave the patient with little privacy.

Cancer patients report a decrease in their desire for sexual intercourse, but an increase in their wish for nongenital physical contact and for emotional intimacy. A central task for the patient and partner is renegotiating the kinds of physical contact and affectional relating that feel good. Needs, wishes, and capabilities change with the patient's condition.

Terminal illness may also have a strong emotional impact on the patient's partner, who may feel anger, anxiety, resentment, exhaustion, fear, aversion, and disgust, as well as love, concern, eagerness to help, and admiration. Male partners of cancer patients appear to be at special risk of not have their affectional needs met.[24]

Coping and Defending

Weisman has described two modes of confronting illness and of preserving psychological equilibrium. In the first mode, the patient *copes*, using active problem-solving approaches to deal with new events, circumstances, and responses:

> You know, I've really been feeling low. They can't seem to stop all this vomiting. But I've decided I'm not going to miss out on things I would like to do just because of it. I want to get out, to see my friends. So, I've been taking my vomit bucket with me when I go out to lunch. If I feel myself getting sick, I go to the ladies room, and come back when it's over.

Defending is the complementary adaptational mode in which the patient attempts to maintain the status quo by not confronting or assimilating new information.[53] Defenses (such as denial, avoidance, minimization, turning negative into positive, and rationalization) are called into action when the patient's anxiety is so great that it threatens his or her ability to cope:

> Oh this? [*pointing to a belly full of ascites*] It's nothing. Or maybe I'm pregnant. I have been eating a lot, so maybe I'm getting fat. When does that show come on?

Denial is a familiar and striking feature of the psychological presentation of terminally ill patients. Denial is the process of negating a fact or a truth, and is a maneuver that compromises the patient's connection with reality. Most dying patients deny some aspects of their illness some of the time. Remarkably, this amalgamation of knowing and not knowing often oscillates rapidly in such a way that seemingly contradictory views of reality will be held within the space of a few moments.[52] The term, "middle knowledge," describes this fluctuating mixture of denial and acceptance or awareness.

Early in the illness, denial may allow the patient to enjoy what still feels like normal daily life. As illness progresses, denial often becomes less and less adaptive: concrete plans need to be made about jobs, finances, vacations, and so on; medical decisions require the attentive weighing of subtle risks and benefits; and family members often need the patient's support and a realistic outlook in order to adjust to the illness. Cancer patients who are able to face problems head-on with an optimistic outlook do better than patients who deny.[51]

An ever-shifting tension occurs between coping and defending. A resilient patient is able to assimilate experiences which a more psychologically brittle patient would need to deny, avoid, or repress. An individual's level of resiliency waxes and wanes with changes in levels of physical distress, emotional support, fatigue, and stress. Many patients think of "coping" as a static process that is begun and completed, as if one adjusts once and for all to dying. Patients are often surprised by their mood fluctuations and by their evolving responses to being ill.

Although day-to-day coping often varies quite dramatically, general coping styles are rather consistent over time. An awareness of the patient's characteristic defenses and of areas of vulnerability is invaluable to the clinician.

In a crisis setting, such as that of terminal illness, respect and support for the patient's defenses is generally a better therapeutic stance for the clinician than trying to challenge or change such patterns. Usually, the patient's defenses represent the best possible solution for the current dilemma, and alternative ways of coping are likely to be more psychologically perilous. The process of helping the patient traverse the treacherous path toward greater awareness is one of the most challenging and rewarding aspects of terminal care.

When the patient's defenses are maladaptive (*e.g.,* interfering with receiving appropriate medical care, adding significantly to the burden on the family), several approaches are available. Recognition and encouragement of the positive aspects of the patient's coping will enhance the patient's sense of personal competence, reduce anxiety, and thus decrease the need for major defensive maneuvers. Often, it is possible to redefine the situation to engage the patient's defenses in a more constructive direction:

> *I know that being a Marine is very much part of you—being strong, tough, not letting things get to you. It takes a tough man to face his sadness . . .*

Sometimes, the patient's supports can be bolstered in order to reduce the anxiety-provoking situations that force the patient to invoke maladaptive defensive maneuvers (*e.g.,* by putting a home-health aid in the home in the evening when a patient tends to get paranoid and frightened).

When denial is maladaptive, gentle confrontation can begin with an exploration of the patient's view of his or her situation. An effective technique is for the clinician to speak to the part of the patient that is aware and is concerned about his or her condition, while acknowledging the other part that needs to avoid being overwhelmed by reality. The clinician should wait and listen for small niches in the armor of denial, and seize these moments to ask a tentative, but gently confrontative question:

> *When you said that you didn't want to go to your nephew's wedding, I wonder if maybe part of you was worrying about whether you'd be well enough to make it to the wedding. . . .*

In urgent situations, forceful confrontation may be necessary, with the goal of helping the patient deal with his or her situation differently:

> *I'm afraid we are going to have to have a difficult conversation. I know you would like to believe that you are getting better, but I think that it is clear that you are getting much sicker and that the cancer is moving rapidly now. I hope we can slow it down, but I am not optimistic. You have three small children and have not made plans yet about who will care for them if we can't turn things around. I am worried that the next week or so may be the only opportunity you may have to decide how you would like them cared for, and to make arrangements.*

Loss and Grief

Grief is the psychological response to loss. Individuals grieve, not only over the loss of their health and their loved ones, but also for normal daily life, for ideas, values, and places. They mourn for lost opportunities, and for such abstract qualities as security and orderliness. Patients also grieve for themselves, for who they were, are, and wish to become.

> MÁRGARÉT, áre you grieving
> Over Goldengrove unleaving?
> Leáves líke the things of man, you
> With your fresh thoughts care for, can you?
> Áh! ás the heart grows older
> It will come to such sights colder
> By and by, nor spare a sigh
> Though worlds of wanwood leafmeal lie;
> And yet you wíll weep and know why.
> Now no matter, child, the name:
> Sórrow's spríngs áre the same.
> Nor mouth had, no nor mind, expressed
> What heart heard of, ghost guessed:
> It ís the blight man was born for,
> It is Margaret you mourn for.

Gerard Manley Hopkins

Grieving may begin when a potentially terminal illness is first suspected; it is recapitulated over and over as further losses occur, solidifying the awareness that death is approaching. The patient's first concrete losses are usually those associated with medical treatments. Surgery, radiation therapy, and chemotherapy involve losses—of bodily integrity, of hair, of privacy. Events that signify the progression of illness—treatment failures, new symptoms, new diagnostic measures—regularly promote a heightened sense of vulnerability, loss, and grief. As the patient becomes more disabled, the circle in which he or she lives narrows. The first losses are usually work (including domestic work) and all that work may stand for. Casual friends and acquaintances—the friendly butcher, the cronies at the bar, the other "beano" afficionados—recede from daily life. Later, closer friends and relatives may be excluded from the patient's life. As death approaches, the patient's circle may narrow to include only intimate family members and health professionals. Severely debilitated or moribund patients may only have energy for the most basic physiologic functions and often become emotionally disconnected from even the few people to whom they are closest.

Grieving takes many forms, since individuals have various styles of handling emotions. Some patients grieve loudly—crying, wailing, and expressing emotion intensely. Others grieve quietly, sharing their sadness only with close family members. Still others grieve privately, reworking and remembering important people, places, and events in their own minds, sharing with no one else. In general, patients benefit from expressing emotions that arise in grieving, because the sharing of their feelings counterbalances the intrinsic loneliness of the dying process.

> Give sorrow words; the grief that does not speak
> Whispers the o'er-fraught heart and bids it break.

William Shakespare,
Macbeth, IV, iii, 209

Reactive Depression

Depression and sadness in response to loss can be thought of as natural consequences of the disruption of a close attachment. Although a dying patient's sadness may be painful for family, friends and caretakers, depression that occurs in response to the losses resulting from terminal illness rarely warrants psychiatric treatment, and usually does not meet the criteria for diagnosis of a major depressive disorder.[36] Although feelings of depression and sadness may be present, they are usually not pervasive and unremitting. Rather, the feeling tends to be focused around a particular loss. A particular feeling or memory may precipitate a wave of grief. The patient retains some capacity to respond with pleasure. The terms, sadness, grief, and reactive depression, are used in this discussion to describe the "normal" feeling state associated with illness and loss; while the term "major depression" is reserved to describe prolonged states of dysphoria associated with feelings of guilt, worthlessness, and low self-esteem, often accompanied by unremitting disturbances of sleep, appetite, energy, concentration, and interest in living.

Hope

"Hope" is the thing with feathers—
That perches in the soul—
And sings the tune without the words—
And never stops—at all—

Emily Dickinson

The terminally ill patient struggles to maintain a sense of hope in the face of an increasingly ominous medical situation. Hope is a precondition for successful coping because it permits the patient to approach new problems with the expectation that they can be overcome and mastered. While it remains unclear whether hopefulness can extend survival, hopelessness and helplessness have been associated with the development of physical illness.[43,44] Although a patient's overall prognosis may be "hopeless," the patient can still hope to achieve short-range objectives.[51]

The clinician can nurture hope in the terminally ill patient by confronting problems directly, by conveying a comforting and confident attitude, by focusing on positive and achievable short-term objectives, and by involving the patient as an active agent of self-care. Direct discussion with the patient about feelings of hopelessness acknowledges their reality as well as their manageability.

Trust

Terminal illness forces the patient to depend on others. To comfortably accept care from others, the patient must be able to trust that help will be competently and respectfully delivered. The patient may need to test old relationships with the burden of new roles, and will scrutinize the ability of new care providers to meet his or her needs.

The development of trust is nurtured by the experience of depending on someone and of receiving appropriate care. It takes time. Availability, consistency, competence, dependability and concern are the basic ingredients the clinician contributes to the development of a trusting relationship. The clinician should consider that a problem with trust is present when the patient's initial anxieties and wariness fail to resolve, when discussions repeatedly go over the same ground, or when other care providers are frequently consulted about management decisions. Distrustfulness may be related to multiple factors, including poor communication between physician and patient, failure of the physician to understand the patient's perspective, and long-standing personality problems within the patient. The etiology of the problem with trust can be elicited by a direct, nonjudgmental confrontation:

I'm concerned that somehow you seem not to feel secure with me. It is very important that we try to find some way of understanding each other. How have you been feeling about the way we work together? What are the problems from your point of view?

The physician's willingness to acknowledge the issue, to consider the possibility that he or she might be inadvertently contributing to the problem, and to solicit the patient's views about the relationship often lead to great improvement in the level of trust and in overall patient comfort. When this technique is not effective, further exploration is needed, and a consultation or mental-health referral may be indicated to further evaluate the problem.

"Appropriate" Dying

Avery Weisman defines an "appropriate death" as one "that a person might have accepted and chosen, had there been a choice."[51] Most patients have some ideas about what kind of death they would choose:

I always thought that I wanted to die on my way up the trail from the Clackamas River with a full basket of fish. I wanted to die suddenly in a place I love, with my heart happy, without having to say good-bye.

Such notions often change as terminal illness progresses and as fears about what it will be like are mastered:

I used to have this idea that I just wanted to die suddenly without knowing it. I couldn't face the idea of knowing I was dying. Well, I've known it—sort of— for awhile, and I can stand it. I wouldn't trade this time I've had, what I've had a chance to learn about my family and friends, for anything. It's odd, but even though I know that I'm dying, this is one of the happiest times of my life.

An appropriate dying allows the patient to maintain a sense of control over the dying process and to be aware of and come to terms with its inevitability. The patient may gather close important people in order to share his or her experience with them, to know what they are feeling, to feel safe and protected, and to preserve a sense of continuity with the living. This sharing of the experience may also make bereavement easier on the survivors, reassuring them that the patient had some satisfaction about how the dying process unfolded, allowing them to grieve with the patient, promoting the resolution of outstanding conflicts, and permitting them both to support the dying person and to be supported by him or her.[6,7]

The physician helps the patient achieve the goal of an appropriate death not only by facilitating emotional adjustment, but also by ensuring that pain and symptoms are well-controlled and by helping the patient work out such questions as where death should occur, how much consciousness is desired, and how far palliative treatments should be pursued.

Dysfunctional Adaptation

"Dysfunctional adaptation" may be thought of as a pattern of behavior that hinders the individual's optimal functioning in the context of terminal illness. Although terminal illness itself generates anxiety (*e.g.*, about "bad news," about facing the unknown) and depression (*e.g.*, normal grieving), most patients manage to live with these feelings without severe impairments in their relationships, sense of self, and view of the world. Many dysfunctional coping patterns that clinicians see in terminally ill patients are lifelong maladaptive traits, which continue in the terminal phase. The following section should alert the clinician to the forms of dysfunctional coping that require intervention.

Rejection of Physician's Advice

When a patient refuses or resists professional advice, he or she is likely to be immediately bombarded with good reasons for following the physician's recommended plan of management. The staff urges, cajoles, begs or threatens the patient to comply. Friends and relatives may be enlisted to influence the patient. A battle between the patient and the staff escalates, and the patient may be labeled a "problem patient." The first step in approaching treatment refusal—understanding why the patient has rejected professional recommendations—is often overlooked.*

A patient's choice to limit or refuse treatment or to seek additional treatments often represents an appropriate, considered, and informed decision that balances the discomfort, inconvenience, or toxicity of the treatment against its potential benefits. For example, a patient may find that the nausea induced by an analgesic is less tolerable than the pain that it relieves. Similarly, an indwelling urinary catheter may be more humiliating and inconvenient than urinary incontinence. For another patient, the need to avoid "giving-up" by continuing to seek aggressive or innovative treatments may outweigh improvements in comfort gained by limiting treatment. The patient's or family's informed evaluation of the risks and benefits of treatment may initially be discrepant from that of the professional caretakers, but open discussion will often lead to a consensus. Sometimes, the physician and patient cannot come to agreement about treatment decisions, and "agreeing to disagree" may be an appropriate resolution.

In other situations, rejection of treatment reflects a misunderstanding about the benefits or toxicity of treatment. For instance, some patients will refuse chemotherapy because of concerns about emesis or hair loss, although the prescribed agent may not cause such side-effects. Narcotics may be resisted because of concerns about social stigma, sedation, addiction, or behavioral changes. In these cases, refusal represents a failure of communication and may be resolved with appropriate explanation.

Refusal is sometimes best understood as an expression of feelings rather than of reason. Patients and families (and even physicians) make all choices under the influence of emotions. Some of these emotional reactions promote compliance. For instance, many patients attribute magical powers to the physician and the treatment, leading them to be exceedingly docile. Similarly, patients harboring feelings of guilt and a need for atonement may view the physician as a judgmental authority who must be obeyed and pleased. On the other hand, anger and frustration about being sick, lacking control over one's life, or needing to submit to the regimens and whims of the

---

*A recent study of "treatment refusals" of medications, tests, and adjunctive care in a general hospital found 0.7 to 11.4 instances per 100 patient days.[1] Failure of doctor–patient communication and lack of trust were cited as common causes, while psychopathology was identified as an important factor in about a quarter of cases. Additional factors included hospital fatigue, idiosyncratic beliefs, objections that the researchers agreed were legitimate, and a wish for "death with dignity."

health professions may be expressed as negativism. The patient may counter a sense of helplessness with defiant assertions of independence, bolstering his or her fragile sense of personal power by constantly sparring with the professional staff.

In order to help patients understand and come to terms with their decisions, the physician must try to avoid entering into a struggle over the proposed treatment. Insofar as possible, the clinician should temporarily suspend a commitment to one treatment course and should direct attention to understanding the patient's perspective. Highlighting and acknowledging the feelings of frustration and anger that underly a particular decision often defuse the feelings and allow the patient to reconsider options. Patients often have mixed feelings, which can be elicited by questions such as, "What is it like for you to be thinking of going ahead with this treatment when your doctors don't think it is a good idea?" Such approaches reframe the struggle as one that exists within the patient, rather than as one between physician and patient, and allow the physician to be seen as an ally rather than an adversary to the patient in the decision-making process. Better decisions can be made by physician and patient working together than by either operating alone.

Refusal can also be a demand for attention, expressing such sentiments as, "What right do you have to do this without discussing the matter more fully with me," or "You can't expect me to go along with you if you're treating me so casually." Argumentativeness and negativism are often effective ways of getting relatives or professional caretakers to pay greater heed to one's personal concerns. The desire for more attention is addressed by validating the patient's right to more information, by continuing attention to the inclusion of the patient in all aspects of decision-making, and by enhancing other, more personal methods of making the patient feel appreciated, involved, and understood.

Depression and anxiety strongly affect treatment decisions. Feelings that color decision-making in depressed patients include heightened guiltiness, fears of becoming an unwelcome burden on others, a sense of helplessness and hopelessness about the possibility of effective treatment, loss of interest in life, an inclination to social withdrawal, and a wish for death as an end to misery. The clinician's assessment of the patient's current mental state, including cognitive capacities, mood and affect, will suggest how depression influences the patient's decision-making. Similarly, patients who are extremely anxious may be so agitated and frightened that they cannot consider choices rationally, fleeing from any discussion that confronts them with the reality of their condition. Panicked decisions are rarely good ones. As discussed in Chapter 5, the physician's efforts to provide support and to give reassurance that addresses the patient's specific concerns can reduce the patient's anxiety and facilitate more reasoned decision-making.

Another category of refusers includes patients who have long-standing eccentricities, major psychiatric disorders (*e.g.*, schizophrenia), or characterologic disorders. Such patients may have a limited capacity for qualities such as trust, closeness, and dependence, which facilitate therapeutic interactions. Under the stress of illness, lifelong character traits such as suspiciousness may blossom into profound distrust or frank paranoia, while a chronic preference for social isolation and independence may develop into an overwhelming need to withdraw from the interpersonal strains attendant to the process of receiving care. Many persons in this category of refusers, if treated respectfully and patiently, can establish limited therapeutic relationships with health professionals and can be helped to die comfortably on their own terms.

Finally, organic brain syndromes, as discussed in Chapter 2, Section K, may lead to negativism or treatment refusal. When impairment of the patient's capacities for attention, understanding or judgment are identified, treatment for potentially reversible causes of the deficit should generally be initiated before management decisions are made final. In some urgent cases, however, the appointment of a temporary or permanent guardian may allow needed medical procedures to be undertaken. Formal evaluation of the patient's competence to make decisions regarding his or her care rests on the patient's capacity to understand his or her condition, the risks and benefits of the proposed treatment, and its alternatives. If the patient is competent by these criteria, he or she has full rights to determine the course of treatment. If he or she is incompetent, family members, the physician, or a court-appointed guardian may make decisions on the patient's behalf, based on what they think the patient would have wanted if he or she were competent.

Anxiety

While moderate anxiety may facilitate adaptation to stress, extreme anxiety can interfere with functioning and pleasure and is clearly counterproductive.[18] Anxiety usually improves rapidly with the intervention of talking and being listened to. Unremitting, severe anxiety that does not respond to therapeutic exploration should be further investigated and treated, as described below.

Increased Alcohol or Drug Consumption

Substance abuse rarely develops for the first time in the setting of terminal illness. Patients who have had alcohol or drug problems in the past, however, commonly respond to the stress of serious illness by increasing their reliance on these substances. Clinical evaluation should include attention to long-standing patterns of substance abuse (e.g., as a general response to stress or as a specific response to depression, anxiety, or family discord). Substance abuse may represent self-medication for chronic pain. Treatment begins with gentle but direct confrontation of the patient, which brings the problem into the open and communicates the physician's concern about it:

> Have you been concerned about your drinking?

> Have you noticed that your family is worried and upset by your drug use?

Physical Distress out of Proportion
to Current Medical Condition

When patients complain of symptoms out of proportion to documented or expectable disease, the clinician should consider psychological etiologies. Long-term patterns of hypochondriasis or somatization may be superimposed on the course of a terminal illness. A past history of multiple somatic complaints, persistent concern with bodily functioning, or failure to respond to appropriate reassurance should alert the clinician to these diagnostic entities. Amplification of bodily sensations is also a well-documented concomitant of physical illness and frequently reflects anxiety, depression, or interpersonal disturbances.[2] The exaggeration of symptoms may serve a useful or a dysfunctional purpose in modulating family discord, communicating intrapsychic distress, or highlighting a problem in the physician–patient relationship.

Absence of Grieving

Patients may try to avoid the natural feelings of sadness that occur during terminal illness, fearing that grief will become overwhelming, that they will go out of control and become crazy, that they will be unable to stop crying, that family members or the medical staff will be unable to bear the onslaught of feelings, and that they will be abandoned for behaving inappropriately. The clinician's task in dealing with inhibited grief is to explore the reasons that the feeling is being avoided, to encourage the patient to test his or her abilities to tolerate sadness, and to help the patient build on experiences with small griefs to become better able to feel and express the larger sadness:

> Last week we talked about how sad you are that your wife will have to go back to work after you die. Saying it out loud was a hard thing for you to do, I know, and I wonder what thoughts you've had about it since we last talked. . . . I imagine that's only one of many sadnesses you feel when you think about leaving her. Can you tell me about other thoughts you've had about your wife and the future . . .?

Patients whose social supports inhibit the expression of the various aspects of grief may experience a truncated, absent, or distorted grieving process. Such patients can sometimes be allowed to grieve by establishing a relationship with a care provider who cares about and is cared about by the patient and who serves as a sounding board for talking about losses:

> Doc, you know I'm all alone. No one will miss me when I'm gone. No family. My life is almost over. There's nothing left. But I'll miss you, Doc. You've been great. You've really been there for me. Thanks.

The patient's need for someone to miss who will also miss him may be a source of the appreciativeness, eagerness to relate, and desire to please seen in the dying.

Depression

As noted previously, the vast majority of depressions experienced by terminally ill patients are reactive depressions that do not generally fulfill the diagnostic criteria for major depression. The following schemata outlines the differences among the types of depression that will be discussed in this chapter. Although there is considerable overlap among these categories (and a confusing and inconsistent use of terms in the psychiatric literature), differentiation among the various types will lead to divergent treatment approaches.

REACTIVE DEPRESSION

A *reactive depression* (or transient depression), which shares many features with a grief reaction, occurs in response to losses associated with terminal illness. Often, such a depression is precipitated by a particular loss or by signs of deteriorating health. In general, reactive depressions tend to be milder than major depressions, and neurovegetative signs are less frequently present. Patients may experience guilt about unfulfilled potential and may wish that death would come quickly. Usually, these depressions last up to several weeks and remit spontaneously, although patients are often helped by the opportunity to talk about their distress with a professional or nonprofessional caretaker. In unusual circumstances, a severe reactive depression may remain intense and unremitting, progressing to become a major depression.

MAJOR DEPRESSION

A *major depression* is characterized by dysphoria, poor functioning, anhedonia, worthlessness, hopelessness, helplessness, guilty preoccupations, recurrent wishes for death, and neurovegetative signs, including psychomotor retardation, poor concentration, attention deficit, sleep disturbance (insomnia or hypersomnia), agitation, anorexia, and weight loss. Psychotic symptoms may also be present, including delusions and hallucinations. A family history of major depressive episodes or a personal history of previous depressions can often be noted in such patients. Without treatment, such a depression may last for months and is associated with an increased risk of suicide. The presence of a major depression demands active therapeutic intervention with psychotherapy and/or medication.

DEPRESSIVE PERSONALITY (OR DYSTHYMIC DISORDER)

A patient with a lifelong *depressive personality* style may appear depressed during terminal illness. Generally, such patients have a history of recurrent prolonged depressive episodes or a sustained depressive style throughout life. They tend to be pessimistic, negativistic, critical, and unsatisfied. The depressive episodes, when they occur, tend to be less severe and are of shorter duration than those characterizing a major depression. They may be accompanied by hypochondriacal preoccupations and are poorly responsive to short-term psychotherapeutic or pharmacologic treatment.

About 25% of advanced cancer patients experience major depressions during their illnesses.[35] The presence of major depression does not appear to be related to overall physical condition or nearness to death.[10,36] Major depression can be disabling and life-threatening. In general, any depression that is sustained for longer than 2 weeks and interferes markedly with social functioning or obtaining appropriate medical care deserves active diagnostic and therapeutic efforts.

Assessment of depression is difficult in terminally ill patients for multiple reasons:

1. Chronic pain and other unremitting discomforts may cause a readily reversible depressive state. Appropriate treatment of such symptoms is the first step in managing depression in terminally ill patients.
2. Organic brain syndromes may cause or mimic depression. In one study, 26% of cancer patients thought to be depressed by their medical doctors received diagnoses of organic brain syndromes from psychiatric consultants.[25] In severely ill patients who appear depressed, a careful mental status examination is essential to identify patients with cognitive and attentional impairments, which may mimic depression.
3. Although neurovegetative symptoms are usually present in depression, they are also commonly seen during terminal illness. In particular, anorexia, weight loss, insomnia, decreased libido, fatigue, and drowsiness are each experienced by at least one third to one half of all terminally ill patients (see Table 2-1). Thus, the clinician must rely on other signs of major depression, including hopelessness, helplessness, worthlessness, guilt, agitation, inability to relax, psychomotor retardation, diminished concentration, and early-morning awakening (which are not caused by pain or discomfort). Frequent crying spells, persistent unremitting sadness, social withdrawal, noncompliance, anger, and irritability may also be signs of a major depression, but these findings, in themselves, do not make for a diagnosis of major depression.
4. Anger, social withdrawal, and preoccupation with one's health all occur to some degree in most terminally ill patients, but can also be indicators of an "atypical" depression. Atypical depressions are a subset of major depressive disorders, which may respond to specific pharmacologic treatment.

5. Normal grief, like depression, involves feelings of sadness in response to losses. However, the patient who is experiencing an intense grief reaction with reactive depression, in contrast to the patient with a major depression, tends to respond to the environment in affectively appropriate ways—laughs at jokes, becomes excited at the prospect of a grandchild's visit, or cries when saying good-bye to a loved friend. In contrast, the depressed patient's mood is autonomous, monotonous, pessimistic, and generally unresponsive to environmental stimuli.

In addition, while grieving patients may experience and express great sadness and despair, feelings of guilt, self-reproach, and low self-esteem may appear transiently but are generally not prominent. When such feelings are present and persistent, the physician should explore whether they are acute (*i.e.*, representing a depression) or chronic (*i.e.*, representing a preexisting personality disturbance or chronic depressive disorder).

Suicide

Fifteen percent of newly diagnosed cancer patients have suicidal thoughts at the time of diagnosis.[27,56] Consideration of suicide may provide the patient with a sense of not being helpless in the face of a rapidly advancing cancer. However, terminally ill patients rarely kill themselves. Many people who are not near death think that they would kill themselves if they had end-stage cancer, but the vast majority of dying patients choose to keep on living as long as reasonably possible, even when life is accompanied by significant physical or emotional distress and when methods of committing suicide are readily available. Suicide in terminally ill patients is most commonly related to loss of support from significant others, reflecting how the psychological equilibrium of the terminally ill patient depends heavily on the emotional connection with loved ones.[51]

A patient's mention of suicide can initiate a valuable discussion of sadness, frustration, fears about inappropriate life-sustaining measures, and so on. Such a discussion may reduce the patient's suicidality. Depressed patients, in particular, should be carefully questioned about suicidal thoughts and plans. Any patient who expresses more than passing suicidal preoccupations should be referred for immediate mental-health consultation.

THE FAMILY'S ADAPTATION

The family's response to terminal illness is important in itself as an indicator of personal distress and as a predictor of the response to bereavement, and is also a mediator of the patient's adaptation.

Tasks Confronting the Family of a Terminally Ill Patient

The family faces a number of psychological tasks in dealing with the impending death of a loved one.

Renegotiating Roles

As discussed in Chapter 4, illness often necessitates dramatic role shifts in a family. As dying patients become sicker, they surrender their usual roles within the family. In addition, the patient's care needs create new roles, which family members must fill. Rearrangements of usual patterns (*e.g.*, who does the shopping or cares for the children) occur, for better or for worse. Whereas some patients may struggle to retain old roles, others surrender them readily. Family members vary in their abilities to fill these newly created roles. Some roles are never filled, and the family lives with important lacunae. For example, when the patient has been the family mediator or emotional weathervane but can no longer perform these functions, family members may be left feeling disconnected from each other, unable to acknowledge their feelings, and angry at the patient for abandoning them. Other roles may be filled only too readily, leaving the patient feeling extraneous and irrelevant, as when an eager daughter takes over financial decisions before the patient feels ready to relinquish this role. New responsibilities may also be frightening. Taking care of the patient involves the possibility of making mistakes, saying the "wrong thing," seeing terrible sights, and becoming overwhelmed with emotion. Preparing family members for what is likely to happen, demonstrating methods of care the family will use, and exploring fears often makes these seemingly overwhelming responsibilities feel more manageable. Identification of the role changes occurring in a family can provide information about stresses and strains, and can lead to interventions such as renegotiating problematic roles or providing extra support.

Maintaining Stability

The disruption of life caused by a terminal illness challenges the family unit to maintain a sense of stability and order. A sense of predictability and structure is particularly important to small children. Anxieties that "nothing will ever be the same" can be countered by maintaining familiar rituals and patterns, which affirm a sense of continuity (*e.g.*, sitting down to dinner in the patient's bedroom or having a birthday celebration in the hospital). The clinician should be alert for families in which the framework of daily life is shattered by terminal illness, since the inability to maintain some stable patterns may be a sign that the family is being stressed beyond its limits.

Restitution and Mending

In caring for a terminally ill relative, the family has a wonderful opportunity for restitution of past failures and mending of old conflicts and differences. By mastering the tasks and anxieties associated with taking care of a terminally ill patient, the family can develop a sense of pride, of healing, of "paying-back," and of "coming-of-age." Knowing that one did a good job and eased the death of a family member can be a source of strength in coping with the long-term grieving process, assuaging old guilt, and allowing the resolution of some ambivalence in the relationship. Family members who have the opportunity to care for a dying relative in a hospice-style program have been found to have less anger, guilt, and health problems in the bereavement period than relatives of patients who experienced conventional care during the terminal illness.[6]

Anticipatory Grieving

Anticipatory grieving is the process by which family members prepare for the patient's death. The long process of letting go while also incorporating and retaining parts of the relationship begins when a potentially terminal illness is first diagnosed, when life without the loved one is first imagined. Early grief, however, tends to be conditional ("What if . . .?") and is held in abeyance while the patient is doing well;

it intrudes itself as a palpable and unavoidable issue when the patient begins to fail. Even then, anticipatory grief poses a paradoxical experience for many family members. On the one hand, taking care of a sick, vulnerable, and often helpless terminally ill patient evokes and strengthens intense "attachment" feelings and behavior, similar to those that develop in parents taking care of a newborn infant.[4,5] On the other hand, anticipatory grieving produces a loosening of and withdrawal from the connection with the dying person, a sense of renunciation and of being able to go on alone.

Neither patients nor family members traverse a clear sequence of emotional stages in anticipation of death. Rather, many feelings and levels of awareness are present simultaneously, and are constantly reappearing in varying intensity and sequences. Early on, shock and disbelief generally predominate—the impending loss is denied as the family "buys time" to begin to come to terms with the gravity of the patient's illness. Later, a period of numbness and restlessness may occur. Family members may also become very active, "doing what needs to be done," a phenomenon called "exaggerated coping"—a preoccupation with the details of care, financial arrangements, and so on both acknowledges the new situation and serves as a defense against sadness and helplessness. Various forms of identification with the patient may be noted—for example, family members may develop new physical symptoms or assume ways of coping similar to those of the patient. Separation anxiety may also develop, including an extreme fear of leaving the patient's side even briefly, as if leaving itself could cause death or being present could prevent it. Reminiscing, either solitary or shared, may be intensified—old pictures and letters may be reexamined, or old friends invited for a visit to mull over the past.

As the terminal illness progresses, family members may more fully acknowledge or experience the feelings associated with loss. A sense of sadness and heaviness develops. Anger about the loss may be expressed as irritation over the failure of treatments, the uncaring health professionals, the failure of research to cure cancer, or the costs of the illness. Promises for cure may be desperately sought and embraced. As the patient becomes more withdrawn, sick, and emotionally unavailable, the family may become resentful about being abandoned. Family members may become preoccupied with how the end will come and what it will be like after the patient dies. They anticipate that matters will get much worse, and they may be unable to imagine getting through their grief. Family members are often exhausted, both from the care needs of the patient and from the emotional process of grieving.

The impact of successful anticipatory grieving on the eventual adjustment of family members to the loss is controversial.[15] Some investigators[17,32] have found that anticipation of the loss improves adjustment following a loss; other investigators, however, have found no relationship between anticipatory grief and postmortem adjustment.[9,28] In any case, anticipatory grief is a useful concept, which describes a significant element of the family's emotional experience during a terminal illness.

Approaching the Moment of Death

Like patients, family members often have a sense of the conditions under which they want the death to occur. They may have clear ideas of who they want to be present, of whether the patient should be conscious or unconscious, or of when they want the death to happen. These ideas may significantly influence their behavior during the patient's last days.

As the end approaches, family members may immerse themselves in clinical tasks—checking the pulse, monitoring the respirations—as a means of reducing the unimaginable (death) to a series of more comprehensible and logical steps:

> I know if she doesn't eat that she can't possibly have the strength to throw off this infection. Her pulse is weaker, and she seems to be breathing faster. I guess that means she's going. . . .

The moment of death may be rehearsed in advance, as a way of preparing for the reality of the loss.

Often, at the very end, the patient's care needs decrease, offering the family an opportunity to sit quietly, reminisce, talk, and cry. At the same time, with fewer tasks to occupy energy and attention, relatives may feel lost, and be unable to deflect their grief with concrete tasks. The full force of the loss becomes more apparent.

Sometimes, the patient is no longer conscious, yet death has not come. This state of limbo may last much longer than family members anticipate. A hope that death will come soon mingles with dread and frustration. The waiting is difficult, but seems to allow the family to feel more ready when death finally arrives.

No matter how much the family has prepared themselves, the moment of death comes as a shock. There is also often a considerable sense of relief that the patient is no longer suffering, that the uncertainty is ended, and that it is finally possible to move on to the next phase.

Bereavement

Goals of Grieving

Lindemann defined three outcomes of "successful" grieving: letting go of the deceased and accepting the reality of the loss; adapting to life without the loved one; and developing new relationships.[26] More specific tasks include being able to acknowledge realistically the pleasures and disappointments in the relationship with the deceased; discovering aspects of the self that the relationship with the deceased inhibited; incorporating into a changed identity meaningful identifications with the person who died; and reestablishing a trusting and secure relationship with the world.

To the acutely bereaved, these tasks may appear to be both insurmountable and undesirable. In the early phases, all the mourner may want is to have the loved one back.

Phenomenology of Grief

NUMBNESS.   After the patient dies, family members who have oriented much of their time, energy, and attention toward the dying person may feel empty and directionless. Although they may become caught up in notifying relatives and planning for the funeral, the intense purposefulness of the terminal phase is missing. "What will become of me?" is a central question. The bereaved are usually preoccupied with the past and the future; the present feels dead, empty, and barren:

> You know, we had such wonderful times together when the kids were little. And then when our daughter got married. . . . We were looking forward to Bob's retiring. We thought we'd buy a camper and travel across the country. . . . We had such ideas. I don't know how I'll manage. I look into my future and I see emptiness. There's nothing there. I don't even feel alive anymore.

Generally, this phase, which researchers call "numbness," lasts from a few days to a few weeks, although there is great individual variability in the duration and quality of this phase, and similar feelings resurface periodically.[8,31] The bereaved oscillate between acknowledgment and denial of death:

I know he's gone. I tell myself that a thousand times a day. But I'm surprised each time I walk into the living room and he's not sitting in his chair.

YEARNING AND PROTEST. As the survivor begins to feel the loss, the wish to reunite with the loved one becomes intense and may be manifested in searching behavior: returning to places that had been shared with the deceased, a predisposition to interpret ambiguous or neutral stimuli as reminders of the lost person (thinking one recognizes the loved one in a crowd or sees his or her car in traffic), preoccupation with thoughts of the loved one, and crying for the loved one. Agitation, restlessness and irritability, and self-reproach are responses commonly seen in the "protest" phase, probably reflecting inner feelings of anger at being abandoned, and guilt about some aspects of the relationship with the lost loved one.

SADNESS AND DEPRESSION. Ambivalent feelings toward the deceased are nearly universal, and strongly negative feelings are not uncommon. Depression in response to a loss is thought to develop particularly when the relationship of the bereaved with the deceased has been characterized by predominantly negative or ambivalent feelings. The mourner's negative feelings are thought to make him or her feel unworthy, guilty, and responsible for the death, while guilt over the positive feelings about the death (*e.g.*, "Thank goodness I don't have to listen to her soaps on TV anymore," "Now maybe I'll have a chance to find someone I really love") give rise to self-condemnation for such wishes.[45] As noted before, the sadness and depression of grief are usually painful for family members to bear, but do not signify psychiatric illness.

DISORGANIZATION. A period of apathetic withdrawal and disorganization is common during the bereavement period. In one study, two thirds of all widows were still in this state 13 months after bereavement.[32] The survivor feels the full impact of the loss (in terms of disruption of old patterns of behavior), but remains strongly connected to the person who has died. This continued connection hinders the grieving person from developing a new sense of self, from forming new relationships or developing new ways of living. Loyalty to the lost loved one makes the survivor feel that he or she is betraying the old relationship by changing or forming new attachments. Survivors often feel immersed in their memories of the lost person, but are also painfully aware that they cannot be sustained by these memories alone.

RECOVERY. Many griefs never end, although the intensity of the waves of sadness attenuates, and a bittersweet, wistful quality comes to replace the agonized distress of the early phases of the mourning process. Grieving is the last phase of a relationship. In the process of letting go of the person who has died, the entire relationship is reworked, reinterpreted, and remembered. In this process, the relationship is changed. Indeed, after an important loss, the relationship with the person who has died continues to be redefined and modified intrapsychically for the rest of the survivor's life. At his or her best, the survivor is reassured by sentiments such as these:

> Though nothing will
> bring back the hour
> of splendor in the grass,
> of glory in the flower,
> We will grieve not,
> rather find
> strength in what remains behind.
>
> William Wordsworth

> What one has once loved, one can never lose.
>
> Helen Keller

The recovery from grief, of course, is slowest for those who have lost the most. It is only natural for a spouse to remain preoccupied with the loss long after more distant relatives and friends are healed. This discrepancy in rate of recovery from grief is often misunderstood by the mourner and may be a source of pain and isolation:

> *My friends have been great. They invite me to dinner, and all I can think about is my husband, but nobody mentions him. It hurts me that they seem to have forgotten him already.*

Survivors need to talk about loss in order to recover. Unfortunately, they may confront the ethos of society in which "not talking about it" is thought to make the loss recede, and in which starting a new life ("move down clean cups" [*Alice in Wonderland*]) is best accomplished by plunging ahead. Throughout the bereavement period, social supports are an important facilitator of grieving and recovery.

Although some of the roles that the lost person filled can be occupied by others, a loved person is irreplaceable. In our society, an elderly widower is more likely to find another wife than an elderly widow is to find another husband. Thus, widows and widowers must have different expectations and adaptations for the future. Although a loss may be "fully" mourned, the lack of someone to fill a valued role remains a persistent source of sadness.

Finally, even when the loss has been accepted and integrated by the survivor, remnants of protest, disavowal, and sadness often persist.

> I am not resigned to the shutting away of loving hearts in the hard ground.
> So it is, and so it will be, for so it has been, time out of mind:
> Into the darkness they go, the wise and the lovely. Crowned
> With lilies and with laurel they go; but I am not resigned.
>
> Lovers and thinkers, into the earth with you.
> Be one with the dull, the indiscriminate dust.
> A fragment of what you felt, of what you knew,
> A formula, a phrase remains,—but the best is lost.
>
> The answers quick and keen, the honest look, the laughter, the love,—
> They are gone. They are gone to feed the roses. Elegant and curled
> Is the blossom. Fragrant is the blossom. I know. But I do not approve.
> More precious was the light on your eyes than all the roses in the world.
>
> Down, down, down into the darkness of the grave
> Gently they go, the beautiful, the tender, the kind;
> Quietly they go, the intelligent, the witty, the brave.
> I know. But I do not approve. And I am not resigned.
>
> Edna St. Vincent Millay

Dysfunctional Adaptation in the Family

Successful intervention in dysfunctional family reactions is based on recognizing maladaptive responses to the stress of terminal illness and on differentiating acute decompensations (which tend to be amenable to treatment) from chronic coping styles (which are relatively resistant to treatment). The following probes will elicit material bearing on these issues:

Tell me how your family usually operates.

When times are tough, how does the family manage?

How has the current situation [terminal illness] affected the family?

Both the clinician's threshold for concern and the treatment goals will be different in a chronically chaotic family than they will be in a well-functioning family that becomes acutely disorganized during an illness.

Dysfunctional Adaptation Prior to the Death

DYSFUNCTIONAL ANTICIPATORY GRIEF. Two dysfunctional grieving patterns commonly occur in families of terminally ill patients: absence or denial of grief, and premature grief.

Family members who do not undergo some anticipatory grieving will meet the death of a loved one without emotional forewarning or preparation. In most cases, denial of grief is a reflection of a conflict—between being in control of feelings and feeling overwhelmed by them; between being strong and being weak; between anger and love. Denial of strong feelings may also be a lifelong pattern. Identification of the specific nature of the conflict and acknowledgment of both sides of the feelings is often helpful in facilitating the grieving process. Rather than trying to change the individual's habitual way of coping (*e.g.*, through being the strong one), the clinician can sometimes help the individual redefine what it means to be strong (*e.g.*, from "not showing sadness" to "helping my husband by talking"):

> *It seems like it is very important to you, and to your husband, for you to be the one everybody depends on, the strong one. I imagine that could make it hard for you to let anyone know how downhearted you are about how much sicker he is. I think it might help your husband to deal with what is happening if you could try to talk to him about how sad you are. I think it would help him to know that you can face it and cope with it.*

Sometimes, anticipatory grieving can occur too soon and too well.[26] Achieving congruence between the erratic course of illness and the delicate process of grieving can be an extremely difficult task. Family members who complete much of their grieving before the patient dies may withdraw from the patient. They may even become angry at the patient for "hanging on" too long or feel tricked by the doctors. An unexpected recovery may confront the relative with the need to reestablish ties with someone to whom goodbyes have already been said. Continued withdrawal may be less painful than reattachment and the prospect of another separation. For the patient, however, emotional abandonment causes pain, panic, depression, and, perhaps, even the wish to die.

MAJOR DEPRESSION. Family members, as well as patients, are vulnerable to major depression during terminal illness. The sadness of grief can be differentiated from major depression using the general rules described in previous sections. The stress of a terminal illness and the awareness of impending loss may precipitate full-blown major depressive reactions in individuals with predispositions to depression. More commonly, however, family members are able to cope with the feelings associated with grieving by relying on other family members and friends for support, and do not require specific psychiatric interventions.

WITHDRAWAL AND AVOIDANCE. Family members may avoid involvement with the dying person because of internal conflicts (*e.g.*, guilt toward the patient, fear of being close to illness and death), previous disagreements with the patient, or difficulties in relationships with other family members. In assessing a family's coping, the professional should inquire about who is *not* present, and why. Often, family members can be encouraged to actively involve the absent relative; a telephone call from the physician to update the missing family member about the patient's condition and include him or her in any decisions may also be helpful. Family members who have avoided dealing with the dying person may be particularly vulnerable to developing intense guilt and unresolved grief reactions later on.

EXCESS INVOLVEMENT.   In some families, one person may "give up everything" to be with and take care of the person who is dying. Strong guilt feelings may lead a family member to assume a self-abnegating role. Long-standing rivalries, resentment, tenuous self-esteem, or the need to prove something may lead to a competition among family members about who will be the one most devoted to the dying person. While terminal illness is frequently a time for family members to make extraordinary changes in their lives and to reorient priorities, excess involvement can be a sign of dysfunctional coping. When death occurs, the overly involved individual must deal with the loss of structure and meaning that kept him or her going during the illness, as well as with the loss of the loved one.

DEVELOPMENT OF PHYSICAL SYMPTOMS.   Physical symptoms which develop in response to the stress of terminal illness may be viewed variously as manifestations of the inevitable fatigue that arises in caring for a terminally ill relative, as a form of identification with the dying patient, as part of a competition about "who is the sickest," as a component of a major depression, or as part of a preexisting somatization pattern. Symptoms may be used as a communication to significant others (physician, family, friends) that the burden of care is becoming overwhelming. When the clinician becomes aware that an increase in help-seeking behavior—visits to the emergency ward or private physician's office—is occurring, a reevaluation of the family member's role and feelings about caretaking is useful. The clinician may want to encourage the family member to enlist extra help, to reduce his or her level of involvement, or to seek personal support from friends or professionals. In other cases, the clinician can help the family member's physician understand the multiple determinants of the family member's symptoms and requests for help.

INCREASED ALCOHOL OR DRUG CONSUMPTION.   Increased consumption of alcohol, tobacco, and drugs (especially sedatives, tranquilizers, and hypnotics) are common sequelae of bereavement[33] and are often a dysfunctional response to the stress of terminal illness. Family members who have had long-term substance-abuse problems are at extra risk of recurrent problems during the illness or bereavement period. The clinician should approach such issues by asking nonjudgmental questions and by exploring the feelings leading to the behavior. The physician's explicit concern about substance use may sometimes help a family member to "put the brakes on" this behavior. Referral to a treatment program such as Alcoholics Anonymous may be appropriate.

DETERIORATION IN RELATIONSHIPS.   Family members benefit from each others' support when someone they love is dying. One of the poignant features of terminal illness is that families with distant, tense, and difficult relationships often develop greater degrees of closeness and mutual support. Conversely, the multiple stresses of terminal illness may also lead to marked deterioration in family relationships, especially when the family is overwhelmed by the burden of physical care, or by their own psychological responses to the patient's illness and impending death. Conflicts among family members about the patient's medical or emotional management often precipitate familial disputes (as when one family member wants the patient to be told "the truth" about his condition, and another believes that facts should be withheld or distorted). When family conflicts are creating distress, the physician should consider convening the family in order to discuss the underlying issues and to minimize their interference in the care of the patient. Although most family conflicts have a long history, there are sometimes discrete issues that can be resolved, and sustained improvement in family relations can occur.

PRECIPITOUS DECISIONS. Precipitous decisions may be understood as a means of avoiding or denying painful feelings and conflicts or of combating impotence and frustration about being "stuck in limbo" while the patient is dying. New relationships may be sought as replacements for threatened ones or as solace in the face of profound grief. New business or professional ventures may deflect attention away from the terminally ill patient and provide a sense of competence and mastery in the face of helplessness and hopelessness about the loss.

Dysfunctional Grieving Syndromes

Dysfunctional (or unresolved or pathologic) grief occurs when some aspects of the grieving process are inhibited, suppressed, or absent, when symptoms or behaviors are exaggerated or distorted, or when "normal" grieving is prolonged. Dysfunctional grief reactions occur frequently, and are associated with significant psychological and physical morbidity. They are often overlooked or misdiagnosed.

The response to grief is mediated by many factors, including the following:

The length of time since the death
The suddenness/expectedness of the death
The age of the mourner
The relationship to the person who died
The number and quality of other relationships and supports
Past history of losses
The extent of dependency
The number and extent of concurrent stresses
Social negation of the loss
A socially unspeakable loss
Social isolation
Assuming the role of the "strong one"
Uncertainty about the loss (*e.g.,* when the lost one is missing-in-action)
Guilt and ambivalence
Loss representing a severe injury to the survivor's sense of self (*e.g.,* a woman whose only identity is as a mother of a child who has died)
Reawakening of old losses by a current loss
Ego development inadequate to permit mourning
Idiosyncratic resistances to mourning

The diagnosis of a dysfunctional grief reaction often rests on nuances, on accumulations of small bits of evidence, and on the patient's emotional responses to probes about the loss. Table 6-1 lists the signs that may be indicative of unresolved grief. While some of these signs may be present transiently in the early phases of bereavement, a large number of them persisting over time suggests that an unresolved grief reaction may be present.

A physician or other health-care provider who maintains periodic ongoing contact with the close relatives of a patient who has died will usually be in an excellent posi-

TABLE 6-1
Signs of Unresolved Grief*

The absence of sadness (failure to grieve)
Delayed or prolonged grieving
Avoidance of grief (by avoiding the funeral, grave, etc.)
Feelings of extreme guilt and self-reproach
A major depression beginning around the time of the death
Loss of decisiveness and initiative
Self-destructive behaviors
Somatic identifications with the dead person
Vague physical distress (*e.g.*, feeling "choked up") and other forms of somatization
Prolonged searching and overactivity
Recurrence of depressive symptoms at anniversaries of the death
Intense hostility, commonly directed against health professionals
A sense that the death "occurred yesterday" even after considerable time has passed
Unwillingness to move the possessions of the deceased
Deterioration in other relationships after the death
Decreased participation in religious rituals
Inability to discuss the dead person without intense emotion
Recurrent expressions of loss

* After Lazare[23]

tion to identify and respond to problems in the bereavement period. Several reports support the effectiveness of interventions to help family members who are undergoing difficult bereavement reactions.[28,49] Many family members benefit from the opportunity to speak openly with a friend or hospice volunteer. During bereavement, non-professional interventions, such as support groups and widow-to-widow programs have also been shown to be helpful. Relatives who are exhibiting significant problems in coping, especially depression and severe anxiety, should be evaluated by a mental-health professional.

TREATMENT

This section elaborates on strategies for treating specific psychological disturbances—depression, anxiety, insomnia, sexual dysfunction, and dysfunctional grief reactions—among terminally ill patients and their families. It is hoped that the approaches presented here will stimulate the clinician's interest, curiosity, and confidence about managing such psychological problems and will be helpful in understanding the approaches of consultants to whom patients with mental-health disturbances are referred.

General Issues in Psychotherapy with the Terminally Ill

Psychotherapy

While psychotherapy cannot remove the distress of the dying patient, it can provide a relationship in which this distress can be shared and understood. Such an opportunity may be particularly important for patients whose social context does not support the process of expressing and coming to terms with distressing feelings: an old person living alone, a middle-aged mother whose husband and adolescent children do not want to talk about their grief, a husband who has always been the "strong one" in his relationship with his wife and who feels that his masculinity and role in the family are threatened by admitting his grief to them. Here, psychotherapy provides a context for the patient to tell a story to an appreciative listener. The therapist offers insights into current dilemmas. The act of telling, itself, may counter the passivity of sickness, turn helplessness into helpfulness, and allow the patient to achieve some perspective on the meaning of his or her life.

Therapy will also be desirable for patients who seek to resolve specific psychological issues related to their illness or their personal histories, especially those issues that are heightened by an awareness of impending death (*e.g.*, a 20 year old who became ill in the midst of a tumultuous, angry separation from family and who feels tremendous guilt about having given her parents a hard time, or a woman who had deferred her own gratification until "after the kids are gone" and who confronts a terminal illness just at the time she thought she might be free to develop in new ways).

The focus of therapy may be on concrete and practical issues such as how to talk with a retarded child about death or fears about some aspect of death. Old losses become important topics: as death approaches, persistent conflicted feelings toward dead parents may press insistently for understanding and resolution, even decades after the parent's death has occurred. For still others, the dependency and vulnerability experienced by the terminally ill may evoke and intensify concerns about developmental issues that may not have been troubling when the patient was well:

Identity (Am I still a worthwhile person if I can't work?)

Intimacy (How can I let him get close to me when my body is so disgusting?)

Autonomy (What is the point of living if I can't do anything for myself?)

Psychotherapy with dying patients tends to be somewhat different than therapy with other physically and emotionally ill patients. Therapists who work with terminally ill patients report less reliance on neutrality in their therapeutic interactions and tend to focus more on the "real relationship" with the patient. Time is short, and the patient often has a sense of urgency, a wish to complete a piece of personal work before death comes. A working alliance is often more readily established than in traditional psychotherapy, especially when the patient is aware of pressing concerns that need to be addressed. Psychotherapy sessions must be tailored to the needs, energy level, mobility, and attention span of the patient, as well as to the tempo of the illness. Many of the usual logistical procedures of traditional psychodynamic psychotherapy—rigid scheduling, formal office visits, 50-minute sessions—can be set aside. Home visits are often appropriate and are frequently useful for meeting or including family members.

Countertransference

Dying patients commonly evoke strong feelings in the people taking care of them. For instance, a depressed patient tends to evoke hopelessness, indecisiveness, and discouragement in the physician, whereas a "pseudohopeful" or strongly denying patient who pretends that everything is getting better may elicit false optimism and overly aggressive treatment. Some of these reactions are shared by most clinicians, while others are idiosyncratic and reflect the clinician's personal feelings, needs and values about death and terminal care. The phenomenon of clinicians responding emotionally, and often unconsciously, to patients is referred to as "countertransference" in the psychiatric literature. An awareness of countertransference feelings can be a valuable source of information about the state of the doctor–patient relationship, the patient's current emotional state, and the physician's vulnerabilities in caring for the patient.

Countertransference can be a hazard if it is not recognized. A clinician's affection for a favorite patient may make it impossible for him or her to recognize that death is imminent, and may result in inappropriately aggressive medical treatment. A physician who is particularly frightened by death may find himself or herself avoiding visiting a patient who is approaching death. These examples highlight the clinician's responsibility to attend to his or her emotional reactions, to recognize habitual responses to certain situations (e.g., wanting to avoid contact with "hopelessly" ill patients), and to differentiate the patient's emotional responses from his or her own. Introspection and self-analysis should be an ongoing feature of the physician's care of the terminally ill patient.

Management of Specific Syndromes

Depression

The criteria for diagnosis of depression have been extensively discussed in earlier parts of this chapter. Several general points about the treatment of patients with depression deserve emphasis here.

Most patients with reactive depressions respond beautifully to everyday talking with the people who are close to them. For patients with more severe reactive depressions, or for patients who do not have someone with whom they feel comfortable talking about their feelings, counseling or psychotherapy is the treatment of choice. Most patients show a significant improvement in their symptoms of depression soon after beginning therapy. Although waxing and waning of distress will continue while the patient is in therapy, patients usually improve progressively. The diagnosis of major depression should be considered if the patient fails to show some remission in symptoms of depression during several weeks of therapy.

Patients with lifelong depressive personalities (or dysthymic disorders) generally do not experience significant improvements over the short run in psychotherapy. However, some of these patients may find supportive psychotherapy helpful in allowing them to stabilize their levels of functioning.

Both psychotherapy and antidepressants are effective in treating major depression; these two modalities are synergistic with each other for the treatment of major depression.[55]

No studies demonstrate the superiority of any particular antidepressants in this setting. In general, tricyclics are the agents of choice. If a patient has had a good response to a particular drug in the past, this drug should be tried first. Otherwise, begin with a secondary amine (e.g., nortryptiline, desipramine) or one of the "new" agents (e.g., trazodone, maprotiline), which are less likely than the "tertiary" amines (amitryptiline, imipramine) to cause troublesome anticholinergic side-effects and are less sedating to patients who may already be fatigued because of serious illness.[48]

An awareness of the common side-effects of the various tricyclics is helpful in choosing an agent and in switching from a poorly tolerated drug to one less likely to cause toxicity. Some side-effects may actually be desirable for a particular patient (e.g., an agitated, anxious person who lies awake at night might benefit from sedation, and thus amitryptiline or doxepin would be chosen). Orthostatic hypotension is a common side-effect of tricyclics in elderly and bedridden patients, and patients should be advised to rise slowly and to sit down immediately if dizziness develops. Nortryptiline and desipramine are less likely to cause orthostasis than are other agents.[40] The most frequent, troublesome side-effects of antidepressants are related to anticholinergic activity: dry mouth, dizziness, impaired visual accommodation, decreased gut motility, urinary retention, sexual dysfunction, delirium, decreased sweating, and thermal disregulation. Trazodone and desipramine have the least anticholinergic activity.[48] All the antidepressants have cardiac side-effects, and patients who are known to have cardiac disease (especially high-grade ventricular ectopy and supraventricular arrhythmias) should be carefully followed for evidence of increased ectopy and heart failure. There is no clear agent of choice for a patient with cardiac disease; one with less anticholinergic activity (*e.g.*, desipramine) is probably a good choice.

Patients generally develop some tolerance to the side-effects of antidepressant therapy. Warning the patient that these symptoms may occur, but that they usually improve with time, often encourages a patient to pursue a medication trial despite "nuisance" side-effects.

To initiate treatment, begin with a low dosage (Table 6-2). Elderly patients usually require reduced dosage. There is some evidence that cancer patients may respond to lower doses of antidepressants.[29]

If the patient's symptoms resolve satisfactorily, maintain the patient at the same dosage for several months, and then taper slowly, following symptoms. If no improvement or partial improvement occurs, increase the dosage every 2 to 4 days by the incremental dose (see Table 6-2) until the patient (1) has unpleasant or intolerable side-effects necessitating discontinuation of treatment and selection of a different drug with dissimilar toxicity; (2) achieves a full therapeutic effect; or (3) reaches a "standard" full dose. Achieving a full therapeutic response may require several weeks of treatment at a full dose. If the patient reaches a full dose without therapeutic effect, continue the medication at this level for 4 to 5 weeks and check the blood level. If the blood level is low, increase the dose until the blood level is in a therapeutic range. If no response occurs after several weeks at a therapeutic blood level, switch to a different tricyclic.

TABLE 6-2
Antidepressant Drugs

Agent	*Anticholinergic Effect**	*Sedative Effect**	*Initial Dose (and Incremental Dose)*	*Usual Full Dose (Range)*
Amitryptiline	5+	5+	25 mg	75–150 mg
Imipramine	4+	3+	25 mg	150–300 mg
Doxepin	4+	5+	25 mg	75–150 mg
Desipramine	1+	3+	25 mg	100–200 mg
Nortryptiline	2+	3+	25 mg	100–150 mg
Trazodone	1+	2+	50 mg	50–300 mg
Maprotiline	3+	3+	25 mg	50–100 mg

*1+ = minimal; 5+ = marked

Generally, the first symptom that will improve with tricyclics is insomnia (if present). Decreased level of energy, psychomotor retardation, and appetite tend to improve next, whereas dysphoria and the other psychological expressions of depression are usually the last symptoms to improve, sometimes responding only after a full 4 weeks at a therapeutic dose. Drug levels may be helpful in guiding the physician to choose an appropriate dose, especially when a patient has not achieved good results on a reasonable dosage or has experienced toxic side-effects at low dosage.

ADDITIONAL MEASURES.   If a patient clearly meets the criteria for major depressive disorder, and has not responded to a full trial of two or three tricyclics, a trial with monoamine oxidase (MAO) inhibitors may be appropriate. The use of these agents generally requires psychiatric consultation or referral.

Methylphenidate 10 mg bid has been shown to be effective in the treatment of medically ill patients with depression[22] and may be a reasonable drug for use in this setting if immediate onset of antidepressant effect is needed. Similarly, a response to dextroamphetamine 15 to 20 mg qd for 1 to 3 days may predict future responsiveness to tricyclics. These drugs can produce insomnia, and rebound depression may occur when the dosage is reduced.

Finally, electroconvulsive therapy is a safe, effective, and fast treatment for depression and should be considered for seriously ill patients with life-threatening depression.[48]

TREATMENT OF THE SUICIDAL PATIENT.   A mental-health referral is indicated when the wish to die seems out of proportion to the objective realities of the situation or whenever a patient expresses active suicidal wishes, especially when the patient is severely depressed. A distinction can usually be made between those patients who are resigned to imminent death and have rejected life-prolonging procedures and those patients who wish to die when meaningful life remains possible. Although a terminally ill patient may present suicide as a "rational" choice, the clinician should not accept this reasoning at face value, and should firmly insist that the patient explore with a mental-health expert the meaning and implications of an irrevocable decision to end life. A patient who is determined to commit suicide will not be deterred by psychiatric referral, but some patients may be able to identify correctable problems during a consultation. For example, pain, major depression, alcoholism, and withdrawal of social supports are "risk factors" for suicide, but are all potentially treatable. Psychiatric hospitalization with suicide precautions may be indicated for the management of an acutely suicidal patient.

Anxiety

Anxiety is a nearly universal accompaniment to terminal illness. The patient may complain of anxiety or nervousness or difficulty sleeping. Some patients who say they are anxious are, in fact, depressed, whereas some who say they are depressed are actually anxious. Patients also frequently experience anxiety in somatic terms— "I have a stomach ache" or "I'm feeling sick all over," reflecting the manifold physical effects of the experience of anxiety. Pain (or the anticipation of pain) is also frequently associated with anxiety. The presence of somatic symptoms that are disproportionate to objectively documented disease is an important sign of dysfunctional anxiety. Regardless of subjective complaints, the physician may observe signs of tension, restlessness, agitation, uneasiness, or apprehension.

Anxiety may be a symptom of a variety of physical and psychological syndromes. Common physical precipitants of anxiety or of the somatic symptoms associated with anxiety in terminally ill patients include the following:

Drugs (including steroids, antipsychotics, anticholinergics, digitalis excess, stimulants, opiates, bronchodilators, antihypertensives)

Withdrawal syndromes (*e.g.*, alcohol, barbiturates, opiates)

Dietary substances (caffeine)

Systemic illnesses (*e.g.*, anemia, hyperthyroidism, hypoglycemia)

Cardiovascular disease (*e.g.*, angina, arrhythmias, congestive heart failure)

Respiratory disorders (*e.g.*, symptomatic lung cancers, asthma, chronic obstructive pulmonary disease, pneumonia, pulmonary embolus, and other causes of respiratory insufficiency)

Neurologic conditions (*e.g.*, intracranial mass lesion, temporal lobe epilepsy, encephalopathy)

Since advanced cancer can cause multitudinous physical sensations that can be interpreted as anxiety, it is often difficult to differentiate anxiety from symptoms of the underlying disease.

Chronic anxiety or recurrent episodes of anxiety, including phobias, panic attacks, or generalized unfocused anxiety may be a sign of a primary psychiatric disorder. Patients with such anxiety syndromes often have a family history of similar disorders. Vague, diffuse, and acute anxiety may also be a sign of impending psychotic decompensation, manic depressive illness, or organic confusional states and may be associated with bizarre and disorganized thinking, hallucinations, and unusual behavior.

TREATMENT.   The normal, appropriate anxiety caused by serious illness is often readily treated by simple interpersonal interventions, such as exploring and clarifying sources of anxiety, explaining, and reassuring. Involving the patient in constructive thinking about the symptom and its etiology may enhance the patient's sense of personal efficacy and may itself reduce anxiety. Although patients sometimes experience a sense of urgency about their symptoms—"I can't stand it, Doc. Do something. I feel like I'm going to crack up"—anxiety is almost never a medical or psychiatric emergency. By approaching the problem calmly and comfortably, the clinician conveys to the patient the idea that the symptom is manageable, bearable, and understandable. Psychopharmacologic treatment may be useful for patients with primary psychiatric disorders and for patients with severe anxiety unresponsive to discussion and reassurance.

The physician caring for terminally ill patients is often faced with patients who are anxious because of their illness or problems related to it. Short-term treatment with medication should be considered for acute anxiety related to painful or uncomfortable diagnostic and therapeutic procedures or to help the patient function more effectively when incapacitated by overwhelming anxiety. Medications such as benzodiazepines can be used to treat the symptoms of anxiety, but do not treat the underlying condition or cause of the anxiety. Whereas medications have a definite place in the management of acute, short-term anxiety, their role in the long-term treatment of anxiety symptoms is controversial.[42] Symptoms often recur after the drugs are stopped. In prescribing these medications for short-term anxiety, rational therapy is facilitated by clearly identifying target symptoms and then by judging treatment effectiveness in terms of the response of the target symptoms to the medication. Medications should be prescribed with the expectation that they may relieve some, but usually not all, anxiety symptoms. Medication should be discontinued if therapeutic results are not achieved within two weeks.

Benzodiazepines are usually the agents of choice. In general, all the medications in this class are of similar efficacy and have similar drawbacks. However, elderly patients and patients with advanced cancer are probably best treated with drugs such as lorazepam (Ativan) and oxazepam (Serax), which have shorter half-lives and fewer active metabolites. These agents are less likely to cause excess plasma accumulation.[47] Drugs with longer half-lives, such as diazepam (Valium), tend to produce too many unwanted side-effects in debilitated patients. Alprazolam (Xanax) may be favored for the unique antidepressant and antipanic actions accompanying its anxiolytic effects.

Side-effects of benzodiazepines include the following:

Increased depression (especially when combined with alcohol or other central nervous system depressants, including narcotics)
Drowsiness and excess sedation
Impaired memory acquisition
Confusion (especially in elderly patients or patients whose mental functioning is marginal)
Paradoxical agitation and hostility (especially in patients who tend to be impulsive or who are confused)

Side-effects may persist for weeks after the drug has been stopped, especially if a long-acting agent is used. Terminally ill patients are particularly vulnerable to side-effects when they have hepatic dysfunction, reactive depression, or impaired cognitive function, or when they are taking other psychoactive medications, including narcotics.

Drug dependence is a rare problem among terminally ill patients, but benzodiazepines should be used cautiously in patients who have a history of alcoholism or drug abuse. Because withdrawal syndromes occasionally occur if these agents are stopped suddenly, dosage should be tapered slowly when the medication is to be stopped, even when low doses have been given for a short interval. Rebound sleep disturbances also occur after benzodiazepines have been discontinued.

Benzodiazepines should be given at low dosage (*e.g.*, oxazepam 7.5–15 mg po tid, lorazepam 0.25–0.5 mg po bid). Dosages can be increased if no therapeutic effect is obtained at this level.

Major tranquilizers are often the drugs of choice for treatment of anxiety in elderly patients, since they are less likely than the benzodiazepines to cause confusion and agitation. In low doses, major tranquilizers are extremely useful in treating anxiety, agitation, and restlessness in terminally ill patients. Clinical circumstances should dictate which of these agents is used.

While haloperidol (Haldol) produces the highest incidence of extrapyramidal side-effects, especially in elderly patients, it also causes the least sedation and has a powerful antiemetic effect. Additional advantages compared with those of other major tranquilizers include the lack of respiratory depression, the least tendency to produce orthostatic hypotension, and the fewest anticholinergic side-effects. A beginning dose for anxiety or restlessness is 0.5 to 1 mg po bid. Dosage may be increased until therapeutic effect has been achieved. Nonpsychotic patients rarely require more than 20 mg/day, although it is safe to increase doses to as high as 60 to 100 mg/day.
Thioridazine (Mellaril) is the least likely of the major tranquilizers to cause extrapyramidal reactions and may be favored when this side-effect is encountered with other antipsychotics. It is more sedating than haloperidol, but has no antiemetic effects. It has more pronounced effects on cardiac conduction than

the other antipsychotics, and also has prominent anticholinergic activity. A beginning dose for anxiety or restlessness is 10 to 25 mg po tid. The maximum dosage is 400 mg/day; terminally ill patients will rarely require more than 150 mg/day.

Chlorpromazine (Thorazine) is the most sedating of the neuroleptics and, for some patients, may be favored for this side-effect. It produces few extrapyramidal symptoms, is strongly anticholinergic, and has good antiemetic properties. Autonomic side-effects, especially orthostatic hypotension, are a common and occasionally serious problem. A beginning dosage for anxiety or restlessness is 10 to 25 mg po tid. Dosages above 200 mg/day are rarely needed for terminally ill patients.

Akathesia (motor restlessness), photosensitivity, decreased seizure threshold, and impaired sexual functioning may occur in patients taking major tranquilizers, and tardive dyskinesia may develop with long-term treatment.

Beta-blockers (*e.g.*, propranolol [Inderal] 10–20 mg po bid) may be effective in reducing the somatic symptoms associated with anxiety and may be useful in patients who cannot tolerate benzodiazepines or neuroleptics.

Relaxation techniques and hypnosis may be effective "single agents" or adjuncts to the treatment of anxiety. Such behavioral techniques may be used to treat anticipatory anxiety associated with medical procedures, to control accelerating nonspecific anxiety, to relieve pain and pain-associated anxiety (and hence to reduce the use of analgesic medications), to increase the patient's sense of control over emotions, and to reduce the physical symptoms (motor tension, autonomic hyperactivity) that are concomitants of anxiety.[39] These modalities can promote a sense of personal efficacy and control, which can mitigate the terminally ill patient's experience of helplessness. Relaxation techniques and hypnosis lack significant side-effects, but generally require that the patient be highly motivated, alert, and able to concentrate. The patient must be willing to engage actively in treatment and usually must practice daily in order to achieve therapeutic success. The clinician should realistically apprise the patient of the potential successes and limitations of such treatment and help to set reasonable goals.

Insomnia

Terminally ill patients commonly suffer from insomnia. Being awake alone at night may be a time of great loneliness, anxiety, and fear, and patients may come to dread sleepless nights. Simple measures, such as finding companionship or talking about fears and feelings that are preventing sleep, may alleviate insomnia and obviate the need for further treatment. A careful history and documentation of the pattern of the insomnia is useful in evaluating the problem and deciding on treatment. History-taking can be facilitated by asking the patient or attendants to keep a sleep diary in which all sleep episodes are recorded and correlated with the presence of relevant physical and emotional symptoms and with the administration of medication.

In terminally ill patients, several causes of sleep disturbance should be considered:

1. Physical distress—Fifty-six percent of patients with cancer pain have disturbed sleep cycles.[14] Adequate analgesia throughout the night is the first step in managing insomnia related to pain. Other symptoms (*e.g.*, nausea, shortness of breath) may also interfere with sleep. Interventions aimed at palliating these symptoms will often improve the sleep disturbance.

2. Depression—Depressed patients may fall asleep with little difficulty, but they usually awake repeatedly through the night or wake up early in the morning and then have difficulty getting back to sleep. They typically describe morning tiredness, which wears off as the day progresses. Other neurovegetative symptoms may also be present. Tricyclic antidepressants are the treatment of choice when insomnia is part of a depressive syndrome. A more sedating agent (*e.g.*, doxepin) may be particularly useful.

3. Anxiety—Anxious patients often have difficulty falling asleep, although they may get a good night's rest once they finally fall asleep. Anxiety is often worst when the patient tries to go to sleep at night, and worrying about insomnia creates even more tension. Benzodiazepines or neuroleptics may be useful here. Behavioral techniques can often help improve the sleep pattern.

4. Fear of dying—Patients sometimes are afraid of "going to sleep and not waking up," and fight off sleep until they become exhausted. Reassurance from the physician and companionship tend to help this type of insomnia.

5. Nightmares—Patients who are having bad nightmares may avoid sleep to prevent bad dreams. Inquiry about bad dreams, and discussion of the fears that arise in them may often be helpful. Benzodiazepines, tricyclics, or neuroleptics may be useful in reducing nightmares.

6. Excess sleep during the day—Some patients, especially the bedridden, do most of their sleeping during the day, spending nights awake. This pattern is treated by keeping the patient up more during the day and trying to reduce napping and dozing. Benzodiazepines may be used in the evening to foster nocturnal sleep.

7. Medications—Corticosteroids, stimulants (including caffeine and alcohol), chemotherapeutic agents, and other medications may cause nocturnal wakefulness.[3] Changes or reduction in dosage may be helpful.

TREATMENT. Medications may be used for short-term palliation of insomnia, but are rarely effective for long-term treatment. When benzodiazepines are used, the choice of an hypnotic agent will be influenced by the drug's absorption rate and duration of action.

Flurazepam (Dalmane) is absorbed rapidly, but its metabolites tend to accumulate in the blood after 2 to 3 nights, leading to daytime drowsiness and reduced performance.[3]

Temazepam (Restoril) is absorbed slowly and thus is of limited value in inducing sleep unless given 1 to 2 hours before bedtime. Although drug accumulation is less of a problem than with flurazepam, temazepam may be more likely to cause dependence, withdrawal seizures, and rebound insomnia.[19]

Triazolam (Halcion) is absorbed moderately rapidly and has an extremely short half-life, leading to minimal drug accumulation. Like temazepam, however, this drug is associated with an increased risk of dependence, seizures, and rebound insomnia.[19] Furthermore, daytime anxiety and early morning insomnia may also occur.[20] This agent also may have a narrower margin of safety than other drugs in its class, and may be associated with the development of psychiatric symptoms, including restlessness, paranoia, suicidality, and depersonalization.[50]

Although benzodiazepines improve sleep objectively and subjectively, 10%[21] to 50%[13] of patients report daytime drowsiness with these agents. They also cause impairment in REM sleep and may cause anterograde amnesia.[13] Patients quickly develop tolerance.

Appropriate doses of benzodiazepine hypnotics for the terminally ill are generally lower than those recommended for healthy populations: flurazepam 15 mg po hs, temazepam 15 mg po hs, triazolam 0.125 mg po hs.

The more sedating major tranquilizers (thioridazine 25–50 mg hs, chlorpromazine 25–75 mg hs) may also be useful for insomnia, especially for elderly and confused patients. Antihistamines (*e.g.*, diphenhydramine [Benadryl] 25–50 mg po hs) are also effective sedating agents, and may be quite helpful for some patients. They may occasionally produce significant anticholinergic side-effects.

Relaxation techniques, a warm bath, or a drink of warm milk at bedtime may be effective for some patients, either as primary treatments, or as adjuncts to medication for the treatment of insomnia.

Sexual Dysfunction

Sexual dysfunction is common among advanced cancer patients, but is often not identified by the physician. Both patients and physicians may be embarrassed about discussing sexual issues. Beliefs that elderly or sick patients are not interested in or concerned about sex or that sexual problems are untreatable may lead the physician to ignore or to sidestep these issues. Any physician who is not hearing regularly from patients about sexual concerns should consider the possibility that he or she is inhibiting such discussions.

Evaluation begins with a history of the patient's current sexual concerns and past sexual adjustment, including information about the time course of symptoms, precipitants of dysfunction, concurrent physical and emotional problems, and the patient's beliefs about the etiology of the problem.

In terminally ill patients, physical factors are likely to play a prominent role. Physical deformity, extreme weakness, and pain may inhibit sexual interest and functioning. The partner may worry that the patient is too frail, that exertion will enhance the spread of the cancer, or that it is dangerous to be physically close to a person with cancer. Narcotics, antidepressants, antipsychotics, benzodiazepines, beta-blockers, antihypertensives, corticosteroids, stimulants, and some chemotherapeutic agents (especially hormonal agents) may cause alterations in sexual functioning. When clinically appropriate, these agents should be stopped in order to evaluate their impact on sexuality.

Although physical factors may impair sexual functioning, many sexual problems are caused or exacerbated by difficulties in communication and by interpersonal problems. The clinician should inquire about the nonsexual relationship between the patient and the partner, paying special attention to the impact of the illness on the relationship. How have they been getting along since the illness? Are there major communication gaps? How are they coping with the situation? What are the patient's (and partner's) goals in terms of sexual functioning?

TREATMENT. Good symptom control, especially analgesia, will enhance the patient's physical comfort and energy level. Treatment of depression, when present, may enhance libido and self-esteem, making sexual activity seem more possible for and desirable to the patient.

Touching, both sexual and nonsexual, is a basic form of human contact and can be an enormous source of comfort and reassurance to the terminally ill patient. Encouraging patients, family members, and friends to include this in their repertoire of relating may help the patient feel loved and connected.

The physician can assist the patient and his or her partner in acknowledging the importance of closeness and sexuality, and facilitate a dialogue in which they express their concerns and identify their wishes for intimacy and sexual contact. Information and reassurance may reduce unnecessary anxieties about the effects of sexual activity on the patient's illness. The patient and family may need to be encouraged to make arrangements for the patient to have private time during which there will be no inter-ruptions. The physician should question the patient and partner explicitly about wor-ries about odors and cleanliness, symptoms that can often be treated (see Chap. 2, Section H). Attention to aesthetics (*e.g.*, encouraging a woman who is embarrassed about a mastectomy scar to wear a pretty scarf or nightgown) can also reduce barriers to intimacy. Massage and other forms of nongenital touching can be encouraged, either as preludes to or substitutes for other forms of sexual activity.

Organic Brain Syndromes
This topic is discussed in Chapter 2, Section K.

Grief Reactions
Specific goals of therapeutic work with the grieving may include helping the patient to discover feelings about the deceased that may have been kept out of aware-ness; dealing with feelings of guilt and self-reproach that the loss may precipitate; and developing understanding about conflicts that make the bereaved particularly vulner-able to this loss.

TREATMENT OF "NORMAL" GRIEF.   Most people with uncomplicated grief find within their social networks the support necessary for the resolution of grief. In gen-eral, grief reactions are "treated" by a person or persons who have the following basic qualities:

An appreciation of the mourner's personal history and the place of the loss in it
Comfort and warmth
Receptive listening and facilitating questioning
Tolerance of strong feelings
An awareness that coping with loss takes time

For patients with uncomplicated grief and good support systems, a number of addi-tional forms of help with the grieving process are available. Such further interventions should be strongly considered as preventive measures for patients who are felt to be at high risk of developing dysfunctional grief syndromes. The risk factors for the development of pathologic grief are listed in Table 6-3.

Mutual support groups, professionally supervised volunteer services, and profes-sional support by mental-health providers are the most common models of interven-tion for uncomplicated bereavement. The effectiveness of each of these forms of care in reducing dysfunctional adaptation in high-risk individuals has been well-docu-mented.[28,30,37,49] Parkes, an experienced researcher and clinician, feels that the provi-sion of individual support early in the bereavement period (before maladaptive pat-terns of grief are firmly entrenched) is the most beneficial bereavement intervention for high-risk individuals.[34]

Mutual support groups involve bereaved participants in helping each other to come to terms with loss. The basic group processes that help the bereaved get on with their lives include the exchange of experience and information, the sharing of prob-lems and coping mechanisms, and the opportunity for personal involvement with oth-ers. Group members act as role models for each other in the struggle to adapt to this life transition.

Trained volunteers, backed up by professional mental-health staff, provide valu-

TABLE 6-3
Risk Factors for the Development of Pathologic Grief

Young age
Lower socioeconomic status
Social isolation
Anger at the deceased*
Clinging/pining/intense yearning*
Self-reproach*
Clinical impression that the individual will cope poorly[34]
Ambivalent relationship with the deceased*
History of depressive illness
Excess dependency on the bereaved or others*
A history of unusual vulnerability to separations and losses
Alcohol and drug abuse
Concurrent severe stresses (loss of income, moving, illness, or multiple losses)[31]

*All of these phenomena may be seen to some degree in normally grieving individuals; when they appear to be unusually intense, they may be indicators of high risk in adjustment in bereavement.

able help to the bereaved. They act as receptive new members of the mourner's support network, encouraging the mourner's expression of grief and facilitating reminiscences about the deceased.

Professional counseling or psychotherapy, based on similar general principles, is also effective and may be particularly appropriate for patients with psychiatric disorders complicating bereavement or for patients with dysfunctional grief syndromes. Short-term (5–20 sessions) or long-term therapy may be offered.

SPECIFIC DYSFUNCTIONAL GRIEF SYNDROMES. An understanding of the conflicts being expressed in the distorted grief reaction allows the clinician to individualize the approach to the patient with pathologic grief.[34] Two syndromes of dysfunctional grieving have been delineated: chronic grief and delayed or inhibited grief.

CHRONIC GRIEF. In chronic grief, the normal attenuation of intensity of the grieving fails to occur, and the mourner remains "stuck" in the feelings of early grief. The mourner exhibits ongoing preoccupation with the deceased, intense idealization, anger, and protest. The continued intense grief serves to maintain the attachment to the deceased. Such individuals, instead of being helped by encouragement to express their grief, may require efforts to promote security, autonomy, and the development of new behaviors.

Early emphasis in treatment should be on the development of an attachment to the therapist. The attachment is postulated to increase the bereaved person's sense of security. The therapist's support, understanding, and interest contribute to the enhancement of the mourner's self-esteem. Feelings of loss are attended to and respected, but the therapist also encourages the mourner to move beyond them by developing new patterns of behavior that support a growing sense of autonomy and mastery. As the bereaved person's sense of competence develops, the therapist withdraws support that is no longer necessary.[38]

DELAYED OR INHIBITED GRIEF. In delayed or inhibited grief, the feelings about the loss are suppressed, inhibited, or denied. The individual fails to feel the protest, anger, yearning, and despair and does not undergo the normal reminiscing and reworking processes that occur in grief. The pain of the loss is avoided. Ambivalence is seen as the central dynamic in patients with inhibited grief, because the mourner's sense of self-worth is undermined by guilt and self-reproach about negative feelings toward the deceased. Lack of confidence in the capacity to withstand the grief leads to its repression.

For the normal process of mourning to unfold, individuals with delayed or inhibited grief need the therapist's encouragement to confront and cope with their feelings of loss. The therapist supports the mourner in talking about the loss. Helpful questions include the following:

> *Tell me about the time leading up to the death.*
>
> *What was he like?*
>
> *What was your relationship like?*
>
> *How have you been doing since the death?*
>
> *What is it like for you to go on without her?*

The mourner should be encouraged to discuss details of the death, to reminisce, and to understand the emotions attached to the memories. This process makes the loss begin to feel real. The therapist's matter-of-fact belief that the painful emotions of grief can be borne instills in the bereaved person the conviction that he or she can tolerate these feelings.

Acceptance of ambivalent feelings toward the deceased may be facilitated by the therapist's acknowledgment that both positive and negative feelings are present in any relationship. For example, the therapist might say:

> *It's clear that you loved your father and worked extremely hard to take care of him during his illness, but I wonder if there weren't times when you got irritated at him for being so demanding.*

Phrasing negative feelings (such as anger and rage) more gently (*e.g.*, as disappointment, irritation, or frustration) may make these affects more acceptable to the mourner.

Surprisingly, part of the process of facilitating grieving may involve attention to previous losses that have been inadequately mourned. Therapy may need to focus on these old losses before the current loss can be mourned.

A balance is struck in therapy between the individual's need to avoid awareness of the loss and the therapeutic goal of confronting it. The reasons for avoidance (*e.g.*, absence of supports, unresolved previous losses) must be appreciated, respected, and addressed in a manner that avoids threatening the bereaved person's capacity to maintain balance. On the other hand, denial or avoidance of the loss fails to support the individual in the process of adaptation. The therapist should pursue a course of slow, cautious, titrated elicitation of feelings, with attention to signs of emotional overload.

Termination of the relationship with the therapist is a loss for the bereaved person and usually brings up intense feelings about the original loss. Such feelings should be discussed as a means for understanding the individual's characteristic responses to loss and as further opportunity for reworking and assimilating the original loss.

Many grief reactions are extremely gratifying to treat because patients get better and because the relationship with the therapist is clearly instrumental in the success of the treatment. For the clinician, treatment of a grief reaction offers a unique opportunity to witness and be part of a painful but life-affirming healing process, which is a reminder that individuals can bear terrible sadnesses and live through them, and that life goes on.

REFERENCES

1. Appelbaum PS, Roth LA: Treatment refusal in medical hospitals. In President's Commission for the study of ethical problems in medicine and biomedical and behavioral research: Making Health Care Decisions: The Ethical and Legal Implications of Informed Consent in the Patient–Practitioner Relationship, Vol 2: Appendices—Empirical Studies of Informed Consent. Washington, DC, US Government Printing Office, 1982
2. Barsky AJ: Patients who amplify bodily sensations. Ann Intern Med 91:63–70, 1979
3. Berlin RW: Management of insomnia in hospitalized patients. Ann Intern Med 100:398–404, 1984
4. Bowlby J: Attachment and Loss, Vol 1, Attachment. New York, Basic Books, 1969
5. Bowlby J, Parkes CM: Separation and loss. In Anthony EJ, Koupernik C (eds): International Yearbook for Child Psychiatry and Allied Disciplines, Vol 1, The Child in his Family. New York, John Wiley & Sons, 1970
6. Cameron J, Brings B: Bereavement outcome following preventive intervention: A controlled study. In Ajemian I, Mount B (eds): The R.V.H. Manual on Palliative/Hospice Care, pp 387–393. New York, Arno Press, 1980
7. Cameron J, Parkes CM: Terminal care: Evaluation of effects on surviving families of care before and after bereavement. Postgrad Med J 59:73–78, 1983
8. Clayton PJ: Bereavement. In Paykel ES (ed): Handbook of Affective Disorders. London, Churchill Livingstone, 1982
9. Clayton PJ, Halikas JA, Robins M: Anticipatory grief and widowhood. Br J Psychiatry 122:47–51, 1973
10. Derogatis LR, Abeloff MD, McBeth CD: Cancer patients and their physicians in the perception of psychological symptoms. Psychosomatics 17:197–201, 1976
11. Derogatis LR, Abeloff MD, Melisaratos N: Psychological coping mechanisms and survival time in metastatic breast cancer. JAMA 242:1504–1508, 1979
12. Derogatis LR, Kourlesis SM: An approach to evaluation of sexual problems in the cancer patient. CA 31:46–50, 1981
13. Donaldson SR: The benzodiazepine hypnotics. Biol Ther Psychiatry 6(10):37–40, 1983
14. Foley KM: The management of pain of malignant origin. In Tyler HR, Dawson DM (eds): Current Neurology, Vol 2, pp 279–302. Boston, Houghton Mifflin, 1979
15. Fulton RJ, Gottesman DJ: Anticipatory grief: A psychosocial concept reconsidered. Br J Psychiatry 137:45–54, 1980
16. Glaser BG, Strauss AL. Awareness of Dying. Chicago, Aldine, 1965
17. Glick IO, Weiss RS, Parkes CM: The First Year of Bereavement. New York, Wiley Interscience, 1974
18. Janis I: Psychological Stress: Psychoanalytic and Behavioral Studies of Surgical Patients. New York, John Wiley & Sons, 1958
19. Kales A, Soldatos CR, Bixler EO, Kales JD: Rebound insomnia and rebound anxiety: A review. Pharmacology 26:121–137, 1983
20. Kales A, Soldatos CR, Bixler EO, Kales JD: Early morning insomnia and rapidly eliminated benzodiazepines. Science 220:95–97, 1983
21. Kales A, Kales JD: Sleep laboratory studies of hypnotic drugs: Efficacy and withdrawal effects. J Clin Psychopharmacol 3(2):140–150, 1983
22. Katon W, Raskind M: Treatment of depression in the medically ill elderly with methylphenidate. Am J Psychiatry 137:963–965, 1980

23. Lazare A: Unresolved grief. In Lazare A (ed): Outpatient Psychiatry, pp 498–512. Baltimore, William & Wilkins, 1979
24. Leiber L, Plumb MJ, Gerstenzang ML, Holland J: The communication of affection between cancer patients and their spouses. Psychosom Med 38(6):379–389, 1976
25. Levine PM, Silberfarb PM, Lipowski ZJ: Mental disorders in cancer patients. Cancer 42:1385–1391, 1978
26. Lindemann E: Symptomatology and management of acute grief. Am J Psychiatry 101:141–148, 1944
27. Louhivuori KA, Hakama M: Risk of suicide among cancer patients. Am J Epidemiol 109:59–65, 1979
28. Maddison D, Walker WL: Factors affecting the outcome of conjugal bereavement. Br J Psychiatry 113:1057–1067, 1967
29. Massie MJ, Holland JC: Diagnosis and treatment of depression in the cancer patient. J Clin Psychiatry 45(3):25–28, 1984
30. Parkes CM: Bereavement counselling: Does it work? Br Med J 281:3–6, 1980
31. Parkes CM: Bereavement: Studies of Grief in Adult Life. New York, International Universities Press, 1972
32. Parkes CM: The first year of bereavement. Psychiatry 33:449–467, 1970
33. Parkes CM, Brown R: Health after bereavement. A controlled study of young Boston widows and widowers. Psychosom Med 34:449–461, 1972
34. Parkes CM, Weiss RS: Recovery from Bereavement. New York, Basic Books, 1983
35. Plumb M, Holland J: Comparative studies of psychological function in patients with advanced cancer I. Self-reported depressive symptoms. Psychosom Med 39(4):264–276, 1977
36. Plumb M, Holland J: Comparative studies of psychological function in patients with advanced cancer. II. Interviewer-rated current and past psychological symptoms. Psychosom Med 43:243–253, 1981
37. Raphael B: Preventive intervention with the recently bereaved. Arch Gen Psychiatry 34:1450–1454, 1977
38. Raphael B: The Anatomy of Bereavement. New York, Basic Books, 1983
39. Raskin M, Bali LR, Peeke HV: Muscle biofeedback and transcendental meditation: A controlled evaluation of efficacy in the treatment of chronic anxiety. Arch Gen Psychiatry 37:93–97, 1980
40. Roose SP, Glassman AD, Siris SG, Walsh BT, Bruno RL, Wright LB: Comparison of imipramine and nortriptiline induced orthostatic hypotension: A meaningful difference. J Clin Psychopharmacol 1:316–321, 1981
41. Rosenbaum IR, Bullard JS, Bullard D: How you can help cancer patients with their sexual concerns. Your Patient and Cancer pp 45–54, December 1983
42. Rosenbaum JF: The drug treatment of anxiety. N Engl J Med 306:401–404, 1982
43. Schmale AH, Iker H: Hopelessness as a predictor of cervical cancer. Soc Sci Med 5:95–100, 1971
44. Seligman MEP: Helplessness. San Francisco, WH Freeman, 1975
45. Siggins LD: Mourning: A critical survey of the literature. Int J Psychoanal 47:14–25, 1966
46. Sontag S: Illness as Metaphor. New York, Random House, 1979
47. Thompson TL, Moran MG, Nies AS: Psychotropic drug use in the elderly (first of two parts). N Engl J Med 308:134–138, 1983
48. Thompson TL, Moran MG, Nies AS: Psychotropic drug use in the elderly (second of two parts). N Engl J Med 308:194–199, 1983
49. Vachon MLS, Lyall WAL, Rogers J, Freedman-Letofsky K, Freeman S: A controlled study of self-help interventions for widows. Am J Psychiatry 137:1380–1384, 1980
50. Van der Kroef C: Reactions to triazolam (letter). Lancet 2:526, 1979
51. Weisman AD: Coping with Cancer. New York, McGraw-Hill, 1979
52. Weisman AD: On Dying and Denying, pp 122–123. New York, Behavioral Publications, 1972

53. Weisman AD, Sobel HJ: Coping with cancer through self-instruction: A hypothesis. J Hum Stress 5:3–8, 1979
54. Weisman AD, Worden J: Psychosocial analysis of cancer deaths. Omega 6:61, 1975
55. Weissman MM, Prusoff BA, Dimascio A, Neu C, Guklaney M, Klerman GL: The efficacy of drugs and psychotherapy in the treatment of acute depressive episodes. Am J Psychiatry 136:555–558, 1979
56. Whitlock FA: Suicide, cancer and depression. Br J Psychiatry 132:268–274, 1978

Sharing Bad News 7

INTRODUCTION

The communication of distressing information can be difficult for both the doctor and the patient, and few aspects of patient care provoke such wide and heated discussion. Patients, family members, and a host of other commentators speak vehemently about how disturbing news should be handled. Clinicians—novice or experienced—often defend their style of giving bad news with a passion characteristic of discourse for which objective knowledge is limited but personal stakes run high.

While excellent prospective randomized controlled studies of cancer treatments have proliferated in the past few decades, the effect of various approaches to information-sharing (and of most other nontechnologic interventions) on the well-being of the patient or family has largely been a subject for speculation, based on casual observations. A lack of convincing empirical data has not deterred many authors, including the present one, from offering opinions. Excellent essays have been presented by Cassem,[8] Simpson,[57] and Reiser.[53]

This chapter seeks to provide a dispassionate review of the subject of telling disturbing truths to cancer patients. The act of truth-telling is discussed as this task presents itself in clinical work—not as a simple matter of deciding once and for all whether to be honest, but as a complex process of information-sharing, which is concurrently carried on by the physician and patient and others, reflecting multiple and often conflicting personal values, and occurring in the context of relationships that evolve over time. The first sections of the chapter introduce the topic by presenting and interpreting a few relevant studies and by posing and examining some central questions about truth-telling. Next, the psychosocial basis for understanding the communication of distressing information is reviewed. Finally, a clinical approach to breaking bad news is offered.

THE CLIMATE OF OPINION

The Endorsement of Honesty

Physicians' self-reported practices of truth-telling with cancer patients have changed dramatically over the past three decades. Despite the appearance during that period of little significant new data on the clinical value of various patterns of information disclosure, the profession underwent a profound conversion.

In studies reported from the early 1950s to the mid-1960s, roughly 90% of surveyed United States physicians indicated that they preferred *not* to inform cancer patients of the diagnosis.[14,48] Observational studies confirmed that physicians and nurses engaged in tactics of "information control" that kept the true diagnosis from the patient.[17,18,52] Leading journals provided instructions on techniques of dissimulation.[33]

Around the same time, a number of studies indicated that patients and their relatives would generally prefer to know the truth when cancer was diagnosed.[1,16,27,31,55] Aitken-Swan, for instance, reported in 1959 that only 7% of patients disapproved of being told. He noted that patients seemed to receive bad news without "untoward effects."[1] Such reports showed a discrepancy between consumer preference and physician practice and indicated that physicians had a mandate for honesty. However, strong reservations about truth-telling were often evident in these studies. Thus, Aitken-Swan noted that "emotional instability" and disturbances in "placidity" and "cooperation" could result from full disclosure, and he suggested that only "curables" be told their diagnosis.

A later series of papers, appearing first in the mid-1970s, reported that physicians almost uniformly described themselves as preferring and practicing full disclosure.[6,9,22,25,45,47,51] In one survey, published in 1979, 97% of physicians said that they routinely disclosed the diagnosis of cancer.[47] The title of a 1976 conference on terminal illness, "Death: The Conspiracy of Silence," testified to the change in opinion about open discussions of dying.[67] In 1980, an editorial headline in the *Lancet* declared, "In Cancer, Honesty Is Here To Stay."[2]

Exceptions to the Endorsement of Honesty

Despite the dramatically changing climate of opinion, a careful scrutiny of many of the cited studies suggests a significant ambivalence about frankness, evident both in what patients say they want and what physicians say they do in sharing bad news. Hinton, for instance, reported considerable variation in the acknowledgment of and desire for truth among people about to die.[28] In a recent Harris poll, a large proportion of the American public noted definite exceptions to the general rule of favoring full disclosure: 38% of the public felt that a physician could withhold information if disclosure would make the patient unwilling to undergo a treatment that the physician felt was "necessary"; 49% if the family requested that the physician not tell; 52% if the information might make the patient anxious or upset; and 68% if the information might significantly harm the patient's health and well-being.[23] The last two categories might be applied to most patients.

In the same Harris poll, the majority of physicians reported daily or more frequent "conscious and deliberate evaluation" of how much to tell a patient; only half "almost never" withheld information. Remarkably, while physicians reported a variety of reasons for not disclosing information (*e.g.*, respect for the family's wishes or perception of the patient as unable to cope or understand), a mere 25% mentioned the patient's wishes as an influence on how much was told. When bad news was not disclosed, physicians reported in only 23% of situations that they were "often" or "always" acting on the patient's explicit directions.[23]

Why Did Opinion Change?

While the trend toward greater physician honesty has been applauded widely, little evidence suggests that the change in physician behavior reflects either formal instruction in truth-telling or other training that might enhance psychological sophistication or ease in working with the dying. The apparent reversal in practices presumably mirrors broad social movements that have promoted honesty in facing death and have emphasized consumer participation and autonomy in medical decision-making. The "death and dying" movement has brought discussions of mortality into the classroom and living room and has suggested, at least in the popular press, that a good patient, after a period of dysphoria, will face up to the "reality of death," "accept" terminal illness, and maybe even feel challenged by the opportunity for dying well. In addition, medical paternalism has been widely criticized, partially owing to the influence of clinical ethicists. A variety of documents and policies have emerged—patients' bills of rights, package inserts, consent forms, committees to review research and to protect the rights of human subjects, living wills, and state legislation on the provision of information to medical consumers—that are intended to ensure full disclosure to patients, to encourage the assertion of informed personal preferences, and to protect the consumer by relying less on the good will of the physician and more on formal procedures. The dramatic modification of physicians' self-reported truth-telling practices may be remarkable testimony to the flexibility of the profession and to its readiness to take up new social values. Indeed, the adoption of frankness by the medical profession probably reflects a profound change in upper-middle-class values, and the conversion of physicians has been more rapid and complete than that of the society as a whole.

The trend toward frankness also reflects the increased interest in and knowledge about cancer, the development of a clinical subspecialty in oncology, and the remarkable advances in cancer research. Physicians rarely conceal good news, and the development of greater truthfulness parallels the development of a greater sense of hopefulness about cancer. Nevertheless, honesty seems to have won the day in all areas of medicine, even in the management of relatively untreatable conditions.

The dramatic change in physicians' truth-telling behavior over the past few decades can also be viewed in a critical light. Lacking evidence that doctors have been formally trained to communicate better or that they have become more sensitive to patients' wishes, the shift could represent a facile flip from a bland not-telling to an equally unthought-out telling. Indeed, these two stances can be viewed as similar rather than polar opposites, representing a view of truth-telling that relies on *a priori* notions, on formal rules for behavior, rather than on sensitivity to the clinical situation, responsiveness to the individual patient, and a willingness to engage in the difficult, time-consuming process of developing a mutual understanding and negotiated plan.[35–37] Simple opinions about truth-telling suggest an extreme position of paternalism: the doctor has one answer for the good of the patient and readily applies this formula in all situations. The eagerness of so many commentators to settle the issue of honesty once and for all must similarly be viewed with dismay. Preferable to formulas based on the wishes of 60% to 90% of polled subjects are approaches that recognize the individuality of patients and the complexity of sharing information about evolving topics. Also, doctors have personalities! One approach will not be right for all physicians.

FRAMING THE PROBLEM OF TRUTH-TELLING

Methodology

Observational studies or probing interviews about information exchange between doctor and patient are rare. Almost all the previously cited reports rely on survey data. But what kind of situation is the respondent imagining when confronted with survey questions? Healthy respondents can afford to endorse honesty; the truth poses no threat in their immediate lives. How would they answer if they were feeling the terror of anticipated bad news? Even with studies of patients or bereaved family members, survey questions lead to vague, ungrounded, and perhaps self-justifying answers. The usual variables of clinical practice are neglected: the setting; the nature of the disease, treatment and prognosis; the point in time when honesty is being considered; the nature of the relationship between the truth-teller and receiver; and the personal background of the individuals sharing the bad news, including, especially, their general attitude toward frankness.

Furthermore, intended or self-perceived behavior may be quite different from actual or observed behavior. An expressed desire for honesty may not predict truth-seeking behavior, and an intent to be truthful does not ensure truthful action. A reflection of the discrepancy between self-perceived and observed behavior may explain the marked difference, noted by Mount, in what physicians say they do about truth-telling and what they say others do: "I don't have problems, everyone else does."[45]

In addition, whenever communication is carefully studied, the verbal content may be different from powerful nonverbal messages. Our daily clinical awareness of the process of truth-telling may touch only the surface of a deep and complex matter. Certainly, we cannot expect a superhuman performance from physicians, demanding that they always be charismatic explainers, who convey truth in a cheerful and hopeful manner.

Many questions about the substance and effect of doctor–patient communications remain unanswered. How do patients who say they favor or disapprove of discretion behave in the clinical setting, either with nondivulging physicians or with the more frank doctor, and how does this affect information-sharing? When are patients' questions about prognosis actually requests for reassurance—"Tell me I'm doing OK"— rather than requests for fuller disclosure, and how are these inquiries perceived by the physician? Can a person who appreciates being protected from harsh facts unwittingly encourage the physician to be dishonest or unrealistically hopeful? How is the physician's wish to be honest manifested, and how does this affect the patient and the overall outcome of communication?

Why Is Truth Valued?

In appraising any approach to sharing disturbing information, personal values are invoked. Truth-telling may be viewed as a desirable end-in-itself—something so important that it would be sought regardless of the personal preferences of the phy-

sician and patient or of the observed outcome—or it may be seen as having opera-
tional benefits and hazards, as a means for other ends—moral, legal, biomedical, and
psychosocial.

Truth may be a universal value, but some persons value it more highly than do
others. Many persons and cultures hold honesty to be much less important at times
than loyalty, kindness, happiness, and so on. A patient or family member may generally prefer to be forthright, but may also want to avoid being scared or depressed,
especially in the presence of persons who depend on him or her to be strong. In the
setting of advanced cancer, the truth can be scary, and frankness may be perceived as
cruelty. Facts are often less valued than information that offers hope or reassurance.
Truthfulness may be valued because it connotes a desired atmosphere of openness and
trust, yet some forms of honesty can subvert relationships. A physician's detailed
technical exposition on the diagnosis and treatment may be viewed by the patient as
evidence of a lack of personal concern. The physician who endorses a professional
code of truthfulness and full disclosure may, by sharing doubts or alternative plans,
create distressing confusion. How much uncertainty should be forced on people for
the sake of honesty?

In one popular model of the ideal client–therapist relationship, the patient senses
"unconditional" acceptance and is helped to "be oneself."[54] Paradoxically, such
a relationship encourages the patient to acknowledge troubling thoughts and feelings, yet also asks the physician to tolerate the patient's self-deception and fear of the
truth.

If patients were randomized to treatment groups that received different forms of
information, various outcomes could be studied: the content of information revealed
to the patient or family, the information that was retained or recalled, the satisfaction
of the patient and family with the form of treatment, and a variety of consequences at
various points in the course of the illness, including immediate and long-term effects
on mood, physical well-being, survival, quality of life, coping, and sense of autonomy
for both the patient and family, and the quality of the relationships between professionals, relatives, and friends. The optimal course might reflect a compromise
between various outcomes and might include hurtful consequences (e.g., better
informed patients might make a better overall adjustment but experience greater
dysphoria).

Similarly, physicians must negotiate among conflicting clinical goals: being honest and informative, preserving a relationship of confidence and trust, being kind and
shielding the patient from undue stress, providing hope and encouragement, respecting the family's viewpoint when it differs from the patient's, responding to the styles
of practice of other health professionals who share in the care process, and honoring
the law. The physician may feel morally obliged to be truthful and may believe that
honesty is needed both to maintain the doctor–patient relationship and to allow the
patient to act rationally, yet may also hold the impression that the patient cannot bear
the shock of disclosure at this moment or that the patient might flee from good treatment if the news is not presented in a highly favorable form.

The clinical approach presented in the final portion of this chapter embodies the
view that most clinicians and patients value truth-in-itself and that most favorable
clinical outcomes are facilitated by effective, honest information-sharing. Decisions
about the content, setting, and timing of disclosure, however, must be negotiated
among the doctor and patient and others. The physician must respect the patient's
wishes and recognize an optimal information-sharing pattern for each individual and
family.

Which Truth? Whose Truth?

Is an optimistic shading of the truth a distortion? When is a "silver lining" a "white-wash?" How do we distinguish tact, discretion, and good manners from charades, sub-tle concealment, and the defensive use of euphemisms? Whose truth is true?

Even if the truth is viewed as an objective matter, truth-telling must involve more than a recital of facts. Information-sharing entails conveying a complex impression to the patient. But does it mean that the patient understands everything that the doctor knows, including the minutiae and technicalities of care? The 10%, 1%, or 0.1% chance of a complication? Of severe complications or minor ones?

Uncertainties haunt the physician. How sure can one ever be about a diagnosis or prognosis? How does one interpret a laboratory test to a patient? When should the patient be helped to appreciate the probabilities on which the physician depends, and when should the expert simplify matters and reduce anxiety-provoking uncertainty?

What does the patient make of the facts? Bad news, in particular, is not just objec-tive data; fears are attached to the words, and evolving meanings are built around facts. Terms such as "cancer," "malignancy," "tumor," and "growth" have an idio-syncratic representation for the patient, regardless of what they mean to the physi-cian. Each individual develops a personal interpretation of the diagnosis, the prog-nosis, and the uncertainty. Even the appreciation of statistics is subjective: a 30% chance of cure may not be the same as a 70% chance of dying.[30,43,61]

Being told is not the same as understanding or admitting to the truth. In Weis-man's 1976 report, 10% of newly diagnosed cancer patients professed to a researcher–social worker that they neither knew their diagnosis nor needed further information, although all had been told about their condition.[64] In Aitken-Swan's study, 19% of "informed" patients denied they had been told.[1] Patients (and presumably physi-cians) do not entertain simply one view of reality. "Middle knowledge," as discussed in Chapter 6, describes how an individual may nearly simultaneously hold in mind a variety of views about the significance of an illness.[65] At different times, in different settings, and with different people, divergent views will be expressed.

Timing and Context

The truth, then, is not simply conveyed in a word or a diagnosis. Moreover, the mean-ing of facts will change as understanding and attitudes change. When a person first hears he or she has "cancer" or "metastases," the words have quite a different sig-nificance than 6 months later. A fatal illness is still a fatal illness when the patient has lived with it for a day, a week, a month, or a year, but the meaning of "fatal" will have changed for that person. An appreciation of the truth will change over time, and the desire for information evolves similarly. Patients want and can use some data now, other data later.

Information-sharing rarely can be viewed as a single event in which the physician either discloses or fails to disclose a set of facts. Clinically, truth-telling is a process that involves the physician and patient over a period of time and does not begin *de novo* with a laboratory result or pathology report. The patient's process of informa-tion-gathering begins well before the illness and reflects long-standing attitudes about understanding one's world and about dealing with anxiety by obtaining or ignoring information. Indeed, discussions of the process of information-gathering may assign too much importance to the physician's communications. The physician rarely initi-ates the process of learning the truth. The patient has heard about cancer, death, sickness, surgery, and so on for a lifetime, and has developed a personal meaning for these entities at this particular stage of his or her life.

Information-sharing occurs in an interpersonal context. Discussions between strangers (*e.g.*, announcing a sudden death in the emergency ward) pose quite different problems than when bad news is broken in the setting of a long-standing relationship and a long-standing illness. Even before the illness develops, honesty or frankness in information-seeking may or may not be a characteristic of the patient or of his or her relationships with doctors and others. Honesty in relationships does not suddenly develop when a fatal illness is initially considered, when a fatal diagnosis is first seen as likely or is confirmed, when death from the disease becomes highly probable, or when death is imminent.

Similarly, discussions of truth-telling often state or imply that an attitude of hopefulness or hopelessness can be conveyed at will by the physician. Patients are sometimes seen as so dependent and malleable that their attitudes can be easily manipulated. Such untested notions embody fantasies about the power of the physician. Doctors are viewed as so potent (and perhaps so aware of their behaviors and so able to control the effects they have on others) that they can change a patient with a few words in a few moments. In reality, words are important, but information is transferred in a context. The enormity of the effect of any distressing communication is often best understood with an awareness of how the doctor and patient arrived at that point in time, of their personal background, and how they interpret facts.

THE PSYCHOSOCIAL BASIS FOR UNDERSTANDING TRUTH-TELLING

The following section reviews some basic issues in our understanding about the sharing of distressing information, mostly drawn from an extensive, but scattered literature on communication in the doctor–patient relationship.[42,62]

The Value of Information

The uninformed patient lacks the knowledge to make decisions in his or her best self-interest. Dying patients require information in order to engage in rational decision-making. Such information provides "timely notice," allowing the patient to set his or her affairs in order, to plan appropriately for the future in legal, financial, social, and psychological matters.

Insofar as disclosure is inadequate, medical care will be carried out without well-informed consent and without the patient's unique evaluation of the benefits and costs of treatment. Even when the patient delegates decisions to the physician, the doctor still often needs to know how the patient values various treatment options and outcomes.

The use of information-sharing to reduce uncertainty and promote reassurance is a basic strategy in patient care and forms an essential component of emotional support. Good explanations reduce pain and stress and may lead to better tolerance of major and minor procedures (see Chap. 5). Information-sharing has generally improved patient compliance.[24,46]

Lacking accurate information and open discussion, patients make assumptions about the significance of tests, treatment, and the casual comments of the medical staff. They overhear conversations that may include unclear terms and may be only partially understood. They may interpret nonverbal communications without the opportunity to confirm their conclusions. Misunderstandings are commonplace under the best of circumstances, but surreptitiously obtained information may not be subject to discussions that might clarify confusion, resolve ambiguities, and verify facts. Covert information seekers are presumably liable to a great deal of misinterpretation, which, in turn, is likely to promote apprehension. Unacknowledged concerns are usually more troubling than concerns that can be discussed and then either be dismissed as unrealistic or addressed with rational plans.

Indirect evidence of the value of truth-telling is provided by one retrospective study that linked early knowledge of the diagnosis of cancer to good adjustment,[58] and by similar anecdotal clinical reports. Unfortunately, such observations do not distinguish whether frankness is a cause or a consequence of good adaptation. If honesty is merely an expression of good coping, then practicing disclosure will not necessarily improve adaptation.

Patient Knowledge and the Desire for Information

Few systematic observations are available of doctor and patient behavior in situations in which the sharing of disturbing information is a prominent concern.[10,17–19,59] Lidz and Meisel observed doctor–patient communication in a number of inpatient and outpatient settings and described great variations in what patients were told, how they learned about their conditions, what they understood, and how medical decisions were made.[40] The authors noted that the family often tried to stop any information-sharing that might have upset the patient. Legal notions of the consent process seemed to have little resemblance to observed behaviors: "disclosure" did not occur as a single event but rather as a series of events carried out in a somewhat disorganized fashion, involving many persons; "decisions" were not made by patients, but "recommendations" were made by physicians to the patients; and patients did not give "consent" but would either acquiesce or occasionally "veto" the physician's plans.

Whenever the communication of information in the doctor–patient relationship has been assessed, patients' knowledge of their medical conditions and treatment has been disappointingly low.[39,49] Formal educational techniques may improve patients' recall and their satisfaction with the explanations they receive, but doctor–patient encounters seem to be relatively inefficient occasions for learning. Not surprisingly, a common topic in cancer-patient group discussions and in the cancer-patient education literature is how the layperson can remember what the doctor said during a visit and how to ask important questions.

Undoubtedly, patients' anxiety and diffidence play a considerable role in their failure to acquire knowledge, but physicians may be also be faulted for explanations that are brief, unclear, overly technical, and so on. A common complaint about physicians has been that they seem rushed and spend too little time explaining.[62] Indeed, criticisms of physicians generally focus on their manner and nonverbal behavior rather than on their technical competence.[3,11–13,32]

Physicians generally underestimate their patients' degree of knowledge and desire for information.[49] Even the most diffident patients may be actively engaged in acquiring information and formulating their own diagnosis. Patients figure out the truth by various means: reading records and requisitions; overhearing the staff in the hallway; speaking to various health-care workers and to other patients; interpreting the behavior of their family, friends, and medical attendants; reading; and self-diagnosis. With such resources available, total avoidance of the truth may be nearly impossible without the wholehearted collusion of the patient, a condition that, in itself, suggests at least an unconscious desire for nondisclosure.

Preferences for Disclosing Distressing Facts

When laypersons or physicians are asked to imagine being faced with bad news or when cancer patients or other patients facing serious illness are surveyed, a strong preference can be elicited for being told the truth. However, Cassileth, presenting data on different age-groups of cancer patients, noted that 4% to 20% wanted only minimal or good information, while 15% to 40% preferred minimally detailed information.[9] Older, poorer, less well-educated patients were relatively more satisfied with their medical care and were less interested in detailed information or in participation in decision-making.

Dramatic patient testimonies on the value of truth-telling are frequently cited in recent writings on this topic, whereas proponents of discretion have probably not been fairly represented, and their viewpoint has not been brought out forcefully in reports of surveys. In clinical practice, patients' complaints about bluntness and "giving no hope" are as familiar as frustration about the difficulty of acquiring and understanding information.

As described previously, when well persons or patients are asked about disclosing bad news to a close relative, truth-telling is generally favored, but more exceptions are noted than when respondents are asked what they want for themselves. When questions about informing another person are presented with additional data that might favor withholding information (e.g., the patient might be upset or the family objects to disclosure), discretion becomes more acceptable. In clinical practice, the desire to withhold information often comes not from the patient but from a second person—a family member or physician—who wants to protect the patient. Anecdotally, physicians who "identify" or are closely involved with a patient are likely to distort the truth and have trouble giving bad news, thus behaving more like family members than dispassionate professionals.

Well-informed patients also appear to withhold distressing information from others. Hinton found that patients exert a great deal of discretion in disclosing their diagnosis.[29] Cassileth reported that only 52% of cancer patients told most of their friends and neighbors.[9]

Family Expertise and Responsibility

The viewpoint and expertise of the family must necessarily be somewhat different from those of the patient or physician. The relatives usually are said to "know the patient better" than the professional caretakers, but the family's perspective and protective instincts may lead them to favor a management plan that is consonant neither with the patient's wishes nor with the physician's mandate. Moreover, since communication between physicians and the family is generally described as haphazard and hasty, relatives are often not well-informed, perhaps owing to intentional withholding by the staff or simply owing to neglect.[34] The trend away from telling the truth only to the relatives may have left them less informed than in the past.

Occasionally, patients may wish that new information first be discussed with their family and that some or all decision-making responsibility be delegated to relatives. Such a pattern of communication and decision-making is an accepted practice in the care of incompetent patients, but is also a familiar feature in the care of some patients who are elderly or who face a fatal illness. Whereas fairly clear rules have been proposed for identifying the incompetent patient and for how decisions can be made on such a person's behalf,[50,51] some choices made for terminally ill patients by physicians and families seem to fall well outside these guidelines. A competent person with cancer or another terminal illness is likely to be treated at times as incompetent (*e.g.*, to have his or her family consulted on decisions that the patient is entitled to make, including the determination of what the patient is to be told about his or her medical condition).

Physicians' Attitudes and Practice

Physicians in the United States express a strong preference for disclosing the truth to their patients. Actual practice has not been well-characterized, but probably entails considerable use of discretion. Medical students and physicians may exhibit greater than average "fear of death,"[8] and this trepidation may be expressed in a reluctance to confront the truth about terminal illness. Presumably, patients are more likely to be told the truth when the physician judges that such information will improve patient compliance (*e.g.*, a patient who initially refuses a treatment favored by the professional staff is more likely to be informed than a compliant patient).

Clinicians in some countries do not value disclosure to the degree usually reported in the United States. Insofar as can be detected from essays and a few studies on this topic, British physicians favor greater use of discretion (*e.g.*, Hillier[26]), whereas frank preferences for concealing the truth from the cancer patient (but usually not from his or her family) have been reported anecdotally in other Western countries, such as Denmark, Israel, and the Soviet Union, as well as in China and Japan.

The contemporary physician's medicolegal preoccupation with informed consent may have encouraged greater disclosure, but has not been documented to improve patient understanding or to decrease dissatisfaction or even litigation. The mandate for full disclosure has sometimes led physicians to insist that every patient know the most dismal facts. Insofar as physicians respond to a notion of the law rather than serving the interests of the individual patient, the right to obtain information becomes, at worst, a requirement to listen to a hasty lecture and to sign a barely intelligible form.

Awareness of Disturbing Information

The patient's awareness of the truth and desire to pursue greater understanding fluctuates. Truth-seeking and truth-avoidance will vary from moment to moment, depending on the patient's immediate frame of mind, the situation in which information-sharing occurs, and the clinical condition that is being addressed.

Denial, with its many gradations and vicissitudes, is reviewed in Chapter 6. The diagnosis of denial presupposes that the patient has the opportunity to obtain correct information; unwilled ignorance is not a "coping strategy." Denial is largely an unconscious psychological mechanism and may not correspond with the patient's consciously expressed preferences for being told the truth. No studies have examined the relationship between the patient's reliance on this psychological coping style and the manner in which the physician chooses to present bad news. Physicians have various opportunities to exploit denial: they may bolster this defense during periods of extreme stress; they may use their awareness of this coping strategy to manipulate the patient; or they may unwittingly collude with the patient to avoid acknowledging painful facts. Respecting denial—not attempting to force a confrontation with an avoided reality—should not be confused with encouraging denial, a strategy that only rarely deserves consideration. Similarly, respecting denial can be distinguished from withholding the truth when a patient wishes to hear the truth and is psychologically able to appreciate further distressing information.

Denial has been correlated with improved survival and adaptation in at least one clinical setting.[20,21] Avoidance and denial may be successful coping mechanisms for some patients at some times.[38] Most writers, however, view denial as an ineffective or maladaptive defense, especially when it persists beyond an initial brief period of shock over encountering bad news.

As noted previously, terminally ill patients often understand far more about their condition than others realize. Patients whom the medical staff or family think are ignorant of the diagnosis will often know the major facts about their condition.[7,28] Persistent, tactful interviewers can regularly elicit frank or partial acknowledgment of the truth when more casual interviewers find denial or ignorance. Experienced interviewers who favor or feel comfortable with acknowledging painful facts will encounter more honesty among patients than interviewers who are reluctant to confront bad news.

Lying

Lying is difficult. Consistency in telling the truth is relatively simple, but consistent fabrication demands that one remember all one's lies and be ready to defend them. Among a group such as a family, consistency in dissembling is extremely difficult to achieve.

Sociological observers have presented dramatic reports of how nondisclosure tends to isolate the patient,[17-19] and a number of clinicians have anecdotally verified this phenomenon. For family members and medical staff alike, the masquerade of not telling is taxing. Rather than lying unconvincingly, discussion may be avoided or evaded. Pretending causes tension in all contact with the patient, and interferes with easeful, intimate relationships:

> We couldn't joke in the house because we all were keeping the secret that Grandma was dying.

Patients can often sense when the truth is being withheld. Carefulness or reluctance of the family or staff in communicating information is an early clue for the patient that something serious has happened.

The extent to which physicians lose their credibility or displease or seriously mislead patients by withholding information has not been adequately studied in a representative clinical setting. Sociological descriptions of circumstances in which nondisclosure is practiced have generally protrayed withholding as a shabby ruse and a disservice to patients, although more sympathetic reports have been proffered.[41] When lies are discovered, distrust and suspicion may forever contaminate relationships. Both caretakers and the family are subject to this problem.

Shifts from discretion to frankness in information-sharing are also likely to cause difficulties. The abandonment of bland reassurance and excessive optimism may alienate patients:

> I came to see him, and he always told me that I was doing good. Now he tells me that the chemotherapy did no good. I'm confused.

The Hazards of Truthfulness

An often stated or implied disadvantage to sharing bad news is that the truth may provoke anxiety, sadness, and many other disagreeable feelings and may lead to hopelessness and suicide. Cabot, however, wrote of the "innocuousness of the truth,"[4] and other clinicians have generally reported that severely dysphoric affects pass quickly. According to Weisman, no patient responded to truth-telling by becoming "distressed to an unmanageable degree despite transient anxiety, depression, and perhaps some anger."[64] Moderate dysphoria may be considered an inevitable consequence of a serious illness and as a prerequisite to achieving satisfactory psychological accommodation.

Nevertheless, severe dysphoric responses may occur and some may be avoidable. The effects of disclosure on mood and coping deserve further exploration. Extreme cases are often cited—"The lie tormented him"[60]—but the effects of withholding truth require a more dispassionate review. Why should dysphoria be so strongly avoided? Can patients be shielded from painful facts, or does lying merely prevent open expression, perhaps forcing disagreeable affects to be submerged in the patient's private world? Who is being protected by discretion? When do patients become angry with the clinician, leaving treatment or detouring to other physicians or to "quacks" who offer greater hope and reassurance?

Ultimately, hopelessness is usually seen as the worst consequence of hearing the truth—"He'll give up and die if you tell him." A small clinical literature on voodoo death,[5] bone pointing,[44] and similar instances of extreme despair or giving-up supports this concern, as does an extensive literature on helplessness and loss[56] and on survival under extreme stress.[15] Some patients do, in fact, become hopeless.

The frequency, duration, and intensity of despair among patients receiving bad news has not been studied. Clinical experience suggests that the family's warning that a patient will give up is a useful indication of the relatives' feelings but is often inaccurate about the patient. Hopelessness does not appear to be a common or necessary outcome of hearing distressing truths. When hopelessness occurs, it probably reflects as much how the truth was taken as what was told and how it was presented. In general, dying patients who have been content with their life and who continue to enjoy some good health rarely give up, whereas moribund patients seem to resign themselves to death in a manner that seems reasonable. Giving-up may be a reasonable response at some stages of terminal cancer. Resignation or acceptance of a grim reality should be distinguished from inapproprite despair and hopelessness. The notion that hopefulness requires illusion, that ignorance is bliss, seems to rest on a view of reality as rather toxic, an impression that is not surprising in the world of the cancer patient. The fear that the patient will succumb to despair also embodies the widespread feeling that cancer is hopeless and reflects a tendency to depersonalize the cancer patient, seeing him or her as totally overcome by a terrible disease rather than as a person who, like most sick people, naturally wants to live as long as life is meaningful and who continues to have aspirations and hopes, resilience and strengths.

Little clinical information is available to predict who will succumb to despair and why, but there are abundant testimonies that full disclosure and participation in decision-making enhances coping for some people. Knowledge allows for autonomy, self-direction, and empowerment, engaging the patient in his or her own behalf. Hopefulness can be sustained by a firm grasp on reality, by understanding rather than by ignorance. Indeed, hopefulness may be manifested as an eagerness to learn more about one's health and to participate more actively in decision-making. Cassileth reported that higher degrees of knowledge and interest in knowing about one's condition were not associated with loss of hope among cancer patients, although the study design did not allow any conclusions about the outcome of information-sharing on mood.[9] Misunderstandings, unacknowledged fears, isolation, and an atmosphere of cautiousness about speaking freely can be expected to enhance fearfulness and subvert hopefulness.

Although many cancer patients contemplate suicide, actual attempts are uncommon, while completed suicides are apparently rare. Persons with physical illnesses, particularly cancer and other fatal diseases, may be more likely to kill themselves than the general population, but the increased risk is probably small.[63] Weisman has written convincingly about the need to determine factors of "vulnerability," which not only may predict suicide but also may help identify those patients who could benefit from intensive psychosocial intervention.[63] When Weisman used such a screening instrument, he found that a third of newly diagnosed cancer patients would be considered at "high risk" for psychosocial difficulties.[66]

A CLINICAL GUIDE TO SHARING DISTURBING INFORMATION

> The miserable have no other medicine
> But only hope
>
> William Shakespeare,
> *Measure for Measure* III:i

Listening and questioning, not just explaining, are key skills in imparting distressing news. The best intentions to divulge fully or clearly can lead the physician astray if he or she is not guided by an appreciation of the patient's perspective: what the patient understands, is concerned about, and wants to know.

The physician who is familiar with the patient and who has attended to the patient's perspective during history-taking and previous discussions may begin the exposition phase of an interview with a clear sense of what information needs to be transmitted. If such a background is lacking, consider beginning the exposition phase of the interview with questioning and clarification:

> *Let's go back over some of the things we have already talked about. Last week we talked about your blood level being low again. What is your understanding about the significance of the low blood level?*
>
> *We have some important matters to discuss today. What kinds of questions are on your mind?*
>
> *What do you make of all this?*
>
> *What is your understanding about these tests now?*
>
> *What are your thoughts about what lies ahead?*
>
> *What were you hoping I might do for you?*

Patients usually do want to know the broad facts about their condition and its management, but they may want to hear only a little bit at a time. They often ask questions obliquely. They may avoid direct questions because they do not want to appear stupid or suspicious or to be a nuisance. They also fear hearing a blunt, frightening fact. Respect them for their dilemma. The physician who responds only to bold inquiries will miss the intimations and implicit questions with which most patients signal their concerns. At times, the physician must ease patients into frank discussions. Be ready to talk about whatever topics occupy the patient, but use discussions of superficial matters as inroads to issues of greater import, listening carefully for the patient's deepest concerns. The conversation can be gently and firmly moved toward troubling matters, perhaps weaving back and forth between inconsequential and critical topics. Do not balk if the patient puts off difficult subjects awhile. At times, as one family member described it, "handle it in dribbles rather than a big rush."

When the clinician begins having a sense of the patient's understanding, feelings, and wish to learn more, then rational information-sharing can begin. The patient's questions and concerns lead the physician to present information that can best be appreciated and retained. Patients should know that the physician will tell them as much as they want to know, and that their difficulties in comprehension will be greeted with tolerance and an eagerness to help them understand. Encourage all questions and let patients know that you do not consider their search for answers as evidence of distrust, stupidity, or intrusiveness:

> *It's my job to explain these matters to you so that you understand them. Tell me if I haven't made myself clear. Please don't be afraid to ask questions.*

> *You can learn as much as you want to know, when you want. If I'm not explaining what you would like to know, tell me. You can also tell me if I'm saying more than you want to hear.*

In explaining, the physician has the capability of providing vast amounts of information to the layperson. How is one to decide what to say? As discussed in Chapter 5, Feeling Secure, two general principles are useful. First, tell patients what they want to know. Let them guide you to discuss the subjects that currently meet their personal concerns. Second, tell patients what they need to know, in particular, what is necessary for making rational decisions and carrying out self-treatment. Once patients have had a chance fully to explore their concerns, this second category of information has often already been addressed.

Share information rather than thrusting it upon the patient. Unrequested information should be offered when necessary, but skillful explaining is often a process of helping patients request what they need to know:

> *I suspect you and your family need to make some practical decisions based on how your condition develops.*

> *What else do you want to know to consider these alternatives?*

> *I wonder if you have any questions about how the treatment has been going?*

The best explanations are succinct and simple. Only a little new information can be absorbed at one sitting. Information-sharing takes time and often is a gradual process, which is carried out over weeks, not minutes. Let the patient digest the information awhile. Clarify matters in which the patient seems confused or misled. Repeat and review.

Establish a partnership, not a lectureship. Overly precise, technical explanations can be as incomprehensible and unhelpful as vague circumlocution. Avoid the temptation to expound on clinical topics that are familiar to the physician but skirt the emotionally trying but more pressing concerns of the patient.

Answer direct questions honestly and clearly. Avoid the temptation to be overly optimistic. Avoid severe bluntness or brutal confrontation, but also shun saccharin reassurance and frank dishonesty.

As important as what the physician says is what he or she does afterward. Explain briefly, painting a picture with a few broad strokes, then listen again. What is the patient making of the information? Let further questions be a guide to the areas that require elaboration and clarification. Listen for the mental picture you create for the patient. Attend to the feelings provoked by new information:

> *Your examination today seems pretty much the same as last week. How do you think you've been doing?*

> *This pain comes from your ribs. It is caused by irritation from the cancer. I think we should adjust your medication so that you can go on with your business without the discomfort bothering you anymore. What do you think?*

Full understanding (not merely full disclosure) is a goal, but information-sharing is best carried out without strong insistence on what the immediate outcome of the discussion will be. A preference for honesty and full disclosure provides a gentle pressure, directing the process of explanation toward a sharing of important facts. An unswerving determination to convey the "whole truth" without regard to the patient's wishes tends to block effective communication, leaving the patient overwhelmed or wary and less ready to engage in further information acquisition. A watchful, flexible approach is better than a formula. Even if truth is the highest value, guide patients so that they can follow their own path to this end.

Respect denial but, in general, do not exploit it. Treat patients as reasonable and courageous, but appreciate their reasons for not wanting to know everything. In a setting of mutual trust, the patient can most easily pursue the truth, and the physician can most readily promote honesty and understanding. When patients seem to shun the truth, consider distrust and fear as an explanation for their behavior.

Appreciate how a patient's desire for the truth will vary from time to time and from situation to situation. Assist the patient in finding the optimal setting for receiving and reviewing information. Some matters are best discussed with a family member present, whereas others are better handled privately. Groups are helpful for patients who prefer to discuss an illness with peers. Written materials are useful for some persons. A multidisciplinary team can provide the patient with a choice of information sources.

Patients and their families are entitled to the physician's best guesses about the likely course of an illness, and they may need this information to plan their lives rationally. However, physicians cannot foresee the future and should not pose as crystal-ball readers. Physicians' prognostic statements are often taken literally. Avoid false certainty or an overly precise prognosis:

> *If I could tell you for sure, I would, but I just have to wait and see like you. Some people can live for months and months with a problem like this, while for others it quickly leads to more serious problems. If something develops that suggests to me that the illness is moving quickly or slowly, would you want to stay abreast of the facts?*

Some writers have suggested avoiding "specifics," but such a rule might be taken as a justification for evasion. A few commentators have advised that information should not be offered until an evaluation is complete, thus sparing the patient uncertainty and worry over tentative diagnoses. Indeed, some patients clearly prefer to wait until definitive results are available. Others want to be informed about every step in the diagnostic and therapeutic process and will resent having any information withheld, regardless of whether the physician feels ready to offer a final interpretation. Consider waiting until all the results are at hand, but let the patient be your guide in deciding how to disclose information.

Primitive or magical thinking is common when reality is difficult to face. The physician needs to remember that talking about a distressing condition does not create the problem, nor does ignoring it make it less of a problem. Predicaments that necessarily are disturbing are not made painless by our ministrations; physicians can only ease such distress. Doctors like to alleviate discomfort, but truth-telling makes them the vehicles for delivering painful news. Patients are generally relieved when a suppressed concern is tactfully turned into an openly discussed matter. Patients, however, may blame the physician for hurting them with the truth. Eventually, patients usually recognize that the physician has presented reality, not created it. Persistent anger at the physician often reflects a sense of hopelessness and abandonment.

The physician's apology for breaking bad news can be appreciated as an empathic statement when it is offered after a difficult discussion. An apology that introduces bad news, however, tends to divert attention from the patient's to the physician's discomfort, as if to say, "Feel sorry for me for having to say this to you":

> *I hate to have to tell you this but . . .*

> *I'm really sorry to be put in this position. I wish I could give you better news.*

When important information must be conveyed to a reluctant patient, firmness may be required:

> *It seems that you have some very important decisions to make with your family. I wonder if it wouldn't be helpful to make sure you and I both understand what your medical condition is like now? How do you see things going?*

> *Let's take a few moments to consider how you're set up if your condition should worsen rather than continue holding its own. What kind of decisions and plans should you try to make now in case you're not feeling well enough to handle them in the future?*

> *Your mind seems made up. Still, I would like you to at least consider with me some other possibilities and to make sure you have all the facts at hand so that we'll both feel comfortable with your decision as time goes on.*

When speaking to a patient who is avoiding important truths, the physician may want to address the patient as someone with "two minds," speaking to the more receptive "mind" without disturbing the dominant one:

> *I wonder if there isn't a part of you that wonders about some of the worst possibilities?*

> *I can see that you want to look at the bright side of things, but I wonder if you don't also have times when you want to plan for problems that might arise.*

Graded exposure to disagreeable information can help ease the discussion toward full disclosure. Say, "We've found some evidence of cancer" before saying, "You have cancer in your liver." Say, "The cancer is affecting your bowels" before saying, "The cancer has blocked your bowels completely."

An attitude of hopefulness—cautious optimism—seems desirable. Hope is not a distortion but an optimistic shading, a disposition to confidence, a sense of security about the future. Insofar as possible, new problems are viewed as challenges, invoking new strategies that promise the best possible outcome. Hopefulness is not easily prescribed for the patient or the doctor. Moreover, the physician's sense of optimism or pessimism is likely to be communicated regardless of overt intentions. Professional caretakers promote morale largely through an unspoken attitude that conveys an acceptance of the situation and an eagerness to do the best with it:

There's no guarantee this will work, but I certainly think it's worth a try.

An active, positive approach to the care of terminally ill patients is suggested throughout this book. There are many opportunities for the patient to feel well, to get help, and to make the best of the situation. Many difficulties can be tolerated, and both physical and emotional distress can be managed. The truth may be bad, but it need not be overwhelming. Until the time to die has come, self-worth can be sustained and life can be cherished.

Notes on Breaking Bad News

The following suggestions and considerations are offered for when very distressing information—a death, the initial diagnosis of cancer, a serious complication—is first broached:

1. Setting—Choose a place to talk that allows for privacy and comfort. Everyone should be seated. There should be ample time for discussion and freedom from interruptions.
2. Telephone conversations are rarely satisfactory for breaking bad news. Unless the physician is very familiar with the person to whom he or she is talking, the lack of face-to-face communication will make information-sharing difficult. Ask the patient or family to meet you in the hospital, office or home. If a telephone discussion is necessary, follow it up with a personal interview when feasible. Similarly, letters and wires are poor substitutes for a personal exchange of information.
3. When a bad event has suddenly occurred, the physician should make a special effort to be calm and composed before presenting the information.
4. Involve the family. Consider who should be told first and who should be on hand when the patient hears the news. Who will be with the patient when the bearer of bad news leaves? Are separate interviews needed to discuss information with various family members?
5. Neither evasion nor harsh bluntness is desired. Be hopeful—"The good news is . . ."—but avoid premature reassurance, euphemisms, or false encouragement. Eagerness to allay discomfort should not hinder getting the basic message across.
6. Bad news is best broken gradually. Build up to the truth by reviewing the diagnostic findings or historical sequence that led to the conclusion:

    You've had a seizure. . . . We did some tests to figure out why. . . . The tests show. . . . We concluded. . . . This means. . . .

7. Be simple and clear. Start with a few plain statements. Little new information can be appreciated under stress. Talk slowly. Set limited goals for the first discussion. Listen for concerns and encourage questions.

8. Ask: What does this patient want to know now? What does this patient need to know now? Let the patient's reactions guide the discussion toward further elaboration.
9. Listen for the way the news is interpreted, for its personal significance. Nonverbal communication may convey powerful meanings independent of the intended message and may be misinterpreted, especially when open discussion is lacking.
10. Listen for how this person and family value honesty and "facing the facts" or how they avoid upsetting news. How have they handled truth-telling in the past? How have they responded to bad news?

    Have you ever been through a bad time like this before? What happened? How did you hear about it? What was it like? Did you get depressed? How did your family take it? What helped you through it?

11. Review what has been said.
12. Don't drop the diagnosis and run. The physician should assure the patient and family of his or her availability for discussion and continuing involvement in care.
13. Enlist the help of others for explanation and support.

Suggestions for Involving the Family

Ask the patient how to involve the family. A competent patient is entitled to choose how information is to be disseminated and how others are to be included in decision-making. Should the family be present for important discussions between the doctor and the patient? If not, who will transmit information and answer their questions? May the physician freely discuss the case with any relatives who call? Friends? Does the patient wish to delegate some responsibility for decision-making to the family?

If possible, the initial discussion with the patient on any important new topics should be either carried out in the family's presence or handled privately but then reviewed with the family by the doctor and patient. The physician who participates in major presentations of information between the patient and family can accurately monitor the content and affective tone of the family's information-sharing and avoid the need for repeatedly asking the patient and family how they have presented information to each other. Group meetings sometimes facilitate open discussion of both information and feelings. However, family members will not always be able to talk freely in front of each other. Individual conferences may help family members feel more comfortable with their personal questions and concerns and may perhaps encourage greater honesty in public discussions.

The primary caretaker—the family member who takes principal responsibility for organizing services and for communicating with the professional caretakers about the details of medical management (see Chap. 4, The Task of Physical Care)—may also assume the responsibility of informing family members about the patient's condition. Such a method of disseminating information is easy for the physician, but will often leave some of the family misinformed or feeling neglected. Periodic individual or group meetings should be offered to anyone wishing to stay abreast of the details of the illness and should be considered whenever a major change in the patient's condition occurs. Children particularly need special attention (see Chap. 9).

When family members want information to be concealed from the patient, their feelings should be explored:

Tell me more about why you feel this way? How do you think he will react to this information?

What do you think he knows now? What does he think is going on? Why do you think he doesn't know?

How does he feel about truth-telling? Has he expressed a preference to be told or not to be told? Does he want you to protect him from the pain of bad news? Could we ask him more about it? Could I help you ask him?

How has the patient taken bad news in the past? How have others in the family responded?

What do you think he should not be told? How would he react? What would you want him to know?

At times, a few encouraging statements from the physician about the value of honesty and the strength of the patient will help the family discuss the illness more openly:

Most patients know the greater part of the truth even if they are not told directly. Don't you think he is wondering? Suspicious? Worried? I would not want him to fret needlessly because he has been kept in the dark.

When I talk with him, he seems rather eager to learn more, and he asks many of the same questions you bring up. I have already discussed many of these matters quite frankly with him.

Is the patient emotionally disturbed? Incompetent? I am struck by his eagerness to understand his illness, his interest in making the best of a bad situation, his ability to handle bad news in the past, as evidenced by. . . .

Undoubtedly, he will find this news depressing, but I wonder if we are helping him by trying to avoid matters that must be quite apparent to him and about which he is asking questions.

Among families who insist on withholding major and often obvious facts, two patterns commonly emerge when their motives are explored. First, bad news has always been handled with concealment in this family or community. Such longstanding patterns can be modified, but will not easily admit to major change. Second, the family is deeply troubled by a sense that the patient will be overwhelmed by grief or despair, that emotional control may be lost, and that the patient may give up. The second pattern can be seen in families that ordinarily manage bad news with some frankness. In the second case particularly, the desire to conceal the truth can be partly understood as a symptom of the family's anguish and hopelessness: as a projection of their own sense of being overwhelmed, of their own desire to avoid painful feelings, and of their difficulty in witnessing distress in the patient. Feelings of this sort are rarely well managed by confrontation or reasoning. Caretakers who focus on the symptom—the withholding of facts—may end up in useless arguments about the value of truth or about how information-sharing should be managed. Such arguments alienate the family, deflect attention from the underlying problem, and further aggravate the family's distress. The symptom should be recognized as arising from deep unhappiness and insecurity, as a desperate attempt to avoid pain and an awkward plea for help in dealing with a painful reality. Such problems are addressed directly by psychosocial counseling and support, a process that often begins with an elicitation of underlying feelings, an appreciation of personal strengths, and a recognition of hopefulness amidst despair. As adjustment improves over time, the intensity of the feelings diminishes and the symptom—avoidance of frank discussion—lessens and often resolves.

Respect for the family's feelings does not preclude a firm insistence on honesty, especially in responding to the patient's questions and concerns:

> *I appreciate your explaining these things to me. I certainly will not force any-thing upon him or try to tell him something he doesn't want to hear. On the other hand, I would not lie to him, and I must answer all his questions honestly.*

Unfortunately, an occasional family may act as if everything would have been fine had the patient been kept ignorant, and may blame the physician who discloses bad news for causing the patient's depression. Again, rather than arguing about truth-telling and defending ethical behavior, the physician better serves the family by gently, yet firmly, continuing to promote honesty and by focusing attention on the distress that has generated such anger.

Just as family members may want to protect the patient from bad news, the patient may choose to withhold information from relatives and friends. Unlike the family, the patient has the right to control the flow of information. Withholding by either the patient or the family, however, should generally be viewed by the physician as a problem to be explored, gently resisted, and gradually diffused.

Multidisciplinary Teams and Truth-Telling

Multidisciplinary-team conferences will sometimes reveal striking differences in the degree of frankness or discretion exercised by the layperson with various caretakers. Such variability in candor and the expression of feelings can be perceived as a prob-lem: the providers who enjoy less openness with a patient may feel that they have done something wrong or have not developed a good relationship. Team members may feel that discrepancies in a patient's behavior need somehow to be resolved.

The fluidity and situational dependency of frankness, however, is inevitable. Patients do not need to stare at truth constantly. They can have deeply satisfying rela-tionships in which an awareness of their sadness is minimized. The majority of human relationships may not admit to great honesty or a broad range of affect and may be viewed as "shallow," yet can also be profoundly gratifying. Moreover, the patient's encounter with the caretaker who has the ongoing responsibility for break-ing bad news must be tainted by dread. There is no advantage in having all relation-ships colored by this fear of encountering upsetting information. Likewise, one need not decide once and for all whether a patient is being honest or not. Opportunities for full disclosure and frankness should be created, but different sides of the patient may be shared with different persons at different times. Each caretaker should assess how the patient wishes truth-telling to be handled in that particular relationship, and should tolerate the variability of the patient's frankness.

Laypersons who are dealing with a group of professional caretakers may test the team for consistency and may be distressed by the inevitable differences in how care-takers perceive and present both relatively straightforward or objective matters (e.g., how to treat the pain or nausea) and relatively vague or subjective matters (e.g., is everything going well?). Obsessive laypersons may repeatedly review details with each health professional willing to give an opinion. Families may also foster an impression of some providers as either good (or kind or caring or careful or intelligent) or bad (or mean or uncaring or sloppy or stupid) and may play one off against the other. Such "splitting" often provokes suspicion and conflict among team members.

The team should strive for a reasonable degree of mutual understanding of the patient's condition, the goals of care, and the plans for management. Regular team conferences are helpful. When inconsistencies have been particularly troublesome to the laypersons, consolidation of information-sharing may be necessary (e.g., by deferring to one person for presenting explanations or by attempting to handle such discussions in a group meeting during which differences in viewpoints can be recognized and resolved). The team must also appreciate that anger about various aspects of the patient's or family's situation can be expressed as anger at a particular caretaker, and that some families seek scapegoats. Such behavior does not always need to be addressed with the family or resolved, but it needs to be recognized by the team members, lest they encourage or become victimized by it.

Whenever a team is involved in patient care, careful charting of information-sharing can be useful:

> . . . Spoke with patient and her husband about development of jaundice. Mrs. G was well aware of the change in her color and knew it signified a liver problem, despite Mr. G's encouragement to minimize its importance. She assumed that the cancer had spread to her liver. We discussed her notions that liver cancer is painful and a sign of approaching death. I reassured her about pain, suggested that the jaundice might be associated with fatigue, and discussed the range of likely outcomes: "weeks to months" of progression, symptoms of tiredness and drowsiness. I noted that her blood tests had shown evidence of liver metastases for at least 8 months, so slow progression might be hoped for. Mr. G was initially rather restless, but appeared less eager to change the subject when he sensed how calmly his wife took the news. As in the past, the patient desires minimal evaluation and only simple medical management of the problem. I supported this decision. No diagnostic tests or treatment are needed at this time. I agreed to discuss recent findings with their two daughters who will arrange to be here on my next visit.

> Results conveyed to patient and daughter: the "spot on the lung" is definitely cancer. Daughter said she knew it all along and recalled two neighbors with lung cancer, both of whom died quickly but with little distress. The patient wanted to know what to do next. Two options were suggested: radiation or just watching to see if the metastases gives him any trouble. He was eager to say that he felt well. He says he wants to take a trip to California, and doesn't want to bother with something that isn't hurting him. I concurred, expressing hope that no symptoms would develop, and assured them that treatments are available should problems arise. I stressed the need to report new problems, however, and agreed with the patient to enlist his daughter to help handle this task. He is "being tough"; she and I will do the worrying. The patient uses words such as "cancer," "spot," and "tumor" in a matter-of-fact manner and says he knows it is serious but he prefers to "look on the bright side" or "not dwell on it." We agreed to review the diagnosis and management again next week.

REFERENCES

1. Aitken-Swan J, Easson EC: Reactions of cancer patients on being told their diagnosis. Br Med J 1:779–783, 1959
2. Anonymous: In cancer, honesty is here to stay (editorial). Lancet 2:245, 1980
3. Ben-Sira Z: The function of the professional's affective behavior in client satisfaction: A revised approach to social interaction theory. J Health Soc Behav 17:3–11, 1976

4. Cabot RC: The use of truth and falsehood in medicine: An experimental study. Am Med 5:344–349, 1903
5. Cannon WB: "Voodoo" death. Am Anthropologist 44:169–181, 1942
6. Carey RG, Posavac EJ: Attitudes of physicians on disclosing information to and maintaining life for terminal patients. Omega 9:67–77, 1978–79
7. Cartwright A, Hockey L, Anderson JL: Life Before Death. London, Routledge & Kegan Paul, 1973
8. Cassem NH: Treating the person confronting death. In Nicholi AM Jr (ed): The Harvard Guide to Modern Psychiatry, pp 579–606. Cambridge, MA, Harvard University Press, 1978
9. Cassileth BR, Zupkis RV, Sutton-Smith K et al: Information and participation preferences among cancer patients. Ann Intern Med 92:832–836, 1980
10. Comaroff J: Communicating information about non-fatal illness: The strategies of a group of general practitioners. Soc Rev 24:269–290, 1976
11. DiMatteo MR: A social–psychological analysis of physician–patient rapport: Toward a science of the art of medicine. J Soc Issues 35:12–33, 1979
12. DiMatteo MR, Prince, LM, Taranta A: Patient's perceptions of physician's behavior: Determinants of patient commitment to the therapeutic relationship. J Commun Health 4:280–290, 1979
13. DiMatteo MR, Taranta A, Friedman HS, Prince LM: Predicting patient satisfaction from physicians' nonverbal communication skills. Med Care 19:376–387, 1980
14. Fitts WT, Ravdin IS: What Philadelphia physicians tell patients with cancer. JAMA 153:901–904, 1953
15. Frankl VE: Man's Search for Meaning: An Introduction to Logotherapy. New York, Simon and Schuster, 1959
16. Gilbertsen VA, Wangensteen OH: Should the doctor tell the patient that the disease is cancer? CA 12:80–85, 1962
17. Glaser BG: Disclosure of terminal illness. J Health Hum Behav 7:83–91, 1966
18. Glaser BG, Strauss AL: Awareness of Dying. Chicago, Aldine Publishing, 1965
19. Glaser BG, Strauss AL: Time for Dying. Chicago, Aldine Publishing, 1968
20. Hackett TP, Cassem N, Wishnie WA: The coronary care unit: An appraisal of its psychological hazards. N Engl J Med 279:1365–1370, 1968
21. Hackett TP, Weisman AO: Denial as a factor in patients with heart disease and cancer. Ann NY Acad Sci 164:802–817, 1969
22. Hardy, RE, Green DR, Jordan HW et al: Communication between cancer patients and physicians. South Med J 73:755–757, 1980
23. Harris L et al: Views of informed consent and decisionmaking: Parallel surveys of physicians and the public. In President's Commission for the Study of Ethical Problems in Medicine and Biomedical and Behavioral Research: Making Health Care Decisions: The Ethical and Legal Implications of Informed Consent in the Patient–Practitioner Relationship. Volume Two: Appendices—Empirical Studies of Informed Consent, pp 17–316. Washington, DC, US Government Printing Office, 1982
24. Haynes RB, Taylor DW, Sackett DL (eds): Compliance in Health Care. Baltimore, Johns Hopkins University Press, 1979
25. Henriques B, Stadil F, Baden H: Patient information about cancer: A prospective study of patients' opinion and reactions to information about cancer diagnosis. Acta Chir Scand 146:309–311, 1980
26. Hillier ER: Communication between doctor and patient. In Twycross RG, Ventafridda V (eds): The Continuing Care of Terminal Cancer Patients. Oxford, England, Pergamon Press, 1980
27. Hinton J: Facing death. J Psychosom Res 10:22–28, 1966
28. Hinton J: Talking with people about to die. Br Med J 3:25–27, 1974
29. Hinton J: Whom do dying patients tell? Br Med J 281:1328–1330, 1980
30. Kahneman D, Tversky A: The psychology of preferences. Sci Am 246:160–173, 1982
31. Kelley WH, Friesen SR: Do cancer patients want to be told? Surgery 27:822–826, 1950
32. Kelman HR: Consumer criteria of health services quality. In Gallagher EB (ed): The Doctor–Patient Relationship in the Changing Health Scene, pp 215–226. Washington, DC, John E.

Fogarty International Center for Advanced Study in the Health Sciences, DHEW Publication No. (NIH) 78-183, 1978

33. Kline NS, Sobin J: The psychological management of cancer cases. JAMA 146:1547–1551, 1951

34. Krant MJ, Johnston L: Family members' perceptions of communications in late stage cancer. Int J Psychiatry Med 8:203–216, 1977–78

35. Lazare A, Eisenthal S: A negotiated approach to the clinical encounter. I. Attending to the patient's perspective. In Lazare A (ed): Outpatient Psychiatry: Diagnosis and Treatment. Baltimore, Williams & Wilkins, 141–156, 1979

36. Lazare E, Eisenthal S, Frank A: A negotiated approach to the clinical encounter. II. Conflict and negotiation. In Lazare A (ed): Outpatient Psychiatry: Diagnosis and Treatment, pp 157–171. Baltimore, Williams & Wilkins, 1979

37. Lazare A, Eisenthal S, Frank A, Stoeckle JD: Studies on a negotiated approach to patienthood. In Gallagher EB (ed): The Doctor–Patient Relationship in the Changing Health Scene. Washington, DC, John E. Fogarty International Center for Advanced Study in the Health Sciences, DHEW publication No. (NIH) 78-183, 1978

38. Lazarus RS: Denial: Its costs and benefits. In Ahmed P (ed): Living and Dying with Cancer. New York, Elsevier, 1981

39. Ley P, Spelman MS: Communicating with the Patient. London, Staples Press, 1967

40. Lidz CW, Meisel A: Informed consent and the structure of medical care. In President's Commission for the Study of Ethical Problems in Medicine and Biomedical and Behavioral Research: Making Health Care Decisions: The Ethical and Legal Implications of Informed Consent in the Patient–Practitioner Relationship. Volume Two: Appendices—Empirical Studies of Informed Consent, pp. 317–410. Washington, DC, US Government Printing Office, 1982

41. McIntosh J: Patients' awareness and desire for information about diagnosed but undisclosed malignant disease. Lancet 2:300–303, 1976

42. McIntosh J: Processes of communication, information seeking and control associated with cancer: A selective review of the literature. Soc Sci Med 8:167–187, 1974

43. McNeil BJ, Pauker SG, Sox HC, Jr et al: On the elicitation of preferences for alternative therapies. N Engl J Med 306:1259–1262, 1982

44. Milton GW: Self-willed death or the bone-pointing syndrome. Lancet 1:1435–1436, 1973

45. Mount BM, Jones A, Patterson A: Death and dying: Attitudes in a teaching hospital. Urology 4:74, 1974; reprinted in Ajemian I, Mount BM (eds): The R.V.H. Manual on Palliative/Hospice Care. New York, Arno, 1980

46. Myers ED, Calvert EJ: Effect of forewarning on the occurrence of side-effects of discontinuance of medication in patients on dotheipin. J Int Med Res 4:237–240, 1976

47. Novack DH, Plumer R, Smith RL et al: Changes in physicians' attitudes toward telling the cancer patient. JAMA 241:897–900, 1979

48. Oken D: What to tell cancer patients. JAMA 175:1120–1128, 1961

49. Pratt L, Seligman A, Reader R: Physician's views on the level of medical information among patients. Am J Public Health 47:1277–1283, 1957

50. President's Commission for the Study of Ethical Problems in Medicine and Biomedical and Behavioral Research: Deciding to Forego Life Sustaining Treatment. Washington, DC, US Government Printing Office, 1983

51. President's Commission for the Study of Ethical Problems in Medicine and Biomedical and Behavioral Research: Making Health Care Decisions: The Ethical and Legal Implications of Informed Consent in the Patient–Practitioner Relationship. Vol One: Report. Vol Two: Appendices—Empirical Studies of Informed Consent. Vol Three: Appendices—Studies on the Foundations of Informed Consent. Washington, DC, US Government Printing Office, 1982

52. Quint JC: Institutionalized practices of information control. Psychiatry 28:119–132, 1965

53. Reiser SJ: Words as scalpels: transmitting evidence in the clinical dialogue. Ann Intern Med 92:837–842, 1980

54. Rogers CR: On Becoming a Person. Boston, Houghton Mifflin, 1961

55. Samp RJ, Curreri AR: A questionnaire survey on public cancer education obtained from cancer patients and their families. Cancer 10:382–384, 1957
56. Seligman MP: Helplessness: On Depression, Development, and Death. San Francisco, WH Freeman, 1975
57. Simpson MA: Therapeutic uses of truth. In Wilkes E (ed): The Dying Patient. Ridgewood, New Jersey, Bogden and Sons, 1982
58. Slavin LA, O'Malley JE, Koocher GP et al: Communication of the cancer diagnosis to pediatric patients: Impact on long-term adjustment. Am J Psychiatry 139:179–183, 1982
59. Sudnow D: Passing On: The Social Organization of Dying. Englewood Cliffs, NJ, Prentice-Hall, 1967
60. Tolstoy L: The death of Ivan Ilych. In Great Short Works of Leo Tolstoy, pp 243–302. New York, Harper & Row, 1967
61. Tversky A, Kahnemann D: Framing of decisions and the psychology of choice. Science 211:453–458, 1981
62. Waitzkin H, Stoeckle JD: The communication of information about illness. Adv Psychosom Med 8:180–215, 1972
63. Weisman AD: Coping behavior and suicide in cancer. In Cullen JW, Fox BH, Isom RN (eds): Cancer: The Behavioral Dimension. New York, Raven Press, 1979
64. Weisman AD: Early diagnosis of vulnerability in cancer patients. Am J Med Sci 271:187–196, 1976
65. Weisman AD: On Dying and Denying. New York, Behavioral Publications, 1972
66. Weisman AD, Worden JW, Sobel HS: Psychosocial Screening and Intervention with Cancer Patients: Research Report. Boston, Project Omega, Massachusetts General Hospital, 1980
67. Wornham W: Death: The conspiracy of silence [news and notes]. J Med Ethics 2:46, 1976

Existential and Spiritual Concerns   8

Thomas Welch

> Not a week passes in the practice of the ordinary physician but he is consulted about one or more of the deepest problems in metaphysics and religion—not as a speculative enigma, but as part of human agony.
>
> Richard C. Cabot, 1918[2]

ILLNESS AS AN EXISTENTIAL AND SPIRITUAL CRISIS

Sickness disrupts the usual safety and order of a person's world. Often, serious illness is a person's first experience with severe helplessness and hopelessness. A terminal illness particularly threatens a basic sense of security. When one's world is turned upside down by the powerful presence of the threat of death, there is a pervading and chilling sense of powerlessness. Terminal illness can precipitate feelings of utter helplessness and overwhelming vulnerability, not only for the patient, but also for the family and others who are touched by the patient's dilemma.

Most people tend to picture death on an ever-distant horizon. While striving day-to-day to understand and properly guide their lives, they expect that age will bring the wisdom and perspective to make sense of everything in hindsight. The imminence of death puts a "deadline" on one's reckonings.

Everyone must die, yet terminal illness often comes as a surprise, somehow unexpected even by the elderly.

> *I always thought these things happened to other people. Now, I have to face the difficult and lonely fact that, for everyone else, I am that other person.*

Sickness is often seen as an unjust intrusion on one's life-plan. It is judged especially cruel when it comes to the young. They, by every standard of fairness, should have a full life. For the more elderly, illness affronts the expectations of a perfect retirement, when one finally gets to do all the things that were put off until later years.

Even persons who believe in and look forward to a wonderful afterlife are generally in no hurry to get there. The confrontation with the prospect of annihilation has been described as falling down a hole to a place of immediate and overwhelming terror. Each person's journey through this lonely time is his own. There are no road maps. And there is no turning back. "My family came around me right away when we found out about this cancer," shared one woman. "However, there was no comfort for that kind of fear." No one can calm the dread. Some patients feel so hopeless that they believe they cannot go on; thoughts of suicide may give a strange comfort.

RESPONDING TO THE CRISIS

The frantic feeling of free fall, as though one were floating helplessly into an abyss, is quieted by a variety of responses and adjustments. Gaining some measure of control seems to be the reflex. The person confronted with dying tries to understand what has happened and then, somehow, to make the best of it. Frankl suggests that such a "will to meaning" is a basic human drive, and cites Nietzsche's dictum, "He who has a *why* to live can bear with almost any *how.*"[3]

The physician's biomedical formulations—described by such familiar terms as etiology, pathophysiology, diagnosis, prognosis, treatment of choice—provide some sense of order and hope, and are accepted eagerly by most persons. The physician's assurance that all will be done medically to provide appropriate care is terribly important. In the search for meaning, however, the biomedical framework can be rather unsatisfying, especially when sickness and death are seen as simple "facts of life" for which there is no further explanation, let alone curative treatment. Thus, most patients (and their doctors) regularly develop nonscientific perspectives on illness, mingling technical medical explanations with personal viewpoints about the significance of a condition and about how one deals with it. Even with the common cold, patients tell a tale not only of the transmission of a virus, its action on the respiratory mucosa, the interplay of host defenses with the invading agent, the clinical manifestations, and their response to various treatments, but also of "not taking proper care of myself" or "going out when I shouldn't have," of sickness as "a warning" or "a sign" to reconsider values and behavior, of the personal meaning of a disrupted daily life—"being unable to do things as usual," "relying on others," and so on.

When the progression of disease is viewed as inexorable, and the prospect of annihilation presses into awareness, patients regularly seek further understanding and consolation from existential and spiritual viewpoints. Even if the end of life is viewed merely as a biological event, a heightened awareness of death intensifies familiar concerns about the meaning of life: What sense can I now find in my living as it has unfolded, and what can I make of life when it will all end in death? What endures? A host of existential and spiritual concerns surface and must be addressed: Why me? Is there a message or meaning to this illness? What sense can I make of my values and the purpose of living, now and in the future? If I am out of control, does someone hold the power? How can I maintain a sense of self-worth when so much of my body and life have changed? How can I come to terms with this transformation and find the strength to go on?

THE SEARCH FOR MEANING

> She says, "But in contentment I still feel
> The need of some imperishable bliss."
> Death is the mother of Beauty; hence from her,
> Alone, shall come fulfillment to our dreams
> And our desires.
>
> Wallace Stevens,
> "Sunday Morning" [1923][9]

The presence and the universality of the fear of death is what William James called "the worm at the core."[4] Man is unique in that he may live even his happiest day with an awareness of his mortality. Paradoxically, this characteristic is both a gift and a burden: a gift, in that man, unlike crawling life, is conscious and reflective; a burden, in that he anticipates death and feels terror. To rescue his life from the perceived meaningless of death, man has fashioned a larger context, or paradigm, out of which to live life and to assess its events.[1]

Patients often begin their search for meaning in a state of terror and helplessness. An awareness of terminal illness seems to precipitate crises in many areas of one's life and to force one to view differently all one's connections with the world. Patients seek answers to questions that may be deeply sensed yet unarticulated. Each person draws from available social, cultural, emotional, philosophical, theological, or spiritual resources to shed some light. Even those not accustomed to turning toward religion for help will search in that direction. As one elderly gentleman cried out, "This goddam disease makes you religious!"

In the broadest understanding, spirituality embodies one's sense of design, purpose, and meaning in the universe, one's sense of relationship to all things and events, inclusive of an ultimate power. It is as unique from person to person as is one's fingerprints, and is fashioned by organized religion, family traditions, life experiences, and intellectual, emotional, and spiritual capacities, as well as the needs of the moment. Spirituality also describes the degree of energy a person directs toward perceiving order and meaning in life, a quality that is regularly evoked by the confrontation with death. Exactly what do I believe? And, how can it help me? One patient commented, "As surgery and chemotherapy began to change my appearance, I knew I had to rearrange my priorities about what is really important in my life. I had better have more going for me than what shows on the outside."

Many persons recognize an ultimate power, a personal God who is present, affirming, and comforting. "God was important to me right away," stated one woman. "Maybe it sounds like a copout. But, I put a lot into God's hands. I figure that I will do my part to stay alive, like seeking treatment and taking care of myself. However, the final outcome I will leave to Him. It helps me a lot to let go of what I cannot control. I had to learn to do that. Yet to know that God is there is a great comfort to me." She suffered great emotional and spiritual pain along the course to this point in the development of her spirituality. However, she found what worked for her. "I could speak to Him in the middle of the night when I was most lonely," she said. "He could come into that space that no one else could bridge. I don't know what people without faith do at times like that."

Patients who are most comforted by their religion are usually those who feel rooted in a tradition and who share in its communal expression. Just as important as a sense of a nurturing, affirming God is a nurturing, affirming congregation that effectively expresses its concern for the ill person. Healing ceremonies, promises of prayers, and pastoral visits are sources of support as the patient is learning to cope with new terrors. In bereavement, such rituals as wakes, funerals, sitting shivah, visiting the grave, and observing anniversaries provide a structure that helps the bereaved get through a period of turmoil, while also facilitating mourning and mobilizing support.

Many persons who happen to be terminally ill have not chosen to participate in an organized religion or may not find notions of a personal God or an afterlife pertinent to their search for meaning. They may wish that they could have the consolation which others receive from faith, but they must rely on what has worked in the past to sustain their life. "My comfort comes from reading poetry," shared one young man. "I get a sense of my place in the flow of humanity. That helps me enormously." Many patients invoke such values as kindness, generosity, service, loyalty and duty, honesty, love, appreciation of nature or beauty, being strong, being responsible, accepting fate, or facing absurdity and nothingness. In contributions to work and community, and especially to family, the sick person often recognizes a sustaining sense of meaning and purpose.

The strength and value of existential and spiritual resources and other supports come under severe test from the very beginning of a fatal illness. C.S. Lewis learned from his own loss that

> You never know how much you really believe in anything until its truth or falsehood becomes a matter of life and death to you. It is easy to say that you believe a rope to be strong and sound as long as you are merely using it to cord a box. But suppose you had to hang by that rope over a precipice. Wouldn't you then first discover how much you really trusted it?[7]

And hanging over a precipice is what advanced cancer can feel like. In the face of this danger, and while everything is in transition, sorting out one's belief is no easy task. There is no safe place away from the prospect of death nor away from the life-changing effects of the disease. One's image of a healthy self fades under the strain of sickness, increasing dependence, and mounting anxiety. The world of one's relationships changes inevitably. Family ties may be enriched or may become stressed and exhausted. Some friendships become more intimate and helpful, others, strained and marginal. A series of explosions continues, finding new ways to jolt any freshly found supports. Coping becomes a process of finding a way to continue living while the rules are changing. There exists a soap-in-the-bathtub quality in the effort to find answers to the ultimate questions. When we are sure that we have a way of understanding mysteries, the answer slips off somewhere else, only to be discovered again.

EXISTENTIAL AND SPIRITUAL PAIN

Our dying is much like our living. Most patients and family members find some degree of equanimity or resolution as they face death, or at least do not seem greatly troubled by unanswered questions and unfinished business. For others, especially those whose lives have been marked by disappointment and unhappiness, or for whom death continues to seem like an unfair interruption or intolerable loss of control, the search for meaning can be a bitter, frustrating, or profoundly sad process. By whatever personal standards a person invokes, life can at times be viewed, in whole or part, as disappointment or failure.

Spirituality may be a source of conflict, and some believers in a personal God may derive little comfort from their faith. For instance, persons who have not practiced their spiritual beliefs diligently may have feelings of guilt when they turn to religion for strength in a crisis. Finding yourself on God's doorstep when the chips are down is like showing up at home only when you are short of cash. Even more troubling are those situations in which patients view their illness as God's punishment. People often perceive God as sending illness to them. For instance, one woman saw her cancer as divine retribution for an abortion she had had years earlier. "I thought God had evened the score by giving me this disease," she said. "Strangely, I found comfort in it because of my long-standing guilt. 'Well, that's fair,' I thought to myself. 'I've paid my dues.' But, now I have lung metastases. I can't see anything fair about this. It has gone too far."

The notion of an avenging God may contribute to feelings of guilt, rejection, hopelessness, and confusion and may inhibit a sense of any hopefulness about treatment or the quality of remaining life. Patients and families alike wonder about a God who supposedly is responsible for all this. Anger and disillusionment are quite common feelings in response to God's seeming unfairness. "I don't know what I did to deserve this. I have always lived a good life." Such people may express anger at God, or harbor hurt feelings for a long while. Family members commonly drop the practice of their religion. They are offended at what God "has done" or "allowed." "What good does it do to go to church," said one family member. They seem to believe that the living of a good life and the practicing of religion should immunize them against all harm, including disease, suffering, and death. Persons who see God as responsible for all life's events may behave like children in conflict with a parent. Their relationship with God may be loaded with ambivalence; their anger may engender guilt, or they may fear retribution for their feelings of resentment.

Spiritual pain thus compounds the stresses posed by the disease and its effect on the family. However, these moments can also be an opportunity for profound spiritual growth. "I don't know why one person gets sick, and another does not," shares Rabbi Harold Kushner, "But, I can only assume that some natural laws which we don't understand are at work."[6] This sort of statement may assist the patient in letting go of an unhelpful theology, and in expanding his or her sense of the ultimate power.

Illness can be viewed as a catalyst for improving the lives of others. At times, this altruistic interpretation seems a bit narcissistic. "Maybe God sent this cancer to me so that my husband will stop drinking," pondered one woman. "Maybe now he will see what he is doing. That makes sense, don't you think?" She continued to place herself in the role of a victim, thinking that God was striking her as a means of sending a message to her husband. As her husband's drinking continued, she needed to find a new way to understand her disease.

In another instance, a woman refused her pain medication even though she was experiencing a great deal of discomfort. She understood from her early religious training that the sufferings which she bore in this life would earn access to a heavenly reward. Suffering, by divine plan, was a way to rid oneself of eternal punishment for sin. Such an example illustrates how people sometimes bring limited theologies to critical moments in their lives. The patient's physician sensibly referred her to a chaplain who could help her find greater physical and spiritual comfort.

HOPE

No matter how one derives spiritual sustenance to nourish one's perception of life and all its events, there generally remains a strong investment in the moment and a wish for its continuance. Initially, biomedical technology provides the greatest promise: cure, full remission, prolonged survival, or palliation. Later, as the illness progresses, hope is more likely to be directed to feeling better, making the best of the moment, or appreciating a future beyond physical survival.

As the prospect for any physical cure is abandoned, some patients go through a crisis of trust in the ministrations of their physician. There seems to be a correlation between the intensity of the patient's anger toward the medical profession and the professional distance of the physician. "What are they all about?" questioned one woman, as her expectation of a good treatment outcome was not met. As the efforts of the health-care world appear powerless to reverse the course of the disease and to stay death, patients often become more reliant on their faith in God or on other spiritual beliefs. A stronger trust in God or a finer existential resolve can become the source of renewed strength.

In the pursuit of divine intervention, patients will participate in prayer rituals and healing services, enlisting and welcoming the support of others. Patients petition God's favor through private prayer, as well as by promise to become a better person. "I find these religious services very uplifting, even if no cure comes to me from them," shared one gentleman. "Religion has become very important to me." The intensification of religious fervor and practice may provide a feeling of wholeness and safety, of touching a power far beyond the limitation of earthly life. Important in the process of prayerful expression, and in a host of similar secular activities, is the feeling of doing something positive with regard to a frustrating situation.

Hope remains even when one is prepared to make acknowledgment of the inevitability of death. Something fortuitous may happen to improve and extend one's time. Many people retain some hope that God, fate, or advances in medical science may intervene at any moment to produce a miraculous cure. More important, the will to live reflects a strong reluctance to let go of everyone and everything that have become significant and meaningful in one's life. As one minister with cancer commented, "I keep feeling that I should have a better perspective on things. But my emotions get the best of me everytime. I keep fighting to stay in there." Most persons try to make the most of every remaining moment. "Life is so sweet," cried one woman. "I would do anything to live." Paradoxically, the dying person must at the same time finish all business, even say good-bye, lest death catch him or her unaware, with important tasks incomplete. Only when illness so diminishes the quality of one's existence that hoping for a longer life becomes senseless, do patients usually begin to speak seriously of letting go.

RECONCILIATION AND GROWTH

Spiritual and existential efforts to cope with disease can be viewed as measures to quiet the terror of death. Entering treatment and storming the portals of heaven with prayers are attempts, initially, to make it all go away. As the disease progresses, steps in the process of building a new security include facing the terror, exploring and sharing the feelings, sorting out beliefs, and participating in important rituals. From an existential or spiritual viewpoint, coping with advanced cancer is a process of reviewing, revising, enlarging and strengthening one's world view in order to accommodate and assimilate a new experience. Called into question are all the ultimate issues of life and death as one has perceived them to this point, and all the resources of one's personal religion as a way of addressing them. Kierkegaard described this period of crisis as "a school that provides man with the ultimate education, the final maturity. Only when he has confronted this terror of annihilation, the ultimate fear, can self-transcendence begin."[5]

Out of powerlessness often comes a sense of acceptance or of trust in a greater power. Patients begin to let go of a long-standing assumption that life will go on for them just as it always had. At that point, the world and one's place in it begins to feel different—rich in some ways, alien in others. Priorities begin to shift, and life becomes focused on what is clearly important. One woman called this her "gifts of cancer." Frankl writes about the "ultimate freedom" in adversity—"to choose one's attitude in any given set of circumstances."[3]

Patients often claim to have gained the most important insights in life through coping with their illness. "My time and my relationships are most important to me now," shared a cancer patient. Another reported, "My faith is more important to me now than ever before." The crisis of dying and the uncertainty of being ill become a vehicle for joy and thanksgiving, reconciliation and forgiveness; for renewed strength and faith; for a sense of personal control and responsibility; for a deepened awareness of beauty, of small joys, and fond memories; and an intensified appreciation of the meaning and power of love. "There is a more existential focus to my life now," shared another woman. "I don't dwell on the pains of the past, nor do I agonize over what tomorrow might bring. Being with those who are important to me is central. And, I have found another special friend as my self-esteem has grown—myself." Although cancer had clearly diminished part of her world, she became enriched emotionally and spiritually. As old boundaries are abandoned, new awareness and intimacies can emerge. "When I finally acknowledged my mortality, I wasn't afraid of dying. Or living," she added.

Metaphors are essential in conceptualizing the substance of one's faith. One patient likened her life and suffering to the making of a tapestry. "All I touch now are the ugly knots and loose strings of the reverse side," she said. "My trust in God encourages me to know that soon I'll see the beautiful image on the front side, woven from all the threads of my life. Then everything, even this, will make sense."

There comes about for many people an underlying and maturing sense of surviving the death of one's body. "Dying, in my best understanding, is that time when I take a leap of faith," shared one woman. "It is part of the free fall—like a trapeze artist high above the crowd who suddenly falls, and seemingly from nowhere, with split-second timing, his partner below swings out, reaches out, catches him, and saves him. That leap of faith is when I take my last conscious breath. In faith, I believe God will reach out and catch me." Less dramatically, survival is appreciated in good works and other contributions to family and society, in children, and in the memories held by friends and relatives.

THE PHYSICIAN'S ROLE

Patients can be helped in addressing their existential and spiritual concerns. The physician who respects the importance of such quests can readily support the patient in the personal search for meaning. Rather than offering answers or saying that "everything will work out all right," the clinician's role is to provide a forum for exploring concerns. New meanings evolve from "life-review," particularly from examining the realms of love, work, and play. The clinician, by making every effort to understand the patient's feelings during the difficult process of coping, at least does not add to the patient's isolation and, at best, initiates a precious thread of connection to a shaken soul. Henri Nouwen, a spiritual writer, comments:

> We can do much more for each other than we are often aware of. . . . The first and most important aspect of all healing is an interested effort to know the patients fully, in all their joys and pains, pleasures and sorrows, ups and downs, highs and lows which have given shape and form to their life and have led them through the years to their present situation. This is far from easy because not only our own but other people's pains are hard to face. Just as we like to reach our own destination through by-passes, we also like to offer advice, counsel and treatment to others without having really known fully the wounds that need healing.[8]

Rarely do patients spontaneously or directly share with their physicians the substantial emotional investment they have in the private practice of their religion. Patients may dutifully present themselves for treatment in anticipation of a positive outcome, while maintaining an elaborate system of prayerful petitions and expectations of divine favor. Patients may behave as though the effects of medical treatment and spiritual pursuits operate on different tracks. The integration of these separate lifelines occurs within the patient.

A sincere curiosity and nonjudgmental attitude will aid the clinician in appreciating how existential and spiritual concerns are experienced and acted upon by each patient. Usually, careful listening and a bit of questioning on the part of the physician will readily elicit from patients their personal perspective. In addition to reviewing some of the existential and spiritual questions stated above, the clinician might ask the following:

Do you pray?

What have you been saying in your prayers?

Do you participate in any formal religious activities?

What are they like?

How do you feel about them?

What role have some of these beliefs had in your understanding

About getting ill?

About getting help?

About having a fatal illness?

What helped you through past crises?

Where have you found strength and support?

Most patients seek out and find their own spiritual resources, but the physician may facilitate such a "referral." Just as the individual physician is viewed as embodying the healing powers of medicine and science, the clergy represent a larger reality, and their visits are important to patients, especially those who have been active members of a congregation. The encounter with the clergy may readily contribute to a sense of being valued and can provide an opportunity for patients to unburden themselves from the guilt of real or imagined transgressions. For some patients, the gesture of receiving forgiveness for failings in one's life is far-reaching in its effect and can bring a sense of well-being and wholeness even as one's physical condition deteriorates. Pastoral counseling or collaboration with clergy may soften the blow of a harsh theology or alleviate the guilt that alienates a patient from a potentially consoling spiritual viewpoint. The medical staff also has ample opportunity to facilitate meaningful rituals, including prayer and a variety of formal and informal ceremonies, which patients and families desire during illness and around the time of death.

CONCLUSION

Death makes us all aware of our powerlessness. Looking at the interface between powerlessness and control, we can become clearer about our limitations as care-givers. The illusion of control often makes us less anxious in the present, but we pay a price for its use over the long haul. No one enjoys feeling powerless, especially those who see their role as making things better. What many cancer patients learn, sometimes long before care-givers, is that in surrendering illusions of control, new strengths emerge. For many patients, also, comes the realization that only love is important.

REFERENCES

1. Becker E: The Denial of Death. New York, Free Press, 1973
2. Cabot RC: Training and Rewards of the Physician. Philadelphia. JB Lippincott, 1918
3. Frankl VE: Man's Search for Meaning: An Introduction to Logotherapy. New York, Simon & Schuster, 1962
4. James W: Varieties of Religious Experience: A Study in Human Nature. New York, Mentor, 1958
5. Kierkegaard S, cited in Becker E: The Denial of Death. New York, Free Press, 1973
6. Kushner HS: When Bad Things Happen to Good People. New York, Avon, 1981
7. Lewis CS: A Grief Observed. New York, Bantam Books, 1961
8. Nouwen HJM: Reaching Out. New York, Doubleday & Co, 1966
9. Stevens W: Sunday Morning. In The Collected Poems of Wallace Stevens, pp. 66–70. New York, Alfred A. Knopf, 1973

Helping the Children When a Parent Is Dying   9

Margaret Adams-Greenly
Rosemary T. Moynihan
Grace H. Christ
Harriet Slivka

> There are secrets in this family. I don't
> understand and I'm scared! I feel left out, like
> I'm not part of the family anymore.
>
> Carolyn, age 7

Carolyn's well-intentioned parents were overwhelmed with their own grief, and were uncertain about how to talk with her. They wanted to shield her from the painful knowledge of her mother's advancing lung cancer and impending death. Carolyn tells us that this silence is not protective and that, instead, she feels abandoned, alone, and frightened.

The terminal illness and death of a parent will profoundly affect the course of a child's life.[2] Parental loss during childhood may contribute to problems in interpersonal relationships and self-image, and to adult depression and mental illness.[3,5,9,10] Most of the professional literature in this area focuses on the bereaved child and describes intervention after the parent's death. In contrast, we have found it essential to work *preventively* with children and parents throughout the course of the illness in order to minimize later difficulties.

This chapter addresses a series of common questions: How does the physician guide parents in dealing with this sensitive subject? What are the common concerns of parents? How does one actually talk with a child? What should be said, and when? How does a child cope with everyday normal activities while a parent is dying? Should children attend funerals? What resources can the physician enlist as supports? The chapter begins with a discussion of age-related perceptions of illness and death, and then identifies six principles through which the physician can support the family and help the children when a parent is dying.

Portions of this chapter are reprinted, with permission, from an original article, copyright 1983 by the American Orthopsychiatric Association: Adams-Greenly M, Moynihan R: Helping the children of fatally ill parents. Am J Orthopsychiatry 53:219–229, 1983.

AGE-RELATED PERCEPTIONS OF ILLNESS AND DEATH

A child's ability to understand the serious illness and death of a parent changes with age.[8] Some appreciation of this developmental process is essential in order to communicate effectively with the child.

The Preschool Child

Key issues to bear in mind when dealing with preschool children are their lack of abstract thinking about death, their fear of separation, and their concern with guilt.

Children in this age-group are concrete in their thinking, and fantasy plays an important role in their mental lives.[14] They attribute life processes and consciousness to the dead and see death as " a living on under changed circumstances."[13] They may be able to articulate that a person is dead and is buried, but exploration will usually reveal that they wonder what that person eats or whether a dead person is afraid to be in the dark underground.[11,12] They usually think that death is reversible and may feel angry with a dead person for not returning.

It is important to be mindful of one's words and images in talking with children in this age-group. To say that a dead person is "sleeping" may make preschool children fearful of sleep. Likewise, although religious beliefs may comfort someone older, young children may be quite confused by the idea of heaven, and fear that they are being watched. They may feel angry with a God who is presented as loving, but whom they perceive as someone who takes people away and makes others cry, seemingly at His own whim.[7]

The fear of separation is extremely important in this age-group,[6,7] because of their great dependency on their parents. These children perceive their parents as strong and invincible and are alarmed to find that illness and death are more powerful.[1] They may experience even a short separation as an abandonment, to which they may respond with anger, regression, or withdrawal.

Because these youngsters are developing a conscience and may feel unrealistically responsible for events in their lives, they need much reassurance that illness and death are not a result of their negative thoughts, feelings, wishes, or actions. Similarly, they need to know that their positive feelings and good behavior will not make a sick person well again:

> When her mother was hospitalized, Betty (age 3) thought that Mommy had moved to another home. She wondered why Mommy wanted to live in the other home, and concluded that it was because she (Betty) had been bad.

The School-Age Child

Key issues to bear in mind when dealing with school-age children are their expanding intellect, their need for academic success, and their awareness of the social order.

As children grow through the school years and become more intellectually oriented, their capacity for abstract thinking expands.[6] Thus, at the younger end of this age-group, in which thinking is still somewhat concrete, children may personify death in terms of the devil, a monster, a skeleton, or an angel; they tend to perceive death as frightening and dangerous.[12]

Children over the age of 8, however, are able to have a more realistic concept of death as the cessation of the body's functions.[11] They are concerned with the process of dying and the possibility of pain and suffering.[12]

When illness occurs, these children use the age-appropriate defense of intellectualization; they attempt to cope by understanding.[6] Because they are oriented to school, books, and academic mastery, they may research an illness and develop an out-dated or incorrect perception of it. Thus, they must be kept well-informed.

Children in this group are increasingly involved as members of society through their participation in school, clubs, teams, and religious groups. Accordingly, they become interested in the culture and rituals associated with illness and death and need to be involved with them in order to sustain their sense of the social order.[12]

Although these children are maturing rapidly, the stress of a parent's illness may overwhelm them emotionally so much that their ability to cope may be impaired. Because of their involvement outside the home, difficulties may be manifested in several areas. Symptoms of school refusal, daydreaming, somatization, and conflicts with peers or teachers all may indicate difficulties in coping; a referral for mental-health intervention may be indicated in these situations:

> Jordan, age 6, whose parents both have cancer, was disruptive and argumentative in the classroom. Earlier, he had told his teacher that he had just lost his first tooth. She had said, "That's nice" and turned away. Jordan later admitted to the social worker that he felt unimportant and that his disruptiveness was an attempt to get attention.

> Eleven-year-old Louise, a talented gymnast, broke her arm in a fall while performing a stunt she had been warned against by her coach. Her angry defiance of the coach's instructions and the subsequent harming of herself were understood as a cry for more limits, structure, and support from the mother who was preoccupied with caring for her very sick husband and had not attended Louise's recent competitions.

The Adolescent

Key issues to bear in mind when dealing with adolescents are their developmentally normal conflicts with their parents, their intense moodiness, and their concern with preserving normal life activities.

The adolescent is able to use well-developed abstract thinking about illness and death. Whereas the school-age child understands the cessation of the body's functions, he will usually perceive that as a result of something external such as an accident, murder, or sudden illness. The adolescent, in contrast, understands internal processes such as old age, deterioration, and chronic illness, and realizes that everyone must die of something.[12] Just as the adolescent has a greater awareness of the future than the younger child, he also has a greater appreciation of the past; when losing a parent, the adolescent may experience a fuller, more adult sense of the loss and its meaning.

It is not only normal and appropriate, but necessary, for adolescents to struggle with their feelings about dependence and independence related to their parents. Most adolescents undergo a process of separation from, and sometimes devaluation of, their parents and their values. This normal process is profoundly affected by the potential or real loss of a parent.[7] The adolescent may feel guilty about his rejection of the parents or his anger at their restrictions of his freedom. His conflicts about dependence/independence naturally result in some ambivalence. He may attempt to cope with this ambivalence by "splitting"—overidealizing the dead or dying parent and directing increasing hostility toward the surviving parent.[15]

Adolescence is a time of stormy emotions and strong moods. Intense experiences may be alarming to an adolescent, who feels overwhelmed by emotions. Sometimes this results in an inability to cry, an inner emptiness of feeling, since tears would be so overwhelming that the adolescent would feel like a helpless child.[15] Sometimes the adolescent is unable to cope internally with his upset, and so he puts it into some action, such as truancy, experimentation with drugs or sexuality, or stealing.[4] Such "acting out" may express a need to be noticed, to be punished, or (in the case of stealing) to be given to. And, lastly, some adolescents ward off intense emotions by trying to recapture good moods, as if to say "If I don't feel bad, then nothing bad has happened."

Adolescents often value their roles as young adults in the family, and are pleased with the opportunity to help manage situations. They are capable of assuming considerable responsibility. Caution must be exercised to ensure that this burden is not too great, and that these adolescents have time to maintain normal aspects of their lives. It is extremely important for them to feel accepted by the peer group, to feel a sense of belonging, and to conform to group standards of appearance and behavior. At the same time, their maturity and concern for their role in the family may create unnecessary conflict:

> Fifteen-year-old Frank desperately wanted to have a date for the school dance, but chastised himself for being selfish. He felt guilty for thinking of himself when his mother was sick, although his mother was in stable condition and Frank would not be needed at home.

> Seventeen-year-old Beth lay awake at night worrying about quitting school and getting a job to support the family in the event of her father's death. In fact, the family's finances were in excellent condition, and Beth's father had planned for the security of the family as well as Beth's educational needs.

Needs of All Children

In addition to understanding age-related perceptions of illness and death, it is important to recognize the basic needs of children of all ages who are facing the loss of a parent: (1) information that is clear and comprehensible to them, (2) a feeling of being involved and important, (3) help in understanding the grief of adults around them, (4) respect and acknowledgment of their own thoughts and feelings, (5) maintenance of age-appropriate interests and activities, and (6) reassurance that they will not be abandoned. With an understanding of these needs and of the developmental issues, the physician can intervene effectively in helping families cope with the terminal illness and death of a parent.

PRINCIPLES OF SUPPORT

Working Collaboratively with the Parents

The physician plays a primary role in helping parents feel comfortable accepting the assistance of a mental-health practitioner. The physician's approval gives sanction to this involvement and integrates the emotional and physical aspects of care. It may be helpful for the physician and social worker to meet together with the parents at intervals.

Most parents strive to provide the optimal emotional environment for their children but, like the parents of young Carolyn, may become misguided because of their own fear and sadness. Parents should be approached with respect for their need to feel competent and in control of their children's lives and without implicit criticism. An ideal approach focuses on family strengths, supporting rather than usurping the parents' role.

The parents' sense of psychological competency can be strengthened by providing suggestions for their conversations and play with the child. Informal role-playing or discussions can provide helpful ideas and preparation for talking with the child. Children's books and games often provide an entrée to discussions and review of the child's experience of the illness. Previous losses (*e.g.*, of pets) can be reviewed.

Many parents are helped by being given books that provide them with some intellectual mastery over their situation. One parent, who was completing her master's degree in clinical psychology, reflected this need clearly when she said, "I know what to do to help a 3 year old. I just need to hear it again for my own child. It makes our experience more real." Some suggestions of helpful books for parents, as well as books for the children themselves, are provided at the end of this chapter.

We have found three areas of psychological knowledge that are important to share with parents.

First, the well parent should be helped to know that the child's experience of loss is not the same as his or her own; their respective relationships with the sick person are quite different prior to the illness, and remain so throughout. The parent is losing a spouse—a lover, friend, companion, and partner; the child is losing a parent—a nurturer, a protector, an idol. Parents may need help to recognize the unique situation of the child:

> Jill and Tim were the well-educated, competent young parents of 3-year-old Sarah. They faced Tim's long hospitalizations and pending death with great sadness. A close family, they wanted to include Sarah in their complete experience of separation and loss. At one point, when Sarah hugged Tim, he clutched her to himself, sobbing. She became anxious, frightened, and angry; it was clear that, as a 3-year old, she could not bear the intensity of her parents' grief. Clinging together and crying was something the parents needed to do with each other; Sarah needed to cry at times, but also to be herself, a playful little girl with a short attention span and a limited understanding of long-term illness and death.

Some parents may be hindered in appreciating how their children's experiences differ from their own. This may especially be true if there is a personal history of early unresolved loss or separation. For such parents, the projection of their own childhood experiences may interfere and distort their perceptions now of their children's needs. In these instances, a referral to a mental-health practitioner is indicated.

Second, most parents wish to protect their children from emotional pain. Painful feelings, however, are not only normal but inevitable when a child experiences a loss. Parents are relieved to be told that, although they cannot protect the child from difficult emotions, they can help the child to bear them. We emphasize that the parents are the source of greatest warmth, consistency, and proper information for the child. Children will be better able to tolerate painful feelings when they are able to express these feelings in a supportive climate.

> Thirteen-year-old Kim, looking through photographs of her very sick father taken prior to his illness, exclaimed, "I can't believe it! He was always so strong; he told me he was young and could do anything he wanted. It's not fair!" Kim's outrage at the injustice of her father's fate was difficult for her family to appreciate and required an understanding, empathic, and reassuring response.

Children can better cope with traumatic situations when a parent recognizes and accepts their reactions and feelings. For instance, saying, "I'm crying because I'm sad," or "Everyone feels angry when someone we love is sick," may serve to validate the child's experience and help a youngster feel understood.

Finally, at times, parents need reaffirmation of simple facts about the comprehension and expectations of a child. First, children have shorter attention spans than adults, and too much can be expected of them. Second, children need routine in order to feel secure; it may be very important that even such small items as a breakfast cereal or a juice cup remain the same. Third, children need reassurance that, although the situation is serious, they will not be abandoned and their needs will be met. Fourth, children of all ages regress under stress. Such regression is generally temporary and will reverse when the child again feels secure. Rather than focusing on the regressive behavior itself, the parents are advised to provide greater attention and support for the child.

Providing Age-Appropriate Information

Consultation with parents on how information can be provided to a child begins with a discussion of growth and development and with assistance in assessing the child's cognitive abilities. Bearing in mind the issues discussed earlier, a plan for information-sharing can then be developed. We advise parents that they begin their conversations with the child's own thoughts and observations. They can then acknowledge the child's perception, put it into words, and elaborate upon it, clarifying misconceptions. For children of all ages, explanations should be simple, but honest and clear, and based on the child's own experiences:

> A family of siblings, ages 8, 11, and 15, was discussing their mother's disoriented and confused mental status after surgery. Upset but inquisitive, the 8-year-old girl wondered tearfully if this is what it meant to be crazy. A clear, simple explanation was given to her about the side-effects of anesthesia and strong pain medication. It was also emphasized that the mother's mind was still the same as it always had been and that they would be able to talk with her when the medication wore off. They then discussed ways that they could comfort her. Deeply concerned that she had caused her mother's illness, the 15-year-old girl confessed that she felt she brought home germs from her work as a hospital volunteer. She was helped by reassurance that the cause of cancer was unknown and that many people work in hospitals and do not get sick.

> In another situation, the father of 5- and 10-year-old boys was rushed to the hospital and diagnosed with leukemia after a profuse nosebleed that occurred suddenly at home. Drawing on his own experience, the 5 year old was reminded that when people get cut, they usually bleed for a moment, but then stop. He was told that his father had a serious problem, that his blood was not strong enough to do this, and that he would need to see the doctor often to get special medicines to make it stronger. It was emphasized that, although his father had been angry with him just before the nosebleed, this was not the cause of it. The older boy was told the diagnosis and was helped by gaining an intellectual understanding of blood cells and how they worked; he then did a project for school on new developments in the treatment of leukemia.

Arranging Visits When the Parent is Hospitalized

Excluding children from the hospital does not protect them; rather, it may foster feelings of abandonment or the development of frightening fantasies. Children will not be overwhelmed by seeing a sick parent if they have received adequate preparation and support. Simple and specific explanations of what the child will see can lessen fear. Equipment and machines should be discussed in terms of the helpful role they play (*e.g.,* "The tube in Daddy's arm gives him water because he feels too sick to drink," or "The tube in Mommy's nose goes down to her stomach and takes out the sick stuff so she won't throw up"). Equipment such as intravenous tubing, a syringe, gauze, and other supplies can be given to children, so that they become familiar and comfortable with the hospital environment. An opportunity to examine equipment also helps elicit questions and concerns. The child should be encouraged to be physically close to the parent when possible; sitting on the bed, touching, and hugging help to normalize the situation and make it less awesome. After the visit, the child can draw a picture about it, which may serve to further elaborate and clarify the experience, and resolve any misinformation or fears. Emphasize that the sick parent does not want to be away from the child and is hospitalized only because of necessity.

The conduct of the visit must take into account the age of the child, the acuity of the parent's condition, and sociocultural factors. Some options we have developed are illustrated in the five case vignettes that follow:

> Four-year-old Ben was not allowed into the intensive care unit to see his mother because she was undergoing a complicated, lengthy procedure. He was brought to the waiting room where he drew a picture to be put on the wall by her bed. Afterward, he reported to his nursery school class that his mommy was very, very sick, but that his picture would make her feel happy. Ben met his mother's doctor and nurse who assured him that she missed him and that they were taking good care of her.

> Three-year-old Emily visited her sick father in the social worker's office, surrounded by toys and a space for playing. She examined him with a medical kit and diagnosed him to be well. She then had dinner with him in his room and scolded him for not being at home to play with her.

> Three children, ages 6, 4, and $2\frac{1}{2}$, from a very sheltered and unsophisticated family and likely to be quite overwhelmed by the hospital floor, visited their very sick father in a corner of the lobby. Although warm and close-knit, this family was not psychologically oriented and had never emphasized verbal communication. The unstructured arrangement for the visit allowed family life to proceed as usual. The children played together, near the father, and at times included him in their activity or comments. He spoke little, but smiled and clearly enjoyed being near them. Before leaving, they drew pictures of him which demonstrated, without words, that they understood quite well how sick he was. They then pushed him in his wheelchair around the lobby, and told him that they wished he was home.

> A family of older children, ages 9, 11, 13, and 15 met with the social worker and physician prior to seeing their mother. They were given information, and then discussed their discomfort and apprehension about the visit. They were asked to help the staff understand their mother better—to tell what her likes and dislikes were and how she could be more comfortable. Throughout the

mother's 4-month hospitalization, the children were seen together in what they called "planning meetings," and used the sessions to discuss the hospitalization, as well as concerns about life at home. After each meeting, the children reported on their progress to the parents who, in turn, were proud of the younger family members' ability to adapt.

A 7-year-old girl, an only child whose father was dead, visited her dying mother weekly at her hospital bedside. She played on and around the bed and shared school papers and tests to show how well she was doing. After each visit there was a play-therapy session with her mother's social worker, during which she drew pictures of the visit and discussed her anger, fears, and sadness. These sessions continued after her mother's death until the child was adopted by family members living at a distance. A referral was then made for ongoing psychological help.

Interpreting Progressive Deterioration

As the parent becomes sicker, he or she may be hospitalized more frequently and for longer periods; if able to stay home, he or she may sleep more, be more withdrawn, become thinner, weaker, and so on. It is important for the physician and well parent to continue talking with the child about these changes; otherwise, he or she may not be aware of them or may develop mistaken ideas about their cause. As with the provision of information about the diagnosis, the interpretation of progressive disease must first address what the child can observe:

> Have you noticed that your Mommy sleeps more than she used to? Well, that's because her sickness is making it harder for her body to keep working, so she's getting weaker and more tired.

Clarify that sickness is the cause for change in behavior and activity, not anything the child has thought, said, or done. The well parent may be quite overwhelmed during this phase and may vacillate in his or her ability to deal directly with the children. Work to support this parent's relationship with the children and with the ill spouse. Encourage the well parent to accept help from family, friends, and neighbors, so that he or she is not carrying all the burden of managing a home, a family, and the care of a sick spouse.

When there is a major body change in the patient, such as might be caused by radical surgery or a dramatic weight loss, children may have difficulty integrating their perceptions with their previous knowledge of the parent. Discuss the children's fears and reassure them that this person is still their parent, who loves them and wants to see them. Reassure the children that, although the patient is quite ill, their own needs will continue to be met.

In interpreting progressive disease, parents should be cautioned not to use the word "dying" too soon with young children who have a limited concept of time and may expect the death to occur the next day, rather than in a matter of months:

> When 6-year-old Francine's mother was initially diagnosed with a malignant tumor, Francine understood that her parent had a serious illness, but that everyone hoped for improvement with an operation and medication. The mother did get better, returned home, and resumed her normal life until 8 months later, when she developed a recurrence. Her condition steadily deteriorated over the next 3 months. Francine was first told that her mother was

"sicker," then "much sicker," then "so sick that, even though the doctors were doing everything they could, no one was sure it would help," and finally "so sick that she won't get better." At each of these points, Francine's questions were answered until she was ready to hear, "Yes, Mommy's going to die soon, but we will take care of her and be right here with her."

When a parent is dying, the interpretation of progressive disease should also provide some help to the children in knowing what to do. They may have difficulty deciding when to visit the hospital or the sickroom at home, what they should talk about to the parent, how much housework they should do, or whether to continue social activities and sports. In general, as many routines of family life as possible should be maintained through the chronic phase of progressive disease (e.g., meal times, school attendance and activities, etc.). When the situation becomes more acute or death is imminent, however, the children should be informed and involved. They may need to be told that now is the right time to visit; otherwise, should the parent die suddenly, they may feel guilty that they did not spend meaningful time with the ill parent in his or her last days.

Dealing with the Death and Funeral

The surviving parent should inform the children of the death in person as quickly as possible and in simple terms. Questions must be answered, sometimes repeatedly, until the children understand what has happened. Their emotional reactions should be tolerated and acknowledged, not suppressed.

As previously stated, when adults are able to provide a sense of order and to recognize distressing feelings as appropriate, children are better able to cope with emotional trauma. Children of any age need to learn about and understand their feelings of loss. They need reassurance that these painful feelings are normal and that someday they will still be able to remember the parent without it hurting as much. They need to know that the parent loved them and did not want to leave them:

> After her father's death, 3-year-old Janie remarked sadly, "I wish he hadn't gone away." Her 6-year-old sister, looking at the mother for support, angrily exclaimed "Don't say that! He didn't go away! He died. People go away because they want to, but they can't help it if they die."

Likewise, children need reassurance that there will be changes, but that life will go on. They should be reassured that, although the surviving parent is sad and upset, he or she is very strong and will be able to take care of the children. Children should not be sent away; this can only increase fears of abandonment and unrealistic fantasies about what has happened:

> Rachel told her 4-year-old daughter, Molly, "Something very sad happened today. You know that Daddy has been very sick. Well, he was so sick that he got weaker and weaker until finally his heart just could not work anymore, and he died." When Molly asked when he would come home, Rachel said, "He won't come home. When people die, they don't come back, " and, in simple terms, Rachel explained the funeral and burial. Molly then asked again when he would come back, and was told, "When someone dies, his heart and his lungs, and his legs don't work anymore, and he cannot come back." Molly declared that she wanted him to come home, and Rachel responded, "I feel very sad. We will miss Daddy very much, and we will think

of him often, but we will not see him again." Molly, understanding, then said, "You mean, he's never coming back?" She burst into tears and allowed Rachel to comfort her. Later when she asked if they would still be able to go to Disney World, Rachel said, "Yes, you and I will still do many things. We will miss Daddy, but I will take good care of you and me. We will be okay."

Children need to feel included. Rituals such as wakes and funerals help them to structure their experience and decrease their anxiety. All children should be involved in the proceedings to the extent that they are comfortable:

Five-year-old Sam went to the wake, but did not want to go to the funeral. He stayed at home with his grandmother and made sandwiches for the others to eat when they returned.

Three-year-old Betty went to the funeral because she wanted to see and hear what people would say about her mother. Someone was available to take her outside to play when she was made anxious by many people crying.

Seven-year-old Cheryl chose her own special bouquet to accompany her father's casket.

Twelve-year-old Ben played his drum at his mother's grave.

A group of older siblings (ages 12, 14, and 16) took turns telling stories about their father and led the family in a prayer.

Sixteen-year-old Janine wrote a poem, which she read, tearfully but proudly, at her mother's funeral.

Providing Follow-Up Contact

Following the funeral, questions will arise, and references to the dead parent will be made repeatedly. Young children may maintain the belief that the parent will return, while children of all ages struggle to understand what the loss will mean in their lives:

Four-year-old Michelle confided, "My mommy called last night. She said she would be home for my birthday." Her father responded, "We both *wish* that mommy would come home, and it's so hard to believe that she really won't," and comforted her.

Five-year-old Frank asked, "What will I do now about Mother's Day?"

Seven-year-old Judy asked, "What will happen now to my Daddy's bed? Will someone else sleep in it?"

Eight-year-old Suzanne commented, "It's like being in a jigsaw puzzle that will always have one piece missing."

A group of older siblings (ages 10, 13, and 15) were discussing their family makeup. The oldest boy said, "I'm the family comedian!" His two sisters chimed in, respectively, "I'm the scholar" and "I'm the athlete." When asked about their father they said, "Dad—oh, Dad is the bricks and the steel." And, when asked what role their deceased mother had had they commented sadly, "Mom—she was the cement."

Such questions and comments are often very stressful for the surviving parent, who is repeatedly confronted with his or her own loss. However, encouragement for such expressions will help the children sort out their experience.

A follow-up appointment with the surviving parent and children provides an opportunity for them to gain perspective on their experience and for the physician and social worker to assess how they are coping. Goals for such an appointment might include the following:

1. Briefly reviewing the parent's illness
2. Stating, simply, why the parent died
3. Reiterating that illness and death are no one's fault
4. Reviewing the children's roles during the illness, with emphasis on how much they meant to the parent, how helpful they were, etc.
5. Eliciting the children's current questions and concerns
6. Ascertaining the presence or absence of psychological symptoms (*i.e.*, sleeping or eating problems, difficulties at school, difficulty with concentration, nightmares, bedwetting, family fighting, and other changes in behavior)
7. Commenting on the strengths of the family, while at the same time, acknowledging that this is a difficult time for any family
8. Leaving the door open for more discussion in the future

During the follow-up contact, the surviving parent should be alerted that the children may need to test the limits of their new situation and may also be resentful of changes. A period of adjustment must be allowed. At the same time, familial and social expectations of appropriate behavior and responsibility must continue, providing a supportive structure for the child's mourning. The surviving parent should be in close contact with the child's school, allowing for a collaborative effort in helping the child to adjust. The assistance of the pediatrician and clergy may also be helpful.

At the follow-up appointment, surviving parents find it helpful to talk about the effects of the spouse's death on *themselves* as well as on their parenting role. The children will now depend even more on this parent to meet both physical and emotional needs, even though the parent is depleted by his or her own grief and may have less energy to give. Parents need recognition of the importance of their own mourning and of their own return to the normal activities of life. The mental health of the surviving parent is crucial in helping the children, and he or she may need or want counseling separate from them. Sleeping and eating difficulties, a decline in work performance, increased use of alcohol or drugs, and difficulty managing household routines may all indicate greater-than-normal adjustment problems.

At the time of follow-up, an assessment can be made of the desirability of a referral for ongoing counseling or psychotherapy for the surviving parent, the children, or the family as a whole. Many of the psychological symptoms mentioned above are part of normal bereavement and may last a year or two. The presence of severe or multiple symptoms for more than 1 month may indicate a need for early referral, especially if academic or work performance is jeopardized. Mild, but prolonged behavioral and emotional disturbances also suggest the need for referral. Many families, however, undergo a process of appropriate and normal grieving with no further intervention.

AFTERWORD

Children will continue to deal with the loss of a parent many times in their lives as they move through normal developmental levels: school-age children, concerned with fitting in, will feel that their family is different from others; adolescents may be without a sexual role model; young adults may unconsciously search for the lost parent in their struggle to find a close and lasting relationship; and adults may have children of their own who remind them of the lost parent. The parent will be remembered at celebrations, at times of success and failure, and when there are other losses.

The pain of losing a parent cannot be avoided, but children can be helped to cope with loss when their experiences are structured throughout the course of the illness, and when they are provided with careful attention to their perceptions and individual needs. Grief is an arduous and painful process, but it can be eased by anticipatory measures designed to prepare children for the future and foster their long-term mental health.

REFERENCES

1. Anthony S: The Child's Discovery of Death. New York, Harcourt, Brace, Jovanovich, 1940
2. Barnes M: Reactions to the death of a mother. Psychoanal Study Child 19:339–357, 1961
3. Beck A, Sethi B, Tuthill R: Childhood bereavement and adult depression. Arch Psychiatry 9:295–302, 1963
4. Bonnard A: Truancy and pilfering associated with bereavement. In Leonard S, Schneer H (eds): Adolescents: Psychoanalytic Approach to Problems and Therapy. New York, Dell, 1961
5. Deutsch H: The absence of grief. Psychoanal 6:12–22, 1937
6. Erickson E: Childhood and Society. New York, Norton, 1950
7. Furman E: A Child's Parent Dies. New Haven, Yale University Press, 1974
8. Furman R: Death and the young child: Some preliminary considerations. Psychoanal Study Child 19:321–333, 1964
9. Hilgard G, Newman M, Eisle F: Strength of adult ego following childhood bereavement. Am J Orthopsychiatry 30:788–798, 1960
10. Jacobson E: The return of the lost parent. In Schur M (ed): Drives, Affects, and Behavior, vol 2. New York, International Universities Press, 1965
11. Koocher G: Talking with children about death. Am J Orthopsychiatry 44:404–411, 1974
12. Lonetto R: Children's Conceptions of Death. New York, Springer, 1980
13. Nagy M: The child's theories concerning death. J Genet Psychol 73:3–27, 1948
14. Piaget J: The Child's Conception of the World. Patterson NJ, Littlefield, Adams & Co, 1960
15. Wolfenstein M: How is mourning possible? Psychoanal Study Child 33:593–620, 1966

SUGGESTED READINGS

I. For the Professional

Aradine CR: Books for children about death. Pediatrics 57:372–378, 1976
Cook S: Children and Dying: An Exploration and a Selective Professional Bibliography. New York, Health Sciences, 1973
Furman E: A Child's Parent Dies. New Haven, Yale University Press, 1974
Rudolph M: Should the Children Know? Encounters with Death in the Lives of Children. New York, Schocken Books, 1978

II. For the Parent

Agee J: A Death in the Family. New York, Bantam, 1971
Grollman EA: Talking About Death: A Dialogue Between Parent and Child. Boston, Beacon Press, 1976
Stein SB: About Dying: An Open Family Book for Parents and Children Together. New York, Walker & Co, 1974

III. For the Child

Alcott LM: Little Women. New York, Grossett & Dunlap, 1947 (adolescence)

Brown MW: The Dead Bird. New York, Young Scott Books, 1958 (preschool)

Lee V: The Magic Moth. New York, Seabury Press, 1972. (school-age and older)

LeShan E: Learning to Say Goodbye. New York, Macmillan, 1976 (school-age and older)

Miles M: Annie and the Old One. Boston, Little, Brown & Co, 1971 (school-age)

Viorst J: The Tenth Good Thing About Barney. New York, Athenum, 1971 (preschool, early school)

White EB: Charlotte's Web. New York, Harper & Row, 1952 (school-age and older)

Hospice-in-the-Home

Part Three

Why Dying People and Their Families Seek Home Care   10

INTRODUCTION—THE HOSPITAL VANTAGE

For many sick persons and their families, home care offers distinct advantages over institutional care.[4] These advantages may assume greater poignancy when death is imminent, when concerns about the quality of existence in the remaining time gain ascendancy over efforts to cure illness or prolong life.

During the past century in the United States, the management of advanced cancer and terminal illness has increasingly been carried out in institutions. In one Ohio county, for instance, a review of death certificates between 1957 and 1974 indicated that home deaths dropped from 30% to 15% over the course of the study period, and nursing home deaths increased from 7% to 20%, while the proportion of hospital deaths remained stable around 60%.[2]

The institutionalization of dying is a reflection of many societal changes, including the development and widespread acceptance of high-technology modern medicine, the trend toward small mobile "nuclear" families, the relative aging of the population, and the emerging reliance on social institutions in all facets of personal life. A more immediate factor that discourages outpatient management of advanced cancer is a bias against home care among health professionals. Doctors and nurses occasionally act as if good medical care is possible only in an institution. Discharge from the hospital is often equated with giving-up—"nothing more can be done." Also, ironically, death is often viewed as a medical problem, which should occur only under expert supervision.

The professional bias against outpatient management reflects well-meaning paternalism, a certain degree of arrogance, and a lack of training and experience in caring for severe illness at home. Physicians often do not appreciate that well-supported laypersons are able to provide competent care, or that good medical and nursing supervision can be offered in the community. Moreover, the traditional importance of the family in caring for and protecting its members may be overlooked.

Compounding the hospital personnel's lack of exposure to good medical care in the home are their inevitable encounters with the failures of home-based care—patients who are sent out into the community without adequate planning or support, or whose condition changes so that they require institutional management. The readmission of such patients seems to prove that hospital care is better. In fact, high-quality medical care can be delivered at home when adequate supports are available. Severely ill patients who are eager to leave the hospital will often show marked improvement at home: lessening of pain and of other distressing symptoms; an elevated mood and enhanced sense of well-being; improvement in appetite and fluid intake; and greater alertness and participation in the world about them.

Health professionals also tend to overlook the discomfort, unhappiness, overt disease, and other "necessary inconveniences" caused by institutional care itself. Hospitalized patients are at great risk for significant iatrogenic illness—falls, accidents, drug reactions and errors, infections, and psychiatric decompensation.[3,5] Iatrogenic discomfort and unhappiness also deserve attention. For instance, hospital physicians routinely order disagreeable intravenous therapy to "maintain hydration" or to "ensure minimal caloric intake," without asking whether the treatment will add to the patient's comfort or quality of life, and whether it will be worth the physical distress, worry, or need to remain under close professional supervision.

Finally, regardless of concerns about the quality of technical services provided at various sites of care, home-based management meets the personal needs of many patients and families facing the terminal phase of an illness. Health-care professionals in acute care institutions focus their attention on the medical goals of specific diagnosis and treatment (e.g., finding the exact cause of a chest pain, keeping the serum potassium level just right, operating to correct a blocked ureter). Such goals are appropriate for most patients, but may hold less importance for the terminally ill. Moreover, when these medical goals are pursued rigidly, some of the major concerns of the dying patient and family—such as, enjoying a limited life span in a comfortable and a personally meaningful fashion—may be overlooked.

The intense sense of comfort that many sick persons find at home is difficult to appreciate without attending to patients there. This chapter attempts to give voice to such personal values by outlining a number of overlapping reasons for being at home with advanced cancer. The reader who is familiar with the advantages of home care will be better able to appreciate the patient's and family's concerns and to help them articulate and evaluate their personal goals in conjunction with usual medical goals.

ADVANTAGES OF THE HOME

Avoidance of Institutional Care

Frank hostility to institutional care often overshadows any positive feelings about being at home. Many patients feel assaulted in the hospital. They may go home simply in order to be left alone. They want to flee blood tests, waiting for x-rays, being awakened early in the morning for a rectal temperature, strange beds and unfamiliar roommates, and spending long, eerie nights listening to moaning down the hall or to muffled voices in the nursing station.

Patients may feel neglected in the hospital. Tales of long waits for a nurse to answer the call-buzzer are legion. Patients complain that they are treated impersonally. Similarly, doctors and nurses often report that they are too busy to "really sit down and talk" with dying patients, an admission that confirms the priority they give to technical tasks over emotional support. In the hospital, the sick person is one of many patients. A loved one becomes "Mrs. Smith, the cancer in 313," identified by a wristband. At their worst, hospitals seem to dehumanize people, reducing them to faceless, nameless slots in a smoothly functioning machine. Many features of daily life—the meals, the decor of the room, the patient's clothes, the time to go to bed— are determined by the institution. Sometimes lacking are the human relationships that help the sick person feel "special." Such ongoing personal connections reassure dying people that they are valued, that they are not being written off as hopeless, and that they will still be cared for as the illness progresses, and remembered after death.

Such reasons for getting away from the hospital are mirrored in the following reasons for wanting to be at home.

Physical Comfort and Privacy

The home setting can promote the patient's physical comfort. A familiar bed and a favorite chair or couch replace a hospital bed. The patient is surrounded by pleasing photographs and paintings, by treasured trophies and souvenirs. Food is cooked especially for the patient by family members who understand his or her tastes. A favorite main course or dessert is prepared. Meals are served fresh and hot.

While British hospices have favored open wards, which allow patients and families to support each other and to witness the serenity of another's death, many persons resent having sick and noisy strangers as roommates. Even patients who go home to a bustling household where their bed is placed in the living room may view the home as quieter and more private than the hospital. Gone is the parade of hospital personnel who check the body and take the vital signs, draw blood, change the bed, clean the floor, bring the meals, fill out forms, and take the patient to mysterious tests and procedures. Gone are the long waits in hallways, lying on a guerney.

> *Hospitals used to be a place where you could go when you needed a rest. Now you go home to get refreshed.*

Familiarity and Security

Some patients want to be at home because of the security and emotional comfort they find there. They feel "at home." Buffeted by an illness that threatens to cut them off from the pleasures and sustenance of daily life, they grasp for a familiar environment, a refuge.

The fear of abandonment, so pervasive in the dying, can be alleviated at home by the consoling experience of belonging, of being taken in. Rather than the sometimes impersonal routines of the hospital, the patient enjoys those rituals of home life that attest to his or her connectedness to the family's past and future. Ideally, home is where one is always welcomed and valued. Familiar places and familiar faces confirm the importance of the person, providing a secure and continuing identity despite the threat of illness. In contrast, institutional care may be equated with abandonment and neglect.

Continuity with Normal Life

Sick people may feel that they are "no good anymore." Illness compromises their ability to enjoy their lives, to participate in the daily activities that sustain them, and to give to others. Home care may be viewed as an attempt to move toward a life of greater normalcy.

At home, the patient often feels less compromised by illness. Familiar surroundings—photographs, hobbies, furniture, mementos—and familiar relationships support the notion of the patient having a unique identity. Time can be filled with the distractions of daily life rather than with the potentially barren and impersonal routines of institutional existence. The sick person, sharing a meal or merely sitting in the presence of friends, continues to participate in and partake of familiar rituals:

> As long as I can remember, probably ever since we got married, we've slept late on Sunday mornings. My wife would get up a little bit before I did, and she would prepare a special breakfast. When I think about our marriage, it's often those Sunday mornings I think about—the smell of the food, the particular quietness and peacefulness and warmth of that day, reading the paper, perhaps planning something special for the afternoon. It's moments like that I have in mind when I think about leaving my wife and about how good life has been for us. I think of not having many of those Sundays left, and of her being alone sometime, not having me to share the day with, and it makes me sad, but it also makes me want to be at home as much as possible now.

Autonomy

Illness and dying inevitably produce a sense of uncertainty and helplessness, as does the surrendering of so much responsibility for one's life to institutions and professionals. At home, patients may feel in charge of their lives. They decide when to go to sleep, when to arise, what to eat, who enters and leaves the room. Rather than being at the mercy of orderlies, doctors, and nurses, they feel that they can dictate the terms of their daily existence:

> Home is your own turf. Here, I can call the shots.

Closeness of Family and Friends

When a final separation is imminent, the ready access of family and friends may take on enormous value. Patients may simply seek to be home in order to have more time with these people. They may also be concerned with the quality of their personal relationships in the hospital. Visitors in the hospital seem different than in the home. They are dressed up for the hospital, governed by the institution's regulations, sitting in unfamiliar rooms. At home, on familiar turf, people feel and behave less like visitors, more like their usual selves. Family and friends can comfortably remain at hand all through the day and night. Children may come and go. Pets can be enjoyed. The family may sleep in the same room or bed, or they may sleep nearby. Intimacy and sexuality are more readily enjoyed at home.

Family Involvement in Care

For the family, home care provides an opportunity to take an active role in helping the dying person. The family has abundant occasion at home for deeds that demonstrate their affection and devotion. They escape the passivity and frustration often experienced by a hospital visitor who watches strangers assume the caring roles normally assigned to the family. In the hospital, the staff seems to say to the family, "Don't get in our way." At home, the family is again able to feed, clean, serve, and protect its members and to be on hand to make sure everything is done right. Such acts help express to the patient, the family, and others that they have not given up on the sick person, and fulfill an often unspoken promise of family members—to care for each other.

The work of attending to the ill can be particularly meaningful in the face of the inevitable helplessness that is felt when death approaches. The family's involvement in caretaking may secure for them a sense of having clearly communicated their affection when it counted. For years afterward, the family's participation in the patient's care may be remembered as an affirmation of their valued role in the dying person's life until the moment of death, as proof of their devotion.

Availability of Help and Tolerance of Dependence

Patients may feel better attended in the home. Hospitals sometimes seem understaffed, particularly at night. The family may worry that a careless ward nurse will give the wrong pill or that a medication request will be forgotten or ignored. Many patients are reluctant to ask for help from strangers, even from the most kindly nurses. Hospital personnel may seem patronizing, infantilizing, or arrogant. A patient may fear being viewed as a nuisance or may worry that the attendants will become critical or resentful of appeals for assistance. A patient may find dependence disturbing and may avoid those requests for help that confirm concerns about being weak and beholden.

At home, the personal attention of one or two family members may give the impression that adequate help is readily available. Moreover, many patients feel that they can readily ask for help from their family and can comfortably accept such aid. Indeed, some of the most docile or reticent patients in the hospital prove to be entitled and demanding when they are at home.

Convenience

In the hospital, visiting hours may be limited or inconvenient, and trips to the hospital may be difficult for visitors. Care in the home may seem easier for the family. Nobody has to get dressed, find a babysitter, pay for a cab, or search for parking. Time with the patient can be interspersed with the normal routines of life in the home.

Cost

Finally, home-based management may be less expensive than institutional care. Patients who lack third-party insurance that fully covers hospitalization or chronic care may simply feel unable to afford institutional care. Family members may choose to attend the patient in the home rather than continuing to work, preferring a loss of income to facing a large hospital bill:

> *I'd rather do the job myself, even if I break my back, than trying to make the money to pay someone else to do it.*

PATIENTS WHO INSIST ON GOING HOME

Deserving special mention are those patients who insist on going home from the hospital or on remaining home, regardless of the wishes of their family or the advice of the professional staff. Such patients may seem stubborn, fearful, or irrational, but their common feature is an unreasoned determination to be at home. Included in this group are some of the people who avoid or refuse evaluation of their medical problems, who reject treatment, who sign out of the hospital against medical advice, and who never return for follow-up appointments.[1] As discussed in Chapter 6, many of these patients prove to be fairly rational. A significant proportion have chronic emotional problems that are not very amenable to treatment. Still others might benefit from psychological help, particularly those who are acutely anxious or depressed or who become negativistic as a displacement of their sense of anger, frustration, and lack of control over their lives. Organic brain disorders should also be considered as contributing to such behavior.[1]

Such patients present a particular interest and challenge. They may surprise their caretakers by showing how well a person can get along without standard treatment or other medical help. They may demonstrate how a determination to be at home can overcome both physical difficulties and social problems. When patients completely reject all treatment, they teach physicians about the natural course of a disease.

Noncompliant patients tend to alienate their health-care workers, especially when exhortations to follow medical advice are made in vain. Some of these patients will blankly refuse any contact with doctors or nurses, but others will accept help on their own terms. Patience with their idiosyncracies may allow for the development of a satisfying doctor–patient relationship and, at times, may lead to reconsideration of decisions to refuse treatment. When these patients are allowed to dictate the kind of care they want, they may tolerate medical and nursing visits and home-health supports, and they often can be helped to die comfortably. Regardless, the physician who tolerates such "difficult patients" will find a valuable opportunity to know an unusual person and to follow an unusual course of treatment.

ASSESSING PREFERENCES FOR THE SITE OF CARE

A few words from a doctor or nurse implying that home care is not a reasonable alternative can sometimes nearly foreclose for the family any consideration of noninstitutional care. Conversely, a concerned professional can open up a discussion that allows the wishes of the patient and family to be expressed and clarified, and that helps these laypersons acquire the information they need to make a good decision about the preferred site of care.

The patient and family often are unsure about decisions about home-based management. They may seek professional support for their decisions. They may not feel certain what is right for them, or what will work out best. They may wonder about the staff's motives for suggesting home care. The patient and family often need to sort out their feelings and to identify their foremost concerns. They especially need concrete information about the process of care at home and about the availability of help. The choices—whether to go home from the hospital or to stay at home—reflect a complicated calculus, which weighs a jumble of human concerns, particularly the patient's and family's sense about prolonging life and maintaining the quality of the remaining time, and their feelings about comfort, security, convenience, and the allocation of available resources.

The physician who does not regularly ask patients and family members how they feel about home care or hospital management will be slow to appreciate the personal meaning behind choices about the site of care. The following questions are often useful:

> *Have you thought about where you want to be now? At home? In a hospital? In a chronic-care hospital?*
>
> *What problems do you see there? What are the disadvantages?*
>
> *What would be good about it? What are the advantages?*
>
> *What kind of help do you think you need now?*
>
> *What kind of help do you think your family could provide?*
>
> *Are you aware of community services? What difference would it make to have a doctor visit? A nurse? A home health aide? A homemaker?*

Previous experiences with home health care may sometimes strongly influence the layperson's initial view of what care in the home will be like:

Physician:	*Have you had any opportunity to see someone very sick or dying being cared for at home?*
One family member:	*I took care of my mother when she was sick. She stayed in my home, and I did everything for her. I was with her when she died. It was very sad, but very gratifying.*
Another family member:	*My grandfather died in our house when I was about 10. He had cancer, and he was in terrible pain. He screamed all night, and he couldn't control his bowels. I don't think I could face anything like that.*

If the patient and family want to consider home care, they need experienced professional help to assess the sick person's condition and to review the availability of needed resources. The primary question is not just how "sick" the patient is. Many severely ill people, including those on the danger list, may comfortably go home for some or all of the terminal phase of their life. Foremost clinical concerns include the following:

What is essential for comfort and security?
What kinds of problems are likely to arise? How can these problems be avoided or managed in the hospital or the home?
What kinds of services and equipment will help the process go smoothly?
How will the site of care affect the patient and family? How will it influence the quality of life?

CAVEATS—THE ROMANTICIZATION OF HOME CARE

Home care for the terminally ill is commonly undervalued by health professionals, but it also is occasionally touted as a magical balm for the pain and sadness of dying. While this chapter elaborates on the problems of terminal care in the hospital and on the advantages of the home, it does not mean to imply that every patient and family finds the hospital impersonal or dehumanizing.

Not every home is an Alhambra nor every family a devoted, efficient, loving team. Previous chapters have focused on the common barriers to safe passage at home and on the painstaking measures required to ensure comfort and security for the patient and family. Furthermore, no site of care (and no medical treatment or psychosocial counseling) will fully relieve the discomfort and fright encountered by most dying patients and their families. Insofar as life is valued, every death will be sad and painful.

Recent experiences with deinstitutionalization of the mentally ill should also lead physicians to think carefully before committing themselves to forms of care that initially seem cheap and humane, but that may actually inflict greater suffering on patients. Common conditions that make the choice of home care problematic include the following:

1. Poorly controlled pain or other severe symptoms
2. A rapidly changing clinical course
3. A likelihood that symptoms will develop that are considered intolerable at home by the patient or the support network
4. Lack of appropriate home-care services
5. A high level of anxiety in the patient or family
6. Patients and families who, when well informed about the advantages and disadvantages of various sites of care, prefer institutional treatment, especially (a) patients who are reluctant to go home but are pressed into acceptance by the family or health-care team and (b) families who are reluctant to take the sick person home but accede to pressures from the patient or health-care team.

REFERENCES

1. Appelbaum PS, Roth LH: Treatment refusals in medical hospitals. In President's Commission for the Study of Ethical Problems in Medicine and Biomedical and Behavioral Research: Making Health Care Decisions: The Ethical and Legal Implications of Informed Consent in the Patient–Practitioner Relationship. Vol Two: Appendices—Empirical Studies of Informed Consent. Washington, DC, US Superintendent of Documents, 1982
2. Flynn A, Stewart DE: Where do cancer patients die? A review of cancer deaths in Cuyahoga County, Ohio, 1957–1974. J Community Health 5:126–130, 1979.
3. Gillick MR, Serrell NA, Gillick LS: Adverse consequences of hospitalization in the elderly. Soc Sci Med 16:1033–1038, 1982
4. Sampson WI: Dying at home. JAMA 238:2405–2406, 1977
5. Steel KP, Gertman PM, Crescenzi C, Anderson J: Iatrogenic illness on a general medical service at a university hospital. N Engl J Med 304:638–642, 1981

Death in the Home   11

So here it is at last, the distinguished thing!

Henry James[4]

The patient who chooses to be at home as death approaches faces a separate decision of where to die. Some families that are strongly committed to home care may wish to keep the dying patient in the house until "the last moment" or "it's all we can bear," planning from early in the course of the illness to have death occur in the hospital. Even if the family intends for death to take place at home, many circumstances can cause a change of heart or of plans. Furthermore, a few patients will die suddenly or unexpectedly at home, regardless of the plans of the physician, patient, or family.

This chapter is divided into two sections: the first describes the preparation for an anticipated death at home; the second presents a clinical approach to managing death when it actually occurs.

ANTICIPATING DEATH AT HOME

Patient and Family Concerns

Regardless of whether the patient or family articulate their concerns as the illness progresses, they are likely to be thinking about approaching death:

> *When will it occur?*

> *What will it be like?*

> *Will there be physical suffering? Emotional turmoil? New and overwhelming problems to be faced? Ghastly symptoms?*

> *What will I do?*

The behavior of the professional caretakers may be scrutinized for clues: "He's coming back in a few days, so he must be worried," or "He said he would come back in a week, so he must think we'll be safe for awhile, yet he acted as if we're heading for bad trouble."

Long before death is imminent, the physician often gets hints of the patient's and family's concerns from their questions or comments. Will the pain accelerate and become intolerable? Will the patient choke? Will he exsanguinate or become incontinent? Will there be personality changes, restlessness, confusion, or other bizarre behavior? Will the requirements for physical care become unmanageable? Will the sick person be "too much of a burden" to the family or professional caretakers?

Such ideas and concerns about the approaching death are nearly universal and are best addressed directly and prophylactically. The physician can ask:

> Have you been wondering about what it will be like as you get sicker? About approaching death?

More specific questioning may be useful:

> What do you envision happening?

> Do you foresee any problems?

> Do you have any particular concerns?

> Have you ever seen anyone die?
>   What was it like?
>   What do you think it will be like?

> How do you feel about being at home? Would you prefer to be in the hospital?
>   What advantages do you see there? What problems?

Family members share similar concerns, and have their own worries:

> How do you think you'll react when he dies?

> How will you feel about being with him right then? Immediately afterward?

> What will you do?

Patients also have concerns about how they will be treated immediately after death. Fears about being alive in the coffin, crematorium, or autopsy room are common, as are worries about being subjected to injury or neglect.

Addressing Concerns and Rehearsing Plans

Once the patient and family's ideas and concerns are elicited, the physician has a number of options. First, unrealistic notions about death can be acknowledged, then gently corrected. Death is almost always comfortable for the patient:

> I can see how you would be thinking about such matters, but your wife's condition is really very different from the one you're recalling. It seems very unlikely that bleeding will be a problem for us.

> We have good treatment for that sort of pain nowadays, and I can assure you that you won't have to face such suffering.

Secondly, realistic concerns can be addressed by anticipating and rehearsing the management of problems:

Doctor: *What would you do if her breathing got worse?*

Spouse: *I could turn up the oxygen.*

Doctor: *Yes, increase the flow rate by 2 liters per minute. That should help. It's unlikely that her breathing will change suddenly, but you could do that even before calling me.*

Spouse: *What if it doesn't work?*

Doctor: *I think it will help. If her breathing becomes more of a problem, we also have medicine that will help her feel comfortable no matter how bad her lungs get. I don't think she needs anything more now, but I want you to know we have a lot of other things we can do to keep her from suffering.*

Son: *The worst part of it for me is every morning when I peek around the corner into his room to see if he's breathing.*

Doctor: *You think he might be dead?*

Son: *Yes.*

Doctor: *What would you do?*

Son: *I just don't know what I'd do. I guess I'd call you.*

Doctor: *Yes, if you found that he had died, you should just call me and I'll come over. You don't need to do anything else. Does that sound OK?*

Son: *Yeah, that's fine.*

Doctor: *How do you think it would be for you?*

Son: *You mean being alone with him? Well, it would be OK. Of course, I would be upset, but we've been expecting it. I just hope he goes peacefully.*

Doctor: *I don't think he is going to die suddenly and unexpectedly. It could happen, but usually we have some warning. You'll probably see some big changes in his condition first. I'll try to warn you when the time is coming.*

When progressive metabolic derangement or organ failure develops, the time and mode of death often become somewhat predictable. Patients with worsening hypercalcemia, cerebral edema, or hepatic or renal failure can be advised that they will slowly lose consciousness. They can be reassured that while they may be bothered by an inability to think clearly or to remain awake, they will slip away rather quickly and gently. The family needs to be warned about the patient's restlessness, confusion, wandering, meaningless behavior, and inability to talk sensibly, and about the frustration of watching the patient drift into coma. They can be reassured that coma, like a deep sleep, causes no suffering, and that the patient's needs for feeding, medication, and other personal care will change, usually lessening:

> *As his condition worsens, I think you'll find that he will get sleepier and sleepier and less able to do things for himself. He won't be able to eat and there's no point in trying to get him to take food. Let's try to keep giving him the Decadron, but don't worry if he cannot swallow the other medications or even the Decadron. You may notice his breathing getting slow or fast or irregular. Fast or deep breathing does not mean he's suffering from shortness of*

breath. It's just part of his brain centers not working right, and we've done all we should about that. Eventually, he will stop breathing.

The physician should assure the family of the continuing concern and availability of the health-care team, and should reassert confidence in being able to maintain comfort and security. Additional outside help should be considered at such times.

The patient and family may want to review and change the decision about where death should occur. They can be reminded that they may alter their plans anytime, electing hospitalization or perhaps reconsidering home care after an admission. If the family says, "We can't face it," or "We know he is going to die, but we have to live here," or gives other indications of hoping to have care be provided in the hospital, their wishes should be respected, but gentle exploration of their concerns should be undertaken. Initial resistance to the notion of death in the home often changes with time and with the opportunity to explore fears and to develop realistic expectations.

Some families may consider that being at home at the moment of death has a sacred value, or they may have committed themselves to keeping the patient from dying in an institution. When circumstances force a change in their plans or when death occurs unexpectedly during hospitalization, such a family may view the hospital admission as abandonment or as evidence of their incompetence and failure to fulfill important duties. Patients, however, are usually much more concerned about how they are treated in the preterminal period (and before) than in the brief final moments. Eventually, most families also come to view the time of death in such a perspective.

The family should consider how they will respond immediately to the death. The next steps need to be rehearsed:

What will you do if he dies?

Who will you call? Do you have the number handy?

Will you be OK alone? Would you prefer to be with him awhile before calling me?

Have you chosen a funeral director? Have you discussed arrangements? Will there be a wake? What kind of funeral are you thinking about?

The physician's instructions are best provided in writing, and include the following:

1. "All you need to do is call me or speak to whichever of my associates is answering the phone, and we will help you handle everything."
2. "Don't call the police, fire department, or ambulance." Dead bodies should not be resuscitated or rushed to the hospital in an ambulance. The summoning of the police occasionally leads to medicolegal and bureaucratic procedures, which are an annoyance to all involved, including the police and coroner. If a family feels unable to wait for the doctor, an ambulance can transport the patient to an emergency room, but the physician and family should explicitly forbid resuscitative measures.
3. "Call us when you are ready." Quick action by the family is not required, and they should not be encouraged to treat the death as a frightening emergency. They can be told, "If you want to be with the patient, you don't have to call us immediately. We can also wait awhile before calling the funeral director."

Additional instructions on the signs of approaching death and the diagnosis of death may be valued (see Appendix 11-1).

Legal, Financial, and Funeral Planning[2]

Appendix 11-2 lists legal and financial issues that commonly deserve consideration prior to an anticipated death.

Unfortunately, legal and financial planning are occasionally left until the last minute, even when the physician has the foresight to broach these issues earlier in the course of the illness. Without the physician's gentle reminder that the patient should get his or her affairs in order while health permits, families may avoid or postpone such matters indefinitely.

Occasionally, patients and families prefer to make some or all of the funeral arrangements in advance. They may find great solace in handling such details before the death. A number of good reference books are available to guide the family.[1,6,7] Financial problems can sometimes best be resolved when the patient is still alive, especially if adequate time is allowed prior to death. The assistance of a social worker or lawyer may be considered.

Most families will have established an affiliation with a funeral director, either from previous deaths in the family or from attending funerals of friends, neighbors, or members of their church or synagogue. Contact with a funeral director prior to the death may be useful for discussing arrangements.

Family tradition often dictates many of the features of the funeral service. As listed in Appendix 11-3, Personal Directions for the Time of Death, the following topics can be reviewed:

1. Autopsy
2. Donation of the body or organs for transplantation research, medical training, etc.
3. Choice of funeral home
4. Public notices
5. The handling of flowers or donations, including establishment of a memorial fund for a charity, hospital, or research fund
6. Location, duration, and format for services (*e.g.*, wake, funeral service [with the body present] or memorial service [without the body], committal service [at graveside], private or open services, an open or closed casket, and choices about religious personnel, music, and the participation of family and friends)
7. Cremation and the handling of the ashes, or burial with or without embalming
8. The choice of a casket, a plot, or a vault, and of a memorial marker
9. Price range for funeral arrangements

The Moment of Death

For survivors, the moment of death commands a peculiar awe and profound respect. The extraordinary change of a person from being alive to being dead is comparable only to the moment of birth. Family members may attach extreme importance to being with the patient at the moment of death:

> *If he had gone to the hospital last night, all that we had done would have been wasted. We would have wondered what happened, if he had suffered, like when my aunt died at the nursing home.*

Usually, the wish to be present at the death is an extension of a previously evident desire to participate in care, to show loyalty and devotion, and to continue with the beloved as long as possible. Occasionally, a magical belief is attached to the moment of death, and whoever is in the room or is closest to the patient is felt to receive a special power, communion, or blessing from the dying. Jealous battles may develop among family rivals. Regardless of such beliefs, a mystical quality often pervades the moment of death. Years later, the scene of the death is recalled, perhaps revered, while the long preceding months may fade into a blur. The most significant memories for the bereaved, however, are generally based on a long history of interaction with the person who died and less so on a short period of terminal illness. One brief phase or one particular event, including the moment of death, becomes important primarily insofar as it reflects or helps to mend the sustained feeling of a relationship.

When death is imminent, a vigil may be desired by the relatives. The family may vaguely sense that the patient should not be alone, or they may overtly feel a formal duty to be at the bedside, perhaps having promised the patient to be on hand.

In the hospital, appropriate arrangements include at least one comfortable chair at the bedside and, preferably, a reclining chair or bed in which a family member can sleep. Ideally, a number of family members should be comfortably accommodated in the sick room and waiting area. Regardless of whether a vigil is established, the family should be explicitly assured that the staff will continue checking on the patient, and that the dying person will not be neglected or allowed to suffer. When the family members choose to go home or to take a break away from the sick room, they should also be assured that they will be promptly notified of any changes in the patient's condition. Other family customs—songs, burning of candles, or religious ceremonies—should be facilitated. When the moment of death does not occur as intended— the family is away, the ambulance is called and death occurs in the emergency ward, or a ritual is omitted—the physician can emphasize to the relatives how important the previous weeks, months, or years were to the patient.

THE CARE OF THE DEAD
AND THE ACUTELY BEREAVED

> After you're dead, the doctor comes.
>
> Moliere
> (from the farce, "Sgnarelle")

Being Notified

For laypersons, the diagnosis of death is rarely made incorrectly, but it is usually offered tentatively. In calling the physician, relatives often say, "I think he *may* have died."

When the physician is notified of the patient's death, the family is usually in a state of shock. Discussion over the phone should be very brief, simple, and clear:

> I will come right over. The trip will take me about 45 minutes [overestimating the delay] so I will be there at 9:30. Who is there? . . . Are you OK? . . . Just wait for me, and we can handle everything when I get there.

While a death sometimes needs to be treated with the same promptness as an emergency, many families are well-prepared for the event and are comfortable with the presence of the body in the home. They are not calling primarily for psychosocial support but for the physician's medicolegal assistance. The family may even wait for a previously arranged visit rather than calling the physician, or may notify the physician immediately while expecting that the visit may be delayed for the professional's convenience.

Spouse: *[For a 3:00 AM call] John died about an hour ago. We came in to check on him, and his breathing had stopped. Can you come by?*

Physician: *Yes. Do you want me to come by now, or can you wait until early in the morning, say 6:30.*

Spouse: *We're OK here.*

Physician: *Are you sure?*

Spouse: *Yes, we're just sitting and talking.*

Physician: *Call me if you want me to come by sooner. We can take care of everything else when I arrive.*

Certification

The physician has a simple medicolegal obligation: making the diagnosis of death and preparing the death certificate. The determination of death, although technically trivial, deserves a slow, deliberate ritual. While the presumption of death by the family is seldom wrong, a few simple steps ensure that the doctor does not make an erroneous diagnosis in a moment of excitement.

1. Observe for respirations.
2. Listen for a heartbeat.
3. Check for pupillary reaction.
4. Notify the family (*e.g.,* "Yes, he's dead," or "Yes, it's over; he's gone."). The relatives know the patient is dead, yet are often in a state of partial disbelief, waiting for an official pronouncement.

The family should be offered the opportunity to be present during this procedure. The physician should treat the patient gently and respectfully in carrying out these duties (and later in helping with the care of the dead), since the family may still consider the patient alive, as if the body could still experience physical pain or emotional suffering and as if speech in the presence of the body could still be appreciated by the deceased.

The requirements of certification of death vary from community to community. When death is imminent, some hospice physicians will prepare a death certificate in advance, leaving it with a nurse or family member who can determine the time of death. Some funeral directors will remove a dead body without awaiting a physician's certification if they have an understanding that the doctor will complete the necessary papers promptly. Problems with improperly completed death certificates and with delays in the completion of forms have plagued funeral directors and are responsible, in part, for the antagonism toward physicians that is occasionally expressed by this profession. There are also situations in which the physician has no formal obligation to attend the death (*e.g.*, in communities with a medical examiner or a police physician who handles the medicolegal duties) or in which the coroner must be notified.

Immediate Decisions: The Autopsy, Organ Donation, and the Funeral Director

Three important decisions must be made immediately.

The family must decide about an *autopsy.* An autopsy is particularly valuable to the family when they have ongoing concerns about the cause and course of the illness, their own susceptibility to disease, and their ability to prevent such conditions. It occasionally can be important for establishing medicolegal facts that are useful for malpractice, compensation, or insurance claims. In discussing the procedure, the family occasionally assumes that the doctor wants a post mortem examination. They often are not eager to consider the procedure, and they may react defensively. Concerns about inflicting pain or indignity—"He's suffered enough"—and about disfigurement are common. Religious prohibitions are occasionally cited, but rarely are consistent with published theological writings.[3] The physician is obligated to help the relatives consider an autopsy:

> You may have some ideas already about an autopsy, but I think it is important for you to stop and think about it a little. This is your only chance to have one if anyone in your family feels it is needed. The autopsy is a brief operation that the hospital performs without any charge to you. There is no pain for your father, and there will be no visible scars or change in his appearance. There will be no delay in your funeral arrangements.
>
> The autopsy is the best way we have to figure out exactly what happened to your father—to really see how the cancer spread and to know exactly why he died. We will also check him for other medical conditions. Occasionally, there are surprises—problems we were not aware of. We might be able to give you some information about whether he had medical conditions that are likely to run in the family.
>
> If you think you are going to have questions about exactly what happened, this is your only chance to get closer to the facts.
>
> What are your thoughts?
>
> Did your father express any feelings about an autopsy?

In addition to this general discussion, a personal evaluation by the physician may be appropriate:

> I think it is unlikely that anything new or useful will be turned up by the autopsy, and I don't think we have any pressing questions about his death. I hope you will consider an autopsy, but I don't think we are likely to miss anything by skipping it.
>
> We have all been involved with trying to figure out what was wrong and in trying to help your father. I am left with some questions that the autopsy might answer, and the results might be useful to you and me later on.
>
> I think we should respect his wishes not to have an autopsy. He wanted his body to be left alone.

> *The results might help the doctors who are doing this research. It won't help your father, but he seemed pleased to participate in the protocol, and the autopsy might carry on his wish to be of help to others.*

Local variations in the autopsy procedure, costs (especially transportation and pathologist's fees), time constraints, and so on should be noted. At the Massachusetts General Hospital, the autopsy is performed free for registered patients, but costs $1500 for others.

If an autopsy is elected, the family should be promised a discussion of the results. A brief report is often available within a week, and the family can be called then, usually to say that nothing remarkable showed up. A fuller face-to-face discussion should be arranged for a later time, allowing especially for questions about the cause, course, and hereditary nature of the patient's condition.

Organ donation or *donation of the entire body* is best arranged prior to death, but can be considered immediately after death. Cancer or infection may preclude donation for transplantation, but organs may be needed for research, while bodies may be valued for both research and medical training.

A *funeral director* must be chosen and notified. Unless services are conducted in the home, the mortician will pick up the body in the home and deliver it to the morgue or funeral home.

Further Duties in Attending a Death

Remove medical apparatus (*e.g.,* catheters and oxygen masks). The body should be tidied (*e.g.,* by cleaning out the nose and mouth). Jewelry and religious items are occasionally left in place, especially if they are to be worn during a wake or interment.

Position the body. The eyes and mouth can often be closed. If possible, set the body in a position that appears comfortable, placing the bedclothes neatly over the chest, as if the patient were sleeping. The family may want the face covered.

The family should be given the opportunity to sit with the patient and touch the body. Family members may want to be alone with the deceased or to be accompanied by others in visiting the deathbed. This is the last time the patient is seen at home— a time for saying goodbye. Depending on funeral arrangements, this time may also be the last chance for the family to see the patient. Children should be offered the opportunity to participate:

> *You won't ever see him again here, and you won't see him again until the wake. Does anyone here want to spend some time with him now? Does anyone want to be with him alone? Touch him again? Say goodbye? Would you like me or someone else to go with you?*

The family should be encouraged to notify friends and relatives promptly. Withholding of the news should generally be discouraged.

The family's priest, minister or rabbi should be notified and, if desired, be summoned to the home. At times, this person is a stranger who hastily performs a few rites, delivers well-meant but useless solace, and leaves. At other times, this person knows the family and deceased well, has participated in other crises in their lives, is sensitive to the family's feelings and aware of their cultural expectations, has training and experience with counseling the bereaved, and provides continued attention after death, and thus offers great comfort and ongoing support and a meaningful religious structure for the mourning.

A decision should be made about when to summon the funeral director for removal of the body. Further choices about the details of services do not need to be made immediately. Any members of the immediate family who wish to assist in funeral planning should be encouraged to participate in later decisions about services.

Since the patient is still felt, in part, to be alive, helpless, and vulnerable, the family may have concerns for his or her well-being. In the hospital, the physician can say, "We will take care of him now until the funeral director comes." At home, one might say,

> The funeral director will pick him up and take care of him until the service.

The hospital-in-the-home should be dismantled. Some families will be eager to complete this immediately. Rented beds and other equipment should be picked up by the supplier. Medications should be thrown away. Occasionally, the nurse or physician can transfer supplies to other patients, while purchased equipment can be donated to the equipment closet of the local hospice, visiting nurses' association, or American Cancer Society chapter. The family may be grateful that someone else can use leftover medical supplies.

Facilitating Bereavement

The period immediately after the death usually finds the family in a state called "shock." At times, they appear calm, and can talk clearly and rationally, yet at other moments they may be slightly restless or frantic and unable to think clearly. The bereaved are swept up uncontrollably in powerful feelings. They may describe themselves as "not feeling real" or not knowing what to do with themselves. Common phrases include, "I'm just trying to get through it," "I can't believe it," and "I feel lost; I'm in limbo." A person may seem to have diverse reactions over a few minutes or hours: at one moment appearing numbed, awed, shocked, lost, and bewildered; at another, rational, detached, observing, and realistic; still, at another, bereft and overcome with sadness.

In the hospital, some families, much to the distress of personnel who prefer order and control, will wail, scream, wander about, and throw themselves on the patient and each other. Insofar as the comfort of staff and patients allows such behavior in institutions, it should be tolerated; it certainly should not be automatically labeled as pathologic or abnormal.

Two major themes pervade the time immediately after the death: (1) the acknowledgment of loss and its ramifications—"He's gone. It's over"—and (2) the acknowledgment of the continued existence of social supports and of an orderly, intact world—"Life goes on." The funeral service and other mourning rituals embody these somewhat contradictory notions, and the tension is played out more in gestures, implications, and tone than in meaning of the words.[5]

Immediately after death, the physician's role in facilitating coping or bereavement is minimal. The state of shock admits little intervention. Talking often seems useless, although the family may be extremely grateful for the calm influence of the physician's presence, the attention to the duties mentioned above, the sense that whatever needs to be done now is being handled properly. For the physician, this may be a time of awe at the powerful display of emotions, and of gratitude for the privilege of sharing in such a profound moment, but also of feeling helpless or superfluous.

There are a few opportunities to facilitate grieving. The family's responses to the death can be influenced by the physician's manner: frank expressions of sadness; ease in approaching the body and encouragement for relatives to view (and confront) death; tolerance of extreme emotional reactions, including "loss of control" or severe stoicism; encouragement to speak honestly in breaking the news to others; and interest in treating the children (and those persons kept from the center of the rituals of mourning) with a sense of respect for their ability to cope and to choose how they wish to participate. The physician's review of the events around the death may be valued by the family and may facilitate their grieving process:

What happened? How had things been going? What did you notice?

How did you feel?

How are you feeling about it all now?

Encouragement and praise are often appropriate, especially when the physician is familiar with the family and their role in the patient's care:

You were great. You were wonderful for him.

You certainly were there when he needed you.

It was tough. He was lucky to have you.

You will have a lot to look back on with pleasure.

Requests for sedation—often made casually by a person other than the severely bereaved, sometimes on behalf of a relative whom the physician does not know—should be explored, and generally denied. The request usually conveys a wish for help, not specifically for sedation, or a wish for an escape or safety valve in case the pressure of grief becomes excessive. A few tranquilizers are unlikely to cause any harm, but the bereaved are usually better assisted by explaining that they will feel badly, and that sleep may be disturbed but that medication is not very helpful for fending off normal feelings. If problems with anxiety, sleeplessness, anorexia, and so on persist, further medical attention, not casual dispensing of sedatives is required:

You are probably going to feel awful for a while, and you may temporarily lose interest in food or have trouble sleeping. Medication just isn't very good for being sad. You may feel very crazy or bad at times—I'm afraid that's to be expected for awhile. I wish I could help you more with this. If you're finding yourself repeatedly unable to sleep or you're getting very tired or not eating or not taking care of yourself, we should sit down and figure out what is happening and what to do.

What kinds of problems has she had with her nerves in the past? Has she seen a doctor? Taken any treatment?

Does she really want these pills? I think she's doing fine and can handle it without medication. Let's let her know we're concerned, though, and she can call her doctor if she needs more help.

More reasoned appeals for sedation—ones that do not reflect such vague worries or concerns about overpowering emotions (*e.g.,* "I had some Valium to take when my mother died, and they helped me sleep, so I wonder if you could give me a few to have around")—should also be explored. A few tranquilizers are innocuous and may give the patient a sense of security from having them on hand. The medication is often not used.

Initial impressions of the "normality" of each family member's bereavement have limited validity at this point. In order to assess properly the process of mourning, arrangements for a follow-up visit should be made. This later visit also serves to reassure the family of the physician's continued interest and availability:

> *I will be in touch with you, then, in about a week, and we can plan to get together again in 3 or 4 weeks. Please get in touch with me sooner if I can be of any help.*

SELECTED REFERENCES

1. Consumer Reports: Funerals: Consumers' Last Rights. New York, WW Norton, 1977
2. DeSpelder LA, Strickland AL: Last rites: Funerals and body disposition. In DeSpelder LA, Strickland AL: The Last Dance: Encountering Death and Dying, pp 158–189. Palo Alto, CA, Mayfield Publishing Co, 1983
3. Grollman EA ed: Concerning Death: A Practical Guide for the Living. Boston, Beacon Press, 1974
4. James H: Cited in Wharton E. A Backward Glance p 367. New York, Charles Scribner's Sons, 1934
5. Mandelbaum DG: Social uses of funeral rites. In Feifel H (ed): The Meaning of Death, pp 189–217. New York, McGraw-Hill, 1959
6. Morgan E: A Manual of Death Education and Simple Burial, 8th ed. Burnsville, NC, Celo Press, 1977 (available from Celo Press, Route 5, Burnsville, NC 28714)
7. Simpson MA: The Facts of Death: A Complete Guide for Being Prepared. Englewood Cliffs, NJ, Prentice-Hall, 1979
8. Worcester A: Care of the Aged, the Dying and the Dead. Springfield, IL, Charles C Thomas, 1935.

APPENDIX 11-1—SIGNS OF APPROACHING DEATH:

Information for the Family

The following information may help you anticipate and understand the changes that appear as a person approaches death. Not all of these changes will occur, nor do they necessarily occur in any particular order. Call your doctor or nurse when you have questions about what is happening or if you are concerned that the patient is uncomfortable.

1. The patient may become increasingly tired and sleepy and may be difficult to arouse.
2. The patient may become confused about time or may no longer recognize familiar persons, places, or objects. Hearing and vision may become impaired, and speech may be slurred, difficult to understand, or nonsensical. A few patients become restless—they move about frequently in bed, pull at the bedclothes, reach out, and have visions of people or things that do not exist.
3. Less nourishment will be required, and the patient's intake of food and drink will diminish.
4. The patient may lose control of his urine or bowels. If this occurs, you should obtain advice on how to keep the patient clean and dry.
5. Urination may diminish or stop.

6. The patient's mouth may become dry, and thick secretions may accumulate in the back of the throat. Breathing may become noisy because of the gurgling or rattling of these secretions in the mouth or chest.
7. The pattern of breathing may change, becoming slower or faster, deeper or shallower, or irregular. Often, the patient will have periods of rapid breathing, followed by periods in which breathing is very slow or even absent for as long as 15 seconds.
8. The arms and legs may become cool as the circulation slows down. The skin may be pale or mottled, and some parts, particularly the underside of the body, may become a dark color, usually a deep blue or purple.

When death occurs, you may notice the following:

1. Breathing ceases entirely.
2. Heartbeat and pulse stop.
3. The patient is entirely unresponsive to shaking or shouting.
4. The eyes may be fixed in one direction. The eyelids may be open or closed.
5. A loss of control of urine or bowels may occur.

What to do when death occurs:

1. Don't call the police, fire department, or ambulance.
2. Call the physician or nurse. We will help you with the next steps.
3. You do not have to call us immediately. If you want to be with the patient for awhile, you can call us when you are ready. You can also wait to call the funeral director.

APPENDIX 11-2—LEGAL AND FINANCIAL PLANNING*:

A Guide for the Patient

In the event of your death, your survivors may need the following information and documents. Provide the exact names, addresses, and telephone numbers of all important persons and organizations. Indicate the location of all significant papers and how these documents can be obtained.

I. Personal Data

Birth certificate
Name and, if living, address and telephone number of parents, brothers, sisters, children
Citizenship papers
Military service record, Veterans Administration registration
Marriage certificates, divorce records
Birth certificates of children, adoption papers
Memberships, clubs, societies, voluntary organizations
Relatives and friends to be notified in case of death

---

*Adapted from the book THE FACTS OF DEATH by Michael A. Simpson © 1979 by Prentice-Hall, Inc. Published by Prentice-Hall, Inc., Englewood Cliffs, NJ 01632.

II. Financial Data

Will (and its executors), trusts and any arrangements for distribution of assets
Life insurance and other insurance policies
Bank accounts, savings
Investments, securities, property, valuables
Safe deposit boxes
Social Security, pensions, benefits
Title to home and other property
Debts, liabilities, including loans, credit cards, outstanding bills
Tax returns and receipts
Attorney, accountant, broker, banker, social worker or others who are familiar
with your financial status and able to help your survivors.

APPENDIX 11-3—PERSONAL DIRECTIONS FOR THE TIME OF DEATH*

Funeral Plans

Clergyman, Rabbi: Contact _____
_____(church or synagogue)
Telephone number _____
to see my family and to conduct the funeral.

Memorial or Burial Society: _____
_____
_____

Phone: _____

Funeral Director: I prefer that _____
Telephone _____
be asked to deal with the arrangements.

Cemetery Property Owned?
Yes _____ No _____
If yes, cemetery name and address: _____
_____
_____

Spaces purchased _____ Plot number _____ Deed number _____
Location of certificates _____

Instructions for Care of My Body

I wish to be: buried _____ cremated _____
Preferred cemetery: _____

*Adapted from the book THE FACTS OF DEATH by Michael A. Simpson © 1979 by Prentice-Hall, Inc. Published by Prentice-Hall, Inc., Englewood Cliffs, NJ 01632.

I wish my body donated to _____
for medical or anatomical studies. I have signed an agreement,
which is located _____

I want to donate the following of my organs, if suitable arrangements can be
made:
Eyes _____ Kidneys _____ Brain _____ Other _____
Program, Hospital, Institute _____
_____
Location of donor card _____

I give my permission for an autopsy (postmortem examination)
if my doctor considers it useful or necessary _____
I do not wish an autopsy to be performed unless required by law _____

I wish for my body to be embalmed: Yes _____No _____

Services

I would like:

immediate cremation without viewing or service _____
immediate burial without viewing or service _____

cremation: ashes disposed of by crematorium _____
ashes buried in cemetery _____
ashes treated as follows _____
_____

displaying and visiting of the body Yes _____ No _____
a memorial service without my body present at
_____
a funeral service with my body present at
_____
a committal service (at graveside) _____

a private service, limited to my family and close friends _____
an open service _____
no service of any kind _____
closed casket _____ open casket _____

I would also prefer the following arrangements (e.g., choice of scripture, readings,
music or other features of a service):

Other comments on costs, quality of caskets, vaults, services, memorials:

Memorials

I would prefer: No flowers _____

Flowers at the discretion of my family _____

No limitations regarding flowers _____

Donations, instead of flowers, to the following (religious or memorial funds, charities, medical research or hospital funds): _____

_____

_____

Signed _____

Date _____

On Being a Reluctant Physician— Strains and Rewards in Caring for the Dying at Home

> Death destroys a man; the idea of Death saves him.
>
> E.M. Forster[7b]

A sensible person can approach work among dying patients only with some reluctance. Almost instinctively, we shun death and, knowing that we might be hurt, try to avoid being touched by great suffering. Yet most of us who choose a career of caring for persons in distress sense an opportunity, amidst suffering, for satisfying, meaningful work. We are attracted to the practice of a craft that rewards us with remarkable pleasures and delights while also bringing us pain and frustration.

Each professional finds his or her own personal satisfactions in ministering to the dying and encounters his or her own particular distress.[11] In this Afterword, I share my own mixture of feelings, my sense of the strains and rewards of providing hospice care in the home.

I

If I think about my first ventures in hospice care, or if I see another young physician starting to visit dying patients at home, I am dismayed by our lack of preparation and support for such work. Physicians-in-training are rarely exposed to home care or specialized terminal-care programs and may not even be aware that some doctors provide such services. Training in related areas—the psychological care of the sick, dying, and bereaved; the management of pain and other symptoms of terminal illness; home care; family-oriented supportive care; even oncology—is often deficient. Role models are few. Colleagues wonder why I do it. Some suggest by their questions that my interests are a bit bizarre and that perhaps I am misusing my time and training. Other colleagues are not even curious. Why leave the security and familiarity of the office and the hospital to work in a field for which one has neither practical experience nor training, and lacks the encouragement, recognition, and example of colleagues and mentors in the profession?

The compelling reason for providing comprehensive medical care in the home is not the physician's own rewards, but the greater comfort and satisfaction achieved there by so many dying patients and their families. Ultimately, I justify this work as a valuable service, yet the venture has many personal pleasures.

II

A foremost reward is the gratitude of the patient and family—the warm reception in their home, the welcomed involvement in their lives. Repeatedly, I am reminded of the physician's enormous privilege of sharing in a person's private world, of a stranger's readiness to trust me because I am a doctor. I gain entry into their lives at a time of unusual intensity of feelings, participating in special moments of sadness and loss and witnessing their confrontation with the meanings of living and dying. In these moments of crisis, of urgent reflection and reckoning, the protective social masks of everyday life may be put aside. A fraternity of strangers emerges, and I find great opportunities for intimacy with my patients and their families.[2]

My degree of involvement in this drama—my occasional home visit or telephone call, my feelings of concern—cannot approximate the intensity of the ordeal for the patient and family. My part is small. Yet even when there is "nothing more to do," the doctor's presence in the home at a time of crisis can be wonderfully reassuring to the layperson. I have learned to notice how I almost unwittingly bring relief: an intolerable discomfort is already better before my treatment is begun; the frantic crisis has calmed; helplessness and a sense of overwhelming burden give way to a feeling of greater hope and strength. The future is again somehow manageable. An extreme example of the value of the doctor's reassuring presence occurs when I attend a death. Here I take on the traditional priestly and charismatic role of the medicine man, lending my authority and expertise to the event, bringing some sense of order. I assuage my own therapeutic helplessness in the face of death by appreciating the importance of my presence and by providing support, focusing on the well-being of the survivors.

III

The novelty and romance of hospice work—a sense of adventure in doing something different than my medical colleagues, yet also of sharing in an ancient, albeit faltering, tradition of physicians attending to the dying in the home—helped propel me into the field. Even today, I enjoy the mixture of pleasant surprise and bemusement I encounter when acquaintances or patients learn that I "still make housecalls." I relish those times when older physicians reminisce nostalgically about going on home visits.

Standing slightly outside the mainstream of the profession has definite rewards at times. The well-documented neglect of the dying means that I have the field to myself. I can carry the ball. There are no specialists eager to care for these patients. Indeed, I am the specialist in terminal care, establishing my expertise and the value of my services in a manner quite similar to my medical school classmates who became subspecialists. Like the academic cardiologist who consults only on one discrete type of heart problem, applying a special investigative technique or procedure, I focus on terminal care, also a narrow area, but one that satisfies my wish to be an "integrationist," to serve as a general or primary-care internist, to follow my interest in psychosocial aspects of practice, and to master a discipline.

New relationships emerge from this novel subspecialty or hobby: alliance with a local hospice volunteer program; contact with oncologists, psychiatrists, social workers, nurses, clergy, and other professionals who share an interest in the field; and opportunities to talk to both professional and community groups. I can look forward to referrals and consultations in my area of special interest and to being the expert who makes the final decisions.

In the home, I feel unencumbered by the routines of the office and hospital. I am on my own, like a missionary in the jungle. The lack of readily available laboratory tests, reference books, or consultants challenges me to "Make Do" (Allan Gregg's version of the meaning of "M.D."[8]). I must rely on my innate skills, my trained good sense, and the resources at hand. If a dressing needs changing, a medication list is required, or a patient needs to be turned or placed on the bedpan, I do it. There is also a fascination in occasionally watching the natural course of illnesses, the "nontreatment" of potentially remedial conditions such as pneumonia, abscesses, sepsis, bowel obstruction, cerebral edema, and hypercalcemia.

IV

Home care with the dying suits my long-time interest in the psychosocial aspects of medicine, in how families and patients cope with illness and how they can be helped to cope. The importance of addressing emotional and existential concerns in terminal illness needs little justification. I have also found new pleasures in the technical or biomedical aspects of doctoring—the pharmacology of narcotics, the pathophysiology of dyspnea and vomiting, the management of minor distresses. Problems such as nausea, dyspnea, or dry mouth were once "merely symptoms," but now the management of those complaints is the focus of much of my attention. Because there are so many deficiencies in the care of the dying—so much unnecessary pain, poorly controlled symptoms, inadequate communication and support—I have much gratifying work to do. I am not "just holding hands" or contemplating the meaning of life with my patients. The patient has been told that there is "nothing more to do," but there are many concrete tasks and much tinkering to be done. I approach each dying patient with the expectation that I will have a great deal to offer them, that they will soon be better. I am rarely disappointed.

I have a powerful curiosity about how people live, and this curiosity is well-rewarded in my work. I have become familiar with the homes and neighborhoods of persons of many classes and backgrounds. I sit in their bedrooms and kitchens, meet their families, and watch how they live with each other. I leaf through old photographs and hear about special moments, about their pleasures and disappointments, and their fears and hopes for the future.

When I have visited a patient once or twice at home, he or she is always changed in my eyes, even if later visits are in an institutional setting.[5] The person at home can be appreciated as part of a social situation—a family, a neighborhood, a way of life. New problems, new strengths emerge.[6] Concepts such as "poverty" or "handicap," take on finer, concrete meaning. Later, in the office, I see how the patient has dressed up to come to the doctor and how he or she has accommodated to the requirements of public behavior on professional turf, perhaps presenting a healthier, happier face.[15] The view of life from the hospital or office seems parochial, rarified.

Death is radically egalitarian—it comes to one and all. It renders us humble, yet also ennobles us. At times, the wretched are somehow transfigured in their suffering. I am repeatedly touched by the kindness and devotion that families and friends show to the patient. If they are so dedicated and do so well in caring for the patient, I am happy to do my part as a physician. Repeated encounters with death bring to the forefront of one's mind such questions: "What is it all about—my work, my life? Is this how I choose to spend my precious hours?" I learn from my patients, particularly from their sense, often barely articulated, of what is important in a life, how suffering can be borne, and how cherished relationships can momentarily transcend the pain of loss. Struggling against an illness that finally must be seen as hopeless, they often find the strength to tolerate helplessness and frustration, and to enjoy the remaining time. Life goes on, and death is not quite so bad as imagined. An oncologist who, because of her own struggle with cancer, was no longer able to practice medicine, writes to her "Friend-Patient" that,

> From you all I have drawn strength and courage, since you have taught me how one can face serious disease with fortitude and positivity; for this I thank you.[10]

In closing her letter, the oncologist states another lesson, learned repeatedly in confronting illness: " . . . we all know that nature does not respect our desires." Similarly, Ned Cassem paraphrases Woody Allen: "Death is Nature's way of reminding us to grow up."[3] To reflect on death is not necessarily "morbid" or depressing; it helps us appreciate our helplessness and limited time. In taking mortality seriously, I am pushed to clarify my goals in life, to find sustaining meaning in my work and relationships, and to savor passing joys.

V

Hospice work is often described as palliative, as caring without curing. In fact, much of general medical care is also palliative, aimed not at eradicating disease but at living better with it. A more characteristic feature of work with the dying is the prominence in decision-making afforded the personal goals of the patient and family. In the usual acute-care setting, the prolongation of life is taken for granted as a goal, and the physician, acting on the individual's behalf, strives for optimal biomedical care as defined primarily by the professional standards that laypersons generally accept. In the hospice, the technological imperative bows to the idiosyncrasies of the patient and family. From this perspective emerges the often urgent concern for comfort rather than prolonged survival. A half century ago, Alfred Worcester, lecturing to Harvard medical students on the care of the dying, spoke of "surrendering to their prejudices."[14] Personal notions of comfort, of "death with dignity," of an appropriate way to die, guide the work. Prolongation of life may be a goal, but so may be the avoidance of disagreeable measures which promote survival. I find this reshuffling of priorities satisfying and compelling. I am more clearly a subordinate to the patient and family in this work, and I take pleasure in recognizing their values and in helping them find appropriate care.

The choice of how far to go with diagnosis or treatment, how hard to push for a little more time, are among the most difficult professional decisions I have to make. Doing "everything possible" can be easier than responding to personal and social values. In order to achieve appropriate care, limits on interventions must be set. The patient and family need a doctor who respects their expertise and can help them clarify and choose what they want, yet who is authoritative, helping to bring clarity and control by saying, "Let's keep trying" or "Let's face the music, it's time to stop."

VI

A number of practical problems with home-based care deserve mention. First, work with dying patients is very time-consuming. In order to provide good medical evaluation and psychosocial support in the home, a leisurely visit is often required. Time is also necessary to refresh oneself and find personal stamina for such emotionally strenuous work. Pressures for productivity are difficult to balance with the demands of hospice work.

Second, the work can be seen as inefficient. In the doctor's workshop—the office and the hospital—convenient routines are established for processing patients. The home is the family's territory—unfamiliar to the doctor and not readily subordinated to the priorities of providing efficient care. I do the driving, parking, and walking to the visit. No secretary or nurse handles the paperwork or channels the patient into the examining room. The rituals of greeting seem prolonged in the home. Food, alcohol, and various gifts are proferred. Family members come and go, and sometimes too many people crowd into the room. *Their* phone rings, interrupting *my* work. Compared to my office or hospital, I am less efficient in moving through portions of the examination and particularly in wrapping up the visit and getting out.

Third, the work is poorly remunerated. The hourly rates of home care payment from Blue Shield, Medicare, and especially Medicaid are far below the usual rates in the office or hospital. Brief housecalls may be paid for adequately, but there is no mechanism to charge for the long visits (30–120 minutes) which are often required to provide proper care. (Similar economic factors mitigate against meticulous physical and psychological management in the hospital and office.) In addition, the physician must consider the expense and inconvenience of travel and parking. Ironically, the cost of an ambulance ride to and from the hospital is roughly 10 times my payment for a housecall, and is covered by all major insurance schemes. The economic benefits to the health-care system from avoiding ambulance rides and hospital costs are not reflected in the home-care visit rates. A partial solution is to delegate much of the work to less expensive professionals (*e.g.*, nurses), although they too are relatively underpaid for long visits and may be unable to charge for "supportive" or "nontechnical" care.

VII

Hospice work brings the physician a constant parade of suffering, loss, and grief. The care of the patient and family may proceed smoothly and satisfyingly, yet there is a heaviness, an underlying sadness in much of the work. At best, there is a bittersweet quality. My religious beliefs afford me no faith in a life after death nor do they help me make sense of suffering or loss. I have come to expect at least a few days of mild depression after a death. Even when I feel little closeness with the patient or family, or am relieved that the end has finally arrived, I often find myself feeling bored or listless afterwards. Life seems stale. I am restless at work. A stranger on the street, seen out of the corner of my eye, is momentarily mistaken for the patient—a signal of what is on my mind. Sulking, I may be beset by guilt. Could I have done more? Reviewing the case, I focus on the shortcomings. I wonder if the family is disappointed with me. Accomplishments are forgotten, and pleasures are difficult to appreciate. Why subject myself to this pain? If only I had the time or opportunity to do things a little differently. Next time . . .

Suffering and loss are not the exclusive province of the hospice physician, nor are only dying patients depressing. Beginning a general medical practice 9 years ago, I was astounded at the amount of depression I encountered, at the volume of distress brought to the doctor if one pays attention to it. As I drive through the streets of Chelsea, passing here and there a home I once entered, I may be reminded of a family's long ordeal and of their continued grief. As I walk the corridors of the hospital ward, I sometimes sense a multitude of tragedies, which the silent patients might tell if I stopped to listen. I am reminded of George Eliot:

> That element of tragedy which lies in the very fact of frequency, has not yet wrought itself into the coarse emotion of mankind; and perhaps our frames could hardly bear much of it. If we had a keen vision and feeling of all ordinary human life, it would be like hearing the grass grow and the squirrel's heart beat, and we should die of that roar which lies on the other side of silence. As it is, the quickest of us walk about well wadded with stupidity.[7]

If one pays attention to so much distresss, to the sadness and fear, one surely must be scathed.

VIII

The patient, family, and I are buffetted from crisis to crisis. We are swept along toward death. Complications often arise in rapid succession. A problem surfaces, a flurry of attempts at repair is followed by tenuous resolution or wary watching. Then a new crisis occurs. Moments to relax or reflect, or to enjoy the patient's periods of improved or stable health, may be few.

I want to be a helpful friend, but I am constantly the bearer of bad news. One patient put the dilemma this way:

We hate to see you. We don't know what we would do without you.

The patient and family will, at times, be terribly frightened, desperate, insecure. They turn to the physician. They may act entitled or demanding, or be resentful that I cannot do more. They may displace onto me their hostility and frustration about the illness. They may cling to me, calling repeatedly, asking for advice and reassurance over every little problem. Such insecurity is especially common at the early stages of our relationship, when the referral is first made, but it recurs with crises. My task comes to seem formidable, foreboding. The beeper will not stop nagging. The commitment of time and energy comes to seem endless, the responsibility overwhelming. I begin feeling worn down, overextended. I want to be left alone. I secretly hope the family will fire me. I know I am supposed to remain calm and cool, to be endlessly giving, but I am getting annoyed and frustrated. My irritability leaks out a bit with the patient and family, and I berate myself for being insensitive. My frustration also leaks out with friends or colleagues.

Some patients weigh especially heavily on my mind. One man never seems to find a moment of reconciliation or acceptance as death approaches. He never feels comfortable. Miserable over his lot, bitter toward his family, dissatisfied with everyone who tries to help, he drives everyone away except me, and I too am no good—the pills for vomiting don't really work that well, I can't appreciate his suffering, I can't save him from his illness. I begin to doubt my skills. Do I really know anything about pain control?

A second patient lingers on the brink of death. She is not uncomfortable, but she is miserable from her helplessness and her inability to enjoy food or companionship. She has nothing better to look forward to than a vague encompassing feeling of sickness, and perhaps she will face worse. Her husband constantly demeans me, leaving me feeling worthless, untrustworthy. I redouble my efforts, seek consultation, yet am unable to provide the kind of support I want them to feel. The rest of the family is worn out. They have given their best for months; they are eager now to get on with their lives, to bury the dead, but she hangs on and on.

A third patient, her appearance grossly deformed by tumors, paralyzed below the waist, wants to be at home. She begins to develop pressure sores. Her mother, an elderly woman, insists that the family can handle the care, but I watch with exasperation as the ulcers spread and deepen, exposing layers of muscle and bone. Outside help is rejected. The patient is comfortable, but I am aghast at the wounds. And how could I explain this "neglect" to the house officer in the emergency ward, to my colleagues in the hospital?

A fourth patient is admitted to the hospital late one night. Rather than calling me for a seemingly trivial matter, he has been "rushed" to the emergency ward and admitted. I have been struggling to keep him at home, believing he wanted to stay there. In the hospital, both he and the family seem happier. The visiting nurse, too, seems relieved, saying that home care was unrealistic. The family withdraws. Why did I try so stubbornly to keep him at home? What didn't I understand? And if they have given up on home care, why shouldn't I?

IX

There came a week around Christmas when nothing seemed to go right. Too many patients were in crisis, and I lacked the resilience to respond fully to the cries for help. Gratifications were rare. I felt I could give no more. One more late-night call or visit would have been more than I could stand.

I decided to stop accepting new patients, and I did everything imaginable to avoid work that was upsetting. Gritting my teeth, I continued seeing a few remaining terminally ill patients, only hoping to get by, to do a minimally satisfactory job without being touched by their suffering. I relied on my partners to take on some of my responsibilities, and I delegated or traded off whatever duties seemed difficult. I shunned books, movies, lectures, and meetings that dealt with dying. I stopped seeing friends who liked to talk about grief and loss, or I instructed them not to trouble me with such talk.

Slowly, I reconstituted. Within a few months, I began to want to get back into hospice work a little. I was very cautious, not only in terms of my time commitment, but also in terms of my personal involvement. I tested the waters carefully, wading in slowly, but eventually dove in again, perhaps more warily or somehow better able to avoid the treacherous undertow, which had caught me before.

Looking back, I can make three observations about "burning-out." First, the crisis occurred at a time when I was rather heavily invested in hospice work while my non-professional life was rather unsatisfying. I was depending especially heavily on my work for personal rewards, and I lacked the buoyancy, the support in my life outside of work, to nourish and refresh me, to sustain me through disappointments. Seeking unrealistic gratifications from work, I had drifted away from feeling the daily pleasures of practicing my craft well.

Second, in returning to hospice practice over the next months, I found the work rather indifferent if I kept detached and well protected. My initial caution about becoming immersed in the work also prevented me from enjoying it as I had before, and only when I felt safe and secure enough to become involved again were the usual rewards for my labor restored.

Third, I feel that the experience of "burning-out" immunized me partially. I am now better able to bear the strain of involvement with the dying. Perhaps I know the danger signals of overinvolvement better, or I have set my expectations lower and can better appreciate the simple pleasures. I have found a more secure, though always somewhat tenuous, balance in my work and play. In the following section, I have tried to describe this balance as a set of personal rules or principles.

X

First, I limit my work commitment. I gauge my load of patients before accepting new ones, aiming to be able to handle all my direct hospice care in no more than a few full days a week. I try to delegate responsibilities, especially those that are less gratifying or seem too time-consuming. I seek opportunities to consult and supervise, rather than to assume total responsibility for each person's care. I limit the geographic area for my services, making home visits more convenient. I sign out to my colleagues on most nights and weekends. I get completely away from my work, making sure that I can enjoy myself unencumbered by interruptions or even by the thought of being called. I may work hard, but I try to keep up the activities that refresh me—a tennis game or a jog, the theater or a concert, getting out of town, a quiet night to read. I also rely on the gratifications of other parts of my work—the day-to-day practice of office medicine, the pleasures of teaching, research, and other intellectual pursuits, including writing this essay.

Second, I am much readier to admit that things have gotten too hot, that I am bothered, that I need help or relief. Holding out and stubbornly insisting that I can get through has not been helpful. I complain about and puzzle over patients with my friends and colleagues. I share an occasional success, but mostly air my frustration. Although helpful suggestions from a friend or colleague are appreciated, I rarely seek advice. I look for sympathy, pity, consolation, and especially for an opportunity to ventilate. Talking itself is meant to relieve a burden, and insight about what has caused the difficulties can be sought afterwards.[4] Case conferences are excellent forums for discussing problems, although they tend to be too impersonal, too professional. I do most of my important talking in the hallways of our office or muttering to a secretary while standing behind her desk or at the nurses' station. I do it at the dinner table or over the phone with friends. I often begin with my angriest feelings, my meanest thoughts, although I usually end up feeling more generous and accepting toward the patient and family, more confident in the value of my efforts, and eager to try out a new approach.

I sometimes turn to William Carlos William's remarkable short stories about doctoring, such as, "A Face of Stone."[13] The encounter of doctor and patient is portrayed in these tales with remarkable skill and a rare willingness to represent the physician's full range of feelings—not just compassion, tolerance, and empathy, but impatience, anger, curiousity, sexual arousal, competitiveness, prejudicial disdain, and gentle humor. "A Country Doctor," Kafka's nightmare vision of a housecall—the futility of the work, the never-ending demands, the terrible sense of personal loss in being torn away from home—also is a favorite.[9] A few essays about the stress of working with the terminally ill have been helpful.[1,12] For example, White writes,

> . . . opposite of love is not hate; the opposite of love is indifference. Our patients may not need our love, but they cannot stand our indifference. If our weaknesses, our fears and our anxieties make us appear indifferent, then no change in our image of ourselves can make us feel successful. If we can change our view of our role to one of trying to help our patients, we may in the long run help more, may help ourselves to grow, and may find better ways of exercising our profession.[12]

Third, I am more appreciative of my limited successes, and I am more tolerant of my limited failures. I strive to do the very best, but I am pleased with "good enough." When I read medical texts now, I am often struck by the exhortations for perfection, the inordinate expectations that physicians will be forever and faultlessly kind, understanding, and wise. I am also less tolerant of those who hold up this idealized image in order to denigrate it, especially those observers of the profession who have never experienced the physician's responsibilities. I depend less on perfect results, on seeing every dilemma solved neatly and quickly. I am less frustrated when my highest personal goals for a case are not met, and I am more appreciative of meeting the goals of the patient and family.

I try to make every referral an opportunity for a good memory and a good lesson. I look for something special to appreciate about each patient and family, for something I can learn from them or share with them. I also try to come away with a bit of new insight about caring for the dying. When I am feeling harried, I may take a few extra minutes in the home to restore this pleasing connection with the family. A little time can often clear up a misunderstanding or conflict that was making the work unsatisfying.

Finally, patients and families can be a great help if I let them. The family's gratitude is frequently best expressed after the death, making bereavement visits especially beneficial for the physician. Even earlier, despite the strain of the illness, the patient and family are usually quite realistic about the stresses of the work, and quite tolerant of lapses in my professional demeanor. They appreciate that I am trying hard. The voice that always pushes me to do better usually comes from within. Likewise, I hope I am less demanding of my co-workers and better able to support them with my appreciation of their work.

A brief, preliminary version of this essay was presented to the Cabot Society of Harvard Medical School, 28 February 1980.

SELECTED REFERENCES

1. Artiss KL, Levine AS: Doctor–patient relationship in severe illness: A seminar for oncology fellows. N Engl J Med 288:1210–1214, 1974
2. Berger J, Mohr J: A Fortunate Man: The Story of a Country Doctor, pp 62–71. New York, Holt, Rinehart and Winston, 1967

3. Cassem N: Dying and growth in contemporary society. Presented at conference on "Issues of Coping: Illness, Dying and Bereavement," Boston, March 13, 1981

4. Cassem N: Internship, liberty, death and other choices: How to survive life in the hospital. Harvard Med Alumni Bull 53:46–48, 1979

5. Currie CT, Moore JT, Friedman SW, Warshaw GA: Assessment of elderly patients at home: A report of fifty cases. J Am Geriatr Soc 29:398–401, 1981

6. Elford RW, Brown JW, Robertson LR et al: A study of house calls in the practices of general practitioners. Med Care 10:173–178, 1972

7. Eliot G: Middlemarch. Boston, Houghton Mifflin, 1956

7b. Forster EM: Howard's End, p 239. New York, Vintage, 1921

8. Gregg A: Our analysis. In For Future Doctors. Chicago, University of Chicago Press, 1957

9. Kafka F: The Penal Colony: Stories and Short Pieces. New York, Schocken Books, 1976

10. Kelley RM: personal communication, 5 May 1981

11. McCue JD: The effects of stress on physicians and their medical practice. N Engl J Med 306:458–463, 1982

12. White LP: The self-image of the physician and the care of dying patients. Ann NY Acad Sci 164:822–837, 1969

13. Williams WC: The Farmers' Daughters. New York, New Directions, 1961

14. Worcester A: The Care of the Aged, the Dying and the Dead. Springfield, IL, Charles C Thomas, 1935

15. Yates JW, Chalmers B, McKegney FP: Evaluation of patients with advanced cancer using the Karnofsky Performance Status. Cancer 45:2220–2224, 1980

General Index

Note: f following page number refers to information in footnotes. A more specific listing of drugs can be found in the Drug Index, which follows this index.

319

Drug Index